Advances in
Neurochemistry

Volume 1

Advances in Neurochemistry

A Continuation Order Plan is available for this series. A continuation order will bring delivery of each new volume immediately upon publication. Volumes are billed only upon actual shipment. For further information please contact the publisher.

Advances in
Neurochemistry

Volume 1

Edited by
B. W. Agranoff
Mental Health Research Institute and
Department of Biological Chemistry
University of Michigan
Ann Arbor, Michigan

and

M. H. Aprison
Institute of Psychiatric Research and
Department of Psychiatry and Biochemistry
Indiana University School of Medicine
Indianapolis, Indiana

PLENUM PRESS • NEW YORK AND LONDON

Library of Congress Cataloging in Publication Data

Main entry under title:

Advances in neurochemistry.

Includes bibliographies and indexes.
1. Neurochemistry. I. Agranoff, Bernard W., 1926-   II. Aprison,
M. H., 1923-   [DNLM: 1. Neurochemistry — Period. W1 AD684E]
QP356.3.A37   612'.822   75-8710
ISBN 0-306-39221-6 (v.1)

Science

© 1975 Plenum Press, New York
A Division of Plenum Publishing Corporation
227 West 17th Street, New York, N.Y. 10011

United Kingdom edition published by Plenum Press, London
A Division of Plenum Publishing Company, Ltd.
Davis House (4th Floor), 8 Scrubs Lane, Harlesden, London, NW10 6SE, England

Printed in the United States of America

CONTRIBUTORS

SOLL BERL • *Department of Neurology, Mount Sinai School of Medicine of The City University of New York, New York, New York*

PATRICK R. CARNEGIE • *The Russell Grimwade School of Biochemistry, University of Melbourne, Parkville, Victoria, Australia*

PETER R. DUNKLEY • *The Russell Grimwade School of Biochemistry, University of Melbourne, Parkville, Victoria, Australia*

SAMARTHJI LAL • *Department of Psychiatry, McGill University, Montreal General Hospital and Queen Mary Veterans' Hospital, Montreal, Quebec, Canada*

FRANK L. MARGOLIS • *Roche Institute of Molecular Biology, Nutley, New Jersey*

BLAKE W. MOORE • *Department of Psychiatry, Washington University School of Medicine, St. Louis, Missouri*

NORMAN S. RADIN • *Mental Health Research Institute and Department of Biological Chemistry, University of Michigan, Ann Arbor, Michigan*

THEODORE L. SOURKES • *Department of Psychiatry, McGill University, Montreal, Quebec, Canada*

LEONHARD S. WOLFE • *Donner Laboratory of Experimental Neurochemistry, Montreal Neurological Institute, McGill University, Montreal, Quebec, Canada*

PREFACE

The emergence of a new scientific book series requires some explanation regarding how it hopes to compensate the reader for the discomforts it undoubtedly produces both in the realms of informational input–overload and in the financial strain on personal and institutional budgets. This series recognizes that investigators who have entered neurochemistry from the biochemical tradition have a rather specialized view of the brain. Too often, interdisciplinary offerings are initially attractive but turn out to recite basic biochemical considerations. We have come to believe that there are now sufficiently large numbers of neurochemists to support a specialized venture such as the present one. We have begun with consideration of traditional areas of neurochemistry which show considerable scientific activity. We hope they will serve the neurochemist both for general reading and for specialized information. The reader will also have the opportunity to reflect on the unbridled speculation that results from the disinhibiting effects on the author who has been invited to write a chapter.

We plan occasionally also to offer reviews of areas not completely in the domain of neurochemistry which we nevertheless feel to be sufficiently timely to be called to the attention of all who use chemical principles and tools in an effort to better understand the brain.

B. W. Agranoff
M. H. Aprison

CONTENTS

CHAPTER 4

BRAIN-SPECIFIC PROTEINS: S-100 PROTEIN, 14-3-2 PROTEIN AND GLIAL FIBRILLARY PROTEIN

BLAKE W. MOORE

CHAPTER 5

ACTOMYOSIN-LIKE PROTEIN IN BRAIN

S. BERL

CHAPTER 6

BIOCHEMICAL MARKERS OF THE PRIMARY OLFACTORY PATHWAY: A MODEL NEURAL SYSTEM

FRANK L. MARGOLIS

CHAPTER 7

APOMORPHINE AND ITS RELATION TO DOPAMINE IN THE NERVOUS SYSTEM

THEODORE L. SOURKES AND SAMARTHJI LAL

Editors' Note

The term "concentration" is often inappropriately used to refer to the amount of a substance heterogeneously distributed within a complex biological sample. This can be particularly misleading in brain samples, since specific cells or organelle populations may contain magnitude differences in distribution patterns. We have therefore elected to use the word "content" as a general term in place of "concentration" for distributions in heterogeneous systems expressed in units such as μmoles/g brain, etc. in the hope that it will reduce ambiguity.

B.W.A.
M.H.A.

CHAPTER 1

POSSIBLE ROLES OF PROSTAGLANDINS IN THE NERVOUS SYSTEM

LEONHARD S. WOLFE

Donner Laboratory of Experimental Neurochemistry
Montreal Neurological Institute, McGill University
Montreal H3A 2B4, Quebec, Canada

1. INTRODUCTION

1.1. Background

Few would question that one of the most exciting and important developments in biochemistry and physiology in recent years has been the emergence of prostaglandins as a new class of molecules mediating and modulating hormonal, neurohormonal, or other stimuli on most mammalian tissues. In just over ten years the literature on prostaglandins has expanded to over 5000 references, from basic chemistry, metabolism, and pharmacology to clinical trials of natural prostaglandins and synthetic analogues. Although the subject is recent, one can look back at the work of others over the 30 years before the announcement of the structures of the six primary prostaglandins by Bergström and coworkers (Bergström *et al.*, 1962, 1963; review, 1968) and identify principles with biological activities that we now know are mainly due to prostaglandins. Foremost among these were the independent

1

observations of Kurzrok and Lieb (1930), Goldblatt (1933, 1935), and von Euler (1934, 1935a) that human semen and extracts of sheep vesicular glands contained factors that stimulated intestinal and uterine muscle and lowered arterial blood pressure. Von Euler (1935b) showed that these activities were due to acidic lipids and proposed the name "prostaglandin." Slow-reacting substance C (Vogt *et al.*, 1966), Darmstoff (Vogt, 1958; Bartels *et al.*, 1970), intestinal stimulant acidic lipids (Gray, 1962, 1964), irin (Ambache, 1957, 1966; Änggård and Samuelsson, 1964; Waitzman *et al.*, 1967), menstrual stimulant (Clithroe and Pickles, 1961; Eglington *et al.*, 1963), vaso-depressor lipid (Strong *et al.*, 1966; Daniels *et al.*, 1967), medullin (Lee *et al.*, 1965), and an unsaturated hydroxy fatty acid fraction from brain (Ambache *et al.*, 1963) all owe much of their biological activity to the presence of one or more of the prostaglandins. Indeed, if an acidic lipid extract from tissues is found to contract smooth muscle and the uterus, the presence of prosta-glandins can be suspected. Prostaglandins are synthesized by most mam-malian tissues as well as by tissues of lower vertebrates. As more species have been studied, it has become apparent that certain tissues of invertebrates (molluscs, gorgonian coral, coelenterates, arthropods) either contain or are capable of synthesizing prostaglandins that often have different stereo-chemistry from those found in mammals (Weinheimer and Spraggins, 1969; Christ and van Dorp, 1972; Destephano *et al.*, 1974). More recently, prosta-glandin endoperoxides have been implicated in the biological activity of the rabbit aorta–contracting substance released from guinea pig lung (Piper and Vane, 1969; Vargaftig and Dao Hai, 1971, 1972; Gryglewski and Vane, 1972; Nugteren and Hazelhof, 1973) and a labile aggregation-stimulating sub-stance released during human platelet aggregation (Silver *et al.*, 1973; Willis, 1974; Hamberg *et al.*, 1974).

This chapter, after some remarks on basic prostaglandin biochemistry, will emphasize the formation, release, and possible functions of prosta-glandins formed endogenously in nervous tissue whether central or peri-pheral, and the neuropharmacological actions of prostaglandins. Evidence that there may be a prostaglandin component in the disturbance of cerebral bloodflow which follows brain injury will also be discussed. Prostaglandins not only appear to be involved in the regulation or control of normal processes but also are responsible for a number of pathological responses in tissues. The discovery of a number of specific inhibitors of prostaglandin synthesis (Pace-Asciak and Wolfe, 1968; Ahern and Downing, 1970; Downing *et al.*, 1970; Vane, 1971; Ferreira *et al.*, 1971; Wlodawer *et al.*, 1971; Vanderhoek and Lands, 1973; Zipoh *et al.*, 1974) has enabled much more precise determination of which component of a physiological or pathological response involves the prostaglandins.

The pharmacological actions of the various prostaglandins are, to say the least, bewildering (see Bergström *et al.*, 1968; Weeks, 1972; Andersen and Ramwell, 1974), and it is far from clear which of these subserve physiological functions. There is growing appreciation that fundamental features of prostaglandin physiology are that they act locally in tissues influencing many stimulus–secretion coupled processes and are involved together with other hormones in the translation of membrane responses through cyclic nucleotides into intracellular processes. Tables 1 and 2 briefly summarize some of the pharmacological effects of different prostaglandin types and possible physiological and pathophysiological processes in which they are implicated.

The prostaglandin literature is widely dispersed. To simplify the task for the reader who wishes more information, selected reviews and books are listed separately in a General Bibliography section at the end of the chapter. The Upjohn Company, Kalamazoo, Michigan, publishes a complete bibliography of the prostaglandin literature which is updated several times a year.

TABLE 1. Some Pharmacological Effects of Prostaglandins

	Prostaglandin effects by type[a]		
	E	A	F
Gastrointestinal motility	↑[b]	0[c]	↑
Gastric secretion	↓[d]	↓	0
Blood flow in most vascular beds	↑	↑	0 or ↓
Cerebral, nasal, and placental blood flow	↓	0 or ↑	↓
Blood pressure	↓	↓	↑
Bronchial and tracheal smooth muscle	↓	0	↑
Uterine motility	↑	0	↑
Luteolysis	0	0	↑
Induction of labor, termination of pregnancy	↑	0	↑
Platelet aggregation	↑ (E_1↓)	0	0
Natriuresis	↑	↑	0
Allergic responses	↓	↓	0
Adrenergic neurotransmission	↓	0	↑?
Hormone-stimulated lipolysis	↓	0	0
Intraocular pressure	↑	0	0
Cyclic AMP (most tissues)	↑	0	0
Cyclic GMP	0	0	↑?

[a] There are species differences in these effects and also differences between *in vivo* and *in vitro* responses.
[b] ↑ = stimulation or increase in response.
[c] 0 = minimal or no effect.
[d] ↓ = inhibition or decrease in response.

TABLE 2. Some Possible Physiological and Pathophysiological
Roles of Prostaglandins

Control of the activity of involuntary neuromuscular systems
Regulation of central and autonomic neurotransmission
Modulation of stimulus–secretion coupling mechanisms
Intermediates in the mechanism of cellular defense and repair
Intermediates in immune responses
Mediators in pyrogen-induced hyperthermia
Regulation of cell division and differentiation
Acceleration of platelet aggregation
Regulation of the microcirculation and tissue perfusion
Control of intrarenal blood flow and blood pressure
Initiation of parturition
Acceleration of luteolysis
Facilitation of calcium binding to membranes

1.2. Names and Structures

The prostaglandins are a family of oxygenated, unsaturated, twenty-carbon cyclopentane carboxylic acids. They can be regarded as derivatives of a parent cyclopentane acid, prostanoic acid, which forms the basic carbon skeleton. The type designations for the primary prostaglandins are based on the functionality in the cyclopentane ring, i.e., β-hydroxyketone for E-type, 1,3-diol for F-type, α,β-unsaturated ketone for A-type, and so forth. Within each type there are class designations indicated as subscripts one to three, which refer to the number of carbon–carbon double bonds. Most of the primary prostaglandins from natural sources have a single stereoisomeric form with the carboxyhexyl and hydroxyoctyl side chains on the cyclopentane ring in the α-configuration and the carbon-15 hydroxyl in the S or L form (Table 3).

1.3. Biosynthesis

The six primary prostaglandins are formed by the bioconversion of unesterified 8,11,14-eicosatrienoic acid (homo-γ-linolenic acid) to PGE_1 and $PGF_{1\alpha}$, 5,8,11,14-eicosatetraenoic acid (arachidonic acid) to PGE_2 and $PGF_{2\alpha}$, and 5,8,11,14,17-eicosapentaenoic acid to PGE_3 and $PGF_{3\alpha}$ (see reviews by Samuelsson, 1964, 1972, 1973*a,b*). In most mammalian tissues and particularly in man, the essential fatty acid, arachidonic acid, is quantitatively the most important precursor for endogenous prostaglandin bio-

TABLE 3. Structures and Names of Some Prostaglandins Formed from Arachidonic Acid[a]

Structure	Trivial and abbreviated name	Systematic name
	Prostaglandin E_2 PGE$_2$	11α, 15S-dihydroxy-9-keto-prosta-5 *cis*, 13 *trans*-dienoic acid
	Prostaglandin $F_{2\alpha}$ PGF$_{2\alpha}$	9α, 11α, 15S-trihydroxy-prosta-5 *cis*, 13 *trans*-dienoic acid
	Prostaglandin A_2 PGA$_2$	15S-hydroxy-9-ketoprosta-5 *cis*, 10,13 *trans*-trienoic acid
	Prostaglandin C_2 PGC$_2$	15S-hydroxy-9-ketoprosta-5 *cis*, 11,13 *trans*-trienoic acid
	Prostaglandin B_2 PGB$_2$	15S-hydroxy-9-ketoprosta-5 *cis*, 8(12), 13 *trans*-trienoic acid
	Prostaglandin D_2 PGD$_2$	9α, 15S-dihydroxy-11-ketoprosta-5 *cis*, 13 *trans*-dienoic acid
	Prostaglandin G_2 PGG$_2$ Endoperoxide intermediate I	15S-hydroperoxy-9α, 11α-peroxido-prosta-5 *cis*, 13 *trans*-dienoic acid
	Prostaglandin H_2 PGH$_2$ endoperoxide intermediate II	15S-hydroxy-9α, 11α-peroxido-prosta-5 *cis*, 13 *trans*-dienoic acid

[a] All are biologically active compounds except PGD$_2$. The endoperoxide prostaglandins PGG$_2$ and PGH$_2$ may have considerably higher biological potency than PGE$_2$ or PGF$_{2\alpha}$.

synthesis. Table 3 lists the major prostaglandins derived from arachidonic acid with their structures, abbreviated names, and systematic names, which can serve as a basis for naming all types of prostaglandins.

Probably all mammalian tissues except the erythrocyte are capable of prostaglandin synthesis. The synthetase complex is tightly bound to membrane elements and attempts to solubilize the system intact have so far failed. Since the original discovery by Bergström's group in Sweden (Bergström *et al.*, 1964*a,b*) and van Dorp's group in Holland (van Dorp *et al.*, 1964*a,b*) of the biosynthesis of prostaglandins from polyunsaturated fatty acids, sheep vesicular gland microsomal preparations in which the enzyme is particularly enriched have provided the basis for detailed studies of the mechanism of the transformation by Samuelsson, Hamberg, and coworkers (see review by Samuelsson, 1972). The initial reaction is the abstraction of a pro-S hydrogen at C-13 from the polyunsaturated fatty acid precursor through a lipoxygenase-like reaction, the Δ^{11}-double bond isomerizes to the Δ^{12}-position, and molecular oxygen is inserted at C-11 and at C-15 with a shift of the double bond to the Δ^{13}-position and formation of a C-8 and C-12 bond and the 9,11-endoperoxide. The first isolatable product of the prostaglandin synthetase is the 15-hydroperoxy prostaglandin endoperoxide (Table 3). The dioxygenase enzyme(s) that catalyzes this reaction is called fatty-acid cyclo-oxygenase(s) (Hamberg *et al.*, 1974). The reduction of the 15-hydroperoxy group produces the 15-hydroxy prostaglandin endoperoxide which has also been isolated (Hamberg and Samuelsson, 1973; Nugteren and Hazelhof, 1973). This reaction can be catalyzed by glutathione peroxidase, which is present in most tissues. The 15-hydroxyprostaglandin endoperoxide is converted by an endoperoxide isomerase into PGE and by an endoperoxide reductase into PGF prostaglandins (Wlodawer and Samuelsson, 1973). The E prostaglandins can then be converted by dehydration (possibly enzymatic) into PGA-type and then by isomerases into PGC- and PGB-types (Jones and Cammock, 1973; Jones, 1974). These latter prostaglandins and the enzymes that form them are not present in all tissues or animal species. The prostaglandin endoperoxides cannot be formed if the precursor fatty acid is esterified to a triglyceride or phospholipid, but only from the free acid (Lands and Samuelsson, 1968). Thus the release of unesterified precursor acids by acylhydrolases into a specific membrane pool available to the prostaglandin synthetase multienzyme complex could be the rate-limiting step in the endogenous synthesis of prostaglandins. This aspect will be discussed in greater detail later. Figure 1 illustrates the stepwise reaction sequence for prostaglandin biosynthesis from arachidonic acid and some of the known side reactions and chemical transformations. The kinetics of the cyclo-oxygenase reactions are exceedingly complex since product activation occurs initially followed by a self-catalyzed enzyme

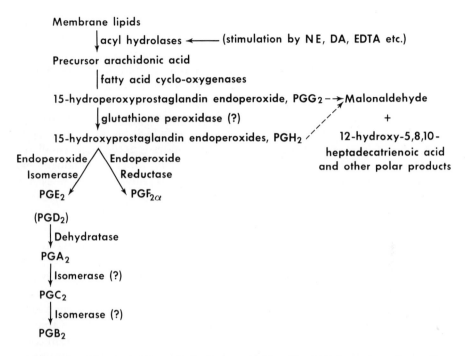

FIGURE 1. Steps in the biosynthesis of prostaglandins. The 15-hydroperoxyendoperoxide intermediate PGG_2 can be converted chemically into $PGF_{2\alpha}$ by stannous chloride or triphenylphosphine; into 15-keto-$PGF_{2\alpha}$ by lead tetra-acetate and triphenylphosphine; into 15-hydroperoxy PGE_2 by aqueous media. The 15-hydroxyendoperoxide intermediate PGH_2 can be converted into $PGF_{2\alpha}$ by stannous chloride or triphenylphosphine; and into PGE_2 by aqueous media. PGE_2 can be converted into $PGF_{2\alpha}$ and $PGF_{2\beta}$ by sodium borohydride; into PGA_2 by acid; and into PGB_2 by base. Malonaldehyde, C-17 hydroxyunsaturated fatty acids, and other polar products may be formed nonenzymatically or by free radical side reactions.

inhibition by hydroperoxides (Lands *et al.*, 1971, 1973). All these studies have been carried out using the vesicular gland oxygenase with added substrate fatty acids. It is far from certain whether these kinetic analyses, particularly the irreversible self-catalyzed destruction of enzyme reported by Smith and Lands (1972) which implies the need for new protein synthesis, would apply to endogenous prostaglandin synthesis. The delivery of specific substrate acids to the fatty acid cyclo-oxygenases may be specifically controlled and compartmentalized and the membrane enzyme complex protected from irreversible inactivation by inhibitory fatty acids and hydroperoxides.

Considerable variability exists in the capacity of tissue homogenates to convert exogenously added labeled substrate into prostaglandins. A number of factors may account for this variability quite apart from the tissue concentration of enzyme proteins, namely: (1) the release of substrate fatty acids through acylhydrolase activity which dilutes the added labeled substrate; (2) the release of inhibitory nonsubstrate fatty acids; and (3) the inhibition of the enzyme by cytoplasmic factors released during the homogenization. Thus measurement of percentage conversion of added labeled substrate fatty acids may not give a true indication of the capacity of the tissue for prostaglandin synthesis from endogenous precursors. As will be seen later, this is particularly true for brain, in which the percentage conversion of added labeled precursor in homogenates is exceedingly small yet endogenous synthesis is considerable (Wolfe *et al.*, 1967). The endogenous precursor fatty-acid pool appears to be compartmentalized and does not mix with exogenously added substrate. Since there is now good evidence that the prostaglandin endoperoxide isomerase and reductase are separate enzymes (Samuelsson, 1973*b*), it is to be expected that different tissues will vary in their capacity to form E- and F-type prostaglandins. In the intact tissue, which prostaglandin type is produced or the balance between them may well be under physiological control. Recent experiments of Nugteren and Hazelhof (1973) have shown that in a variety of homogenate systems a quantitatively important product of prostaglandin biosynthesis from added arachidonic acid is the biologically inactive prostaglandin D_2 (see Table 3), first characterized by Granström *et al.* (1968). It is suggested that this may be an important inactivation pathway of prostaglandins *in vivo*. Caution in interpretation is necessary here since the endoperoxide isomerase could have lost specificity in incubated homogenate or microsomal systems. So far there is no information on the endogenous production of D-type prostaglandins in intact tissue or *in vivo*. Furthermore, in homogenates nonenzymatic formation of F-type prostaglandins from the endoperoxide can occur by reducing agents especially sulfydryl compounds in the presence of ferrihaem. Thus the ratios of the various prostaglandin types formed by tissue homogenates may not reflect the situation in intact tissue.

1.4. Catabolism

Prostaglandins of the E- and F-type are converted extremely rapidly into inactive metabolites when injected into the circulation of experimental animals and man, and the metabolites are excreted principally in the urine. Knowledge of the complex sequence of enzymatic degradations is due almost entirely to the elegant research of the Swedish group, principally by Samuelsson, Hamberg, Granström, Änggård, and Gréen (see reviews by Samuelsson, 1972, 1973*a,b*; Hamberg and Wilson, 1973; Granström, 1973). There are four main types of transformation:

1. Oxidation of the allylic alcohol group at C-15 to the 15-keto-prostaglandins by a specific NADH-dependent 15-hydroxyprostaglandin dehydrogenase present in the cytoplasm. The highest activities of this enzyme occur in the lung, spleen, and kidney cortex, but it is also present with much less activity in many other tissues.

2. The Δ^{13}-*trans* double bond is reduced by a specific reductase to form the dihydro- compounds. Various tissues in the same species and the same tissue in different species have different activities of the reductase. Saturation of the Δ^{13}-double bond does not alter the biological activity to nearly the same extent as oxidation of the C-15 alcohol group. There is evidence that some tissues may possess a 15-keto reductase activity that reconverts the 15-keto- or 15-keto-dihydro-prostaglandins back to the secondary alcohols (Marrazzi *et al.*, 1972). Such an activity may in part account for the prolonged biological activity of prostaglandins on various tissues when administered *in vivo*.

3. β-oxidation occurs in mitochondria to form C-18 (dinor-) and C-16 (tetranor-) prostaglandins. The liver is the principal site of these transformations, and they may occur before or after dehydrogenation and reduction. Prostaglandin E_2 or prostaglandin $F_{2\alpha}$ forms the same metabolites as prostaglandin E_1 or $F_{1\alpha}$, respectively, after the second β-oxidation step because of isomerization of the double bond to the α,β-position before oxidative chain shortening.

4. Microsomal ω-oxidation (principally in the liver and kidney) transforms the E- and F-prostaglandin partial metabolites into dicarboxylic acids, which are rapidly cleared from the blood and appear in the urine as the principal final metabolites. Thus the major urinary metabolites of $PGF_{1\alpha}$ and $PGF_{2\alpha}$ in man are 5α,7α-dihydroxy-11-keto-tetranor-prostane-1,16-dioic acid and its δ-lactone. Analogous metabolites have been identified for PGE_1 and PGE_2.

Many other urinary metabolites have been identified, arising from other transformations (lactonizations, β-oxidation from the ω-position, and so forth) and also transformations in different sequences. Furthermore, different animals frequently have different major metabolites. For example, in the guinea pig the main urinary metabolite of PGE_2 is the 5β,7α-dihydroxy-11-ketotetranor-prostanoic acid, in which there is a reduction of the ring keto-group to a hydroxyl group of opposite configuration to that found in the primary prostaglandins (Hamberg and Samuelsson, 1969).

Knowledge of the catabolic transformations of the A- and B-type prostaglandins is far from complete. Early studies (Hamberg and Samuelsson, 1967; Hamberg, 1968) clearly identified ω-2-hydroxylated (R-stereoisomer) derivatives of the A- and B-type prostaglandins. The A-type prostaglandins are poor substrates for the 15-hydroxyprostaglandin dehydrogenase and appear to be principally metabolized by liver microsomal enzymes to ω-1 and ω-2 hydroxylated compounds. It has been suggested that the A- and B-type prostaglandins may be true circulating hormones because they can escape the inactivation by the prostaglandin dehydrogenase, but evidence is far from conclusive on this point.

Following the determination of the structures of the major urinary metabolites in man and several other laboratory animals, methods based on deuterium-labeled derivatives of the metabolites have been developed to obtain quantitative data on the endogenous *in vivo* production of prostaglandins (Hamberg, 1972, 1973; Samuelsson, 1973*b*). Estimates of the total synthesis in humans in 24 hr for the E prostaglandins are 46–333 μg for males and 18–38 μg for females, and values for the F prostaglandins are 42–120 μg for males and 36–61 μg for females. Analgesics such as aspirin or indomethacin dramatically reduce the amount of metabolites excreted in line with their potent inhibitory action on prostaglandin biosynthesis. These highly interesting studies open the way to measurement of prostaglandin production in normal physiological cycles and particularly in a variety of pathological conditions. Unfortunately, the techniques of purification and quantification involving gas chromatography–mass fragmentography with deuterated compounds as carriers and internal standards are complex and very expensive, and so far they are available only to a few laboratories. Thus advances in the determination of specific changes in prostaglandin production *in vivo* have been slow. The development of specific radioimmunoassay methods for the individual metabolites would be extremely valuable, but their use is dependent on the availability of sufficient quantities of the metabolites.

2. CENTRAL NERVOUS SYSTEM

2.1. Occurrence and Release on Stimulation

Samuelsson (1964) identified $PGF_{2\alpha}$ by chemical methods in ox brain. Subsequent studies by other groups confirmed the presence of prostaglandins in the brain of the ox, cat, dog, rabbit, mouse, and chicken (Wolfe *et al.*, 1965, 1967; Coceani and Wolfe, 1965; Horton and Main, 1967*a*; Holmes and Horton, 1968*a,b*). $PGF_{2\alpha}$ was the predominant prostaglandin, although PGE_2, PGE_1, and $PGF_{1\alpha}$ were identified in some species. Prostaglandin-type determinations were based on silicic acid and thin-layer chromatographic separations following solvent partitions from tissues at variable times after death, and biological activity was determined by a variety of smooth muscle bioassay methods. The quantitative values reported in the earlier literature ($PGF_{2\alpha}$ 10–300 ng/g fresh weight of brain tissue) have little meaning, since biosynthesis from endogenous precursor fatty acids occurs rapidly after death and is stimulated by tissue trauma and other non-physiological factors (Pace-Asciak *et al.*, 1968; Piper and Vane, 1971; Pappius *et al.*, 1974). Furthermore, reports of the presence of PGE_1 and $PGF_{1\alpha}$ in the brains of some mammalian species based solely on chromatographic properties must also be interpreted with caution. The precursor *n*-6 eicosatrienoic acid in complex lipids or as the free acid is undetectable in rat and mouse brain (Lunt and Rowe, 1968; Bazan, 1970; Baker and Thompson, 1972). In ox brain, eicosatrienoic acid is detectable in small amounts, but the proportion of the *n*-9 (not a substrate for prostaglandin synthesis) to the *n*-6 fatty acid has not been determined (Holub *et al.*, 1970). Liquid-nitrogen-frozen cerebral cortex or whole-brain tissue homogenized under conditions to prevent subsequent prostaglandin synthesis, i.e., in 70% ethanol containing indomethacin or eicosatetraynoic acid, has very low

TABLE 4. Endogenous Biosynthesis of Prostaglandins by Cerebral Tissues

Tissue	$PGF_{2\alpha}$	PGE_2	$F_{2\alpha}/E_2$
	ng/100 mg tissue		
A. *Rat cerebral cortex*			
Immediately frozen (liquid N_2)	1.11 (6)	—	—
Slices before incubation	9.00 (4)	—	—
Homogenate before incubation	7.59 (1)	2.02 (1)	3.8
60-min incubations[a]			
Slices	55.70 (5)	12.34 (3)	4.5
Homogenate	70.82 (1)	26.29 (1)	2.7
Indomethacin *in vivo*[b]	14.68 (2)	—	—
in vitro[c]	13.76 (2)	—	—
B. *Cat brain*			
60-min incubations[a]			
Cerebral cortex	152.38 (5)	52.96 (2)	2.9
Cerebellum	51.53 (2)	37.14 (2)	1.4
Caudate nucleus	77.19 (2)	38.42 (2)	2.0
Hypothalamus	74.40 (2)	30.61 (1)	2.4

The prostaglandins were measured following extensive purification by gas chromatography–mass fragmentography of the methyl ester trimethylsilyl ether derivative of $PGF_{2\alpha}$ and the methyl ester benzyloxime trimethylsilyl ether derivative of PGE_2. The tetradeuteroprostaglandins were used as carriers and internal standards. Ions monitored for $PGF_{2\alpha}$ were m/e 423, 427 and for PGE_2 m/e 524, 528.
[a] Incubations in ringer–bicarbonate–glucose medium (RBG) at pH 7.4.
[b] Animal given Indomethacin in two doses of 20 mg/kg intraperitoneally.
[c] Indomethacin added to incubation medium at 3×10^{-4} M.

prostaglandin content (Table 4). This is also true for nonneural tissues (Jouvenaz et al., 1970; Änggård et al., 1972). When these precautions are not taken, the values of prostaglandin contents in whole brain or brain regions mean nothing more than endogenous biosynthetic capacity. Thus the reports of a fairly even distribution of prostaglandins in dog brain (Holmes and Horton, 1968a) or of the presence of prostaglandins in particulate or supernatant subcellular fractions (Kataoka et al., 1967; Hopkin et al., 1968) mean very little. A study utilizing gas chromatography–mass fragmento-graphy methods for specific quantification of the endogenous biosynthetic capacity of brain subcellular fractions from various brain regions has not been done, but it would yield much more specific information on localization of the synthetic enzymes. Also the contributions made by neurons or glial cells to prostaglandin biosynthesis is quite unclear, although the increased release on neuronal pathway stimulation suggests a neuronal localization.

The spontaneous release of prostaglandins (specifically identified or suspected on the basis of chemical and pharmacological properties) into superfusates of various brain regions is now well documented: cerebral cortex (Ramwell and Shaw, 1966, 1967; Bradley et al., 1969); cerebellum (Coceani and Wolfe, 1965); spinal cord (Ramwell et al., 1966; Matsuura et al., 1969; Coceani et al., 1971); and cerebral ventricles (Feldberg and Myers, 1966; Holmes, 1970; Beleslin et al., 1971; Beleslin and Myers, 1971). The release rates for the cat cerebellum (which is fairly representative of other regions) were $1.6–6.4 \, \text{ng/hr/cm}^2$ surface (mean 3.6) in PGE_1 equivalents by the rat fundus strip bioassay (multiply by 5 to convert to $PGF_{2\alpha}$, the pre-dominant prostaglandin in the superfusates). There is a relationship between neuronal activity and increased prostaglandin release. Electrical stimulation of the somatosensory cortex or reticular formation, transcallosal stimulation, and afferent stimulation of peripheral nerves (evoked responses) all increase severalfold the prostaglandin content of cerebral cortex superfusates (Ramwell and Shaw, 1966; Bradley et al., 1969), as does activation of cortical neurones by analeptic drugs (Ramwell and Shaw, 1967). Similar effects have been described for the frog spinal cord (Ramwell and Shaw, 1966; Coceani et al., 1971). Drugs such as barbiturates and chlorpromazine decrease the basal release of prostaglandins in encéphale isolé preparations (Ramwell and Shaw, 1967; Bradley et al., 1969). It seems clear that prostaglandin release from brain can be affected by many different stimuli—neural, hormonal, pharmacological, or traumatic.

Prostaglandins are not accumulated in preformed stores and released from there on stimulation. All the evidence suggests a stimulated biosyn-thesis related to the functional state or the pathological insult. Differences in the types of prostaglandins released from nervous tissue in the stimulated and unstimulated state have been found (Bradley et al., 1969; Ramwell et al.,

1966; Coceani *et al.*, 1971). These could come about in three possible ways: (1) different cell types might be involved in the release (glial cells and neurons); (2) a 9-keto-reductase converting E- to F-type prostaglandins might be more active in the stimulated state; or (3) activities of the 15-hydroxy prostaglandin endoperoxide isomerase and reductase enzymes might be altered during stimulation. The third mechanism is the most likely, but more precise evidence using more specific methods for identification and quantification is required. The conversion of E- to F-type has been reported in guinea pig liver microsomes (Hamberg *et al.*, 1971), and evidence for a 9-keto-reductase based on radioimmunoassay has been given by Leslie and Levine (1973). There is no evidence for this activity in brain, and the interpretation of the radioimmunoassay evidence is not entirely satisfactory.

2.2. Biosynthesis in Brain

The capacity for prostaglandin biosynthesis in tissues is frequently measured by determination of the percent conversion of labeled precursor fatty acids to prostaglandins when incubated with homogenates or microsomal fractions. Tissues fall into various categories, those with high percent conversions (seminal vesicles, renal medulla, lung), those with low capacity (stomach, intestine), and those that show negligible conversion (testes, aorta, brain) (van Dorp, 1966; Wolfe *et al.*, 1967; Pace-Asciak and Wolfe, 1970; Christ and van Dorp, 1973). The kinetics of the biosynthesis are not linear; a rapid formation occurs in the first 5 min which falls off almost completely within 30 min. The exceedingly low capacity for prostaglandin synthesis from exogenous precursors by brain tissue no matter from what region was surprising in view of the numerous reports of stimulated synthesis and release; until recently there had been no attempt to examine endogenous biosynthesis in brain. Pappius *et al.* (1974) have studied the capacity of incubated cerebral cortex tissue to synthesize PGE_2 and $PGF_{2\alpha}$ from endogenous precursors and have shown that there is a considerable capacity for biosynthesis (Table 4). The prostaglandin formation was measured specifically by gas chromatographic–mass spectrometric methods using $3,3,4,4\text{-}^2H_4\text{-}PGF_{2\alpha}$ and $^2H_4\text{-}PGE_2$ as internal standards and carriers (see Axen *et al.*, 1971; Gréen *et al.*, 1973; Gréen, 1973). The cerebral cortex slices whether from cat or rat synthesize predominantly $PGF_{2\alpha}$. However, cat cerebellum, caudate nucleus, and hypothalamus synthesize relatively greater amounts of PGE_2. Thus the activities of the prostaglandin endoperoxide isomerase and reductase differ in various brain regions, a fact that may indicate different functional roles of the prostaglandin types in relationship to specific neuronal pathways. The endogenous formation was linear with

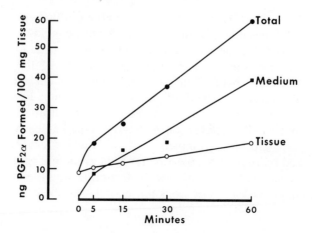

FIGURE 2. Endogenous biosynthesis of prostaglandin $F_{2\alpha}$ by slices of rat cerebral cortex. Each point is the mean of at least three incubations. The prostaglandins were determined following extensive purification by gas chromatography–mass fragmentography of the methyl ester trimethylsilyl ether derivatives. 3,3,4,4-$^2H_4$ $PGF_{2\alpha}$ was added at the end of the incubations as carrier and internal standard. (From Pappius *et al.*, 1974.)

time up to 60 min of slice incubation and was not inhibited by increased prostaglandin content whether from endogenous or exogenous sources (Figure 2). Thus no product inhibition could be found. Indomethacin inhibited prostaglandin synthesis when given *in vivo* or *in vitro*.

In order to compare the synthesis of prostaglandins in slices of brain cortex from endogenous and exogenous precursors, [$^2H_8$]-arachidonic acid was synthesized by reduction of 5,8,11,14-eicosatetraynoic acid with deuterium gas (L. S. Wolfe and J. Marion, unpublished results) and added to the medium before slice incubations. The formation of $^2H_8$-$PGF_{2\alpha}$ was exceedingly small and took place only in the first 5 min of incubation. Exogenous arachidonate does not appear to equilibrate with the arachidonate precursor pool involved in endogenous synthesis (Figure 2). These results offer an explanation for the exceedingly small conversion by brain homogenates of added tritiated precursor fatty acids. During slice incubation, acylhydrolases (specific or nonspecific) most likely liberate arachidonate into a compartment available immediately to the prostaglandin synthetase enzyme complex. It is clear that measurement of endogenous synthetic capacity is a valid procedure to study prostaglandin biosynthesis in brain and should help greatly in answering questions on subcellular localization, regional distributions, and differences among cell types. No information is available on which specific precursor complex lipids are the source of the free arachidonic acid for prostaglandin synthesis in brain or in any tissue.

The biogenic amines, 5-hydroxytryptamine and norepinephrine, are known to stimulate prostaglandin synthesis (Piper and Vane, 1971). These amines also stimulate the liberation of unesterified fatty acids including arachidonate from synaptosomes through activation of phospholipases (Price and Rowe, 1972).

2.3. Catabolism in Brain

Conflicting reports have appeared on the presence in brain of prostaglandin-degrading enzymes. Pig brain has been reported to contain less 15-keto dehydrogenase activity than other tissues but appears to contain the Δ^{13}-reductase (Änggård *et al.*, 1971). Siggins *et al.* (1971*b*), using a histochemical method reported little or no activity in all regions except the cerebellar cortex. On the other hand, incubated homogenates of cerebral cortex and cerebellum of the rat and dog appear almost devoid of the catabolizing enzymes (Nakano *et al.*, 1972), and similar results have recently been obtained with brain slices from rat and cat (Pappius *et al.*, 1974). The data available at present indicate that in general a very low activity of the degradative enzymes is found in brain. Prostaglandins synthesized in brain *in vivo* are probably released into the venous circulation and are degraded principally in other tissues.

2.4. Uptake and Binding Sites

Bito (1972*a,b*) studied the accumulation *in vitro* of tritiated prostaglandins by various mammalian tissues. He found that tissues known to catabolize prostaglandins (lung, liver, kidney cortex) and the choroid plexus, through which active transport of many substances from cerebrospinal fluid to blood occurs, showed large accumulations of tritium from added PGE_1, PGA_1, $PGF_{1\alpha}$, and $PGF_{2\alpha}$. In brain tissue the prostaglandins either appeared to equilibrate completely with the medium (cat) or were apparently partly excluded from intracellular compartments (rabbit, rat). Bito interpreted his results as indicating that cell membranes in general are impermeable to prostaglandins but that specific carrier-mediated mechanisms exist in certain tissues. Pappius *et al.* (1974 and unpublished observations) found that with cerebral cortex slices from rat, whether incubated aerobically or anaerobically, the ratio of counts between tissue and incubating medium with 9-$[^3H]$-$PGF_{2\alpha}$ was always greater than unity (about 1.3) over a wide range of concentrations (8 pg to 333 ng/ml medium). Contrary to Bito's results, it was concluded that some uptake or binding occurs in slices of cerebral cortex.

The reason for the discrepancy may be related to differences in experimental procedure—Bito counted his samples without purification steps, whereas Pappius and co-workers partially purified the prostaglandins by solvent extraction and Amberlite XAD-2 chromatography. Also brain tissue was not defined in Bito's papers and may not refer only to cerebral cortex. Direct measurements have been made of $PGF_{2\alpha}$ in slices from cat and rat cerebral cortex and in incubation media, with and without added $PGF_{2\alpha}$, utilizing gas chromatographic–mass spectrometric methods. The concentration of $PGF_{2\alpha}$ in the tissue expressed in terms of final tissue volume was always higher than in the medium and was unaffected by the absence of glucose. Added $PGF_{2\alpha}$ distributed in the same way as the endogenously synthesized $PGF_{2\alpha}$ which amounted to 60 ng/100 mg tissue/hr. The tissue-to-medium ratio was about 2.3 over a concentration range of 20–250 ng $PGF_{2\alpha}/100\ \mu l$ medium, considerably greater than the 1.3 ratio obtained when tritiated $PGF_{2\alpha}$ was used (H. M. Pappius and L. S. Wolfe, unpublished results). This discrepancy suggests that there is a considerable pool of tissue $PGF_{2\alpha}$ which does not exchange with the labeled prostaglandin. At concentrations of $PGF_{2\alpha}$ below 20 ng/ml in the medium, the tissue-to-medium ratio increased considerably again in contrast to the experiments using added labeled $PGF_{2\alpha}$. It was concluded that the distribution of $PGF_{2\alpha}$ between slices of cerebral cortex and incubating medium was not a simple equilibration and was unlikely to be an active process. Rather, binding must occur, but the binding sites are unsaturated only at concentrations below $5 \times 10^{-8}\ M$. It also appears that $PGF_{2\alpha}$ can cross brain cell membranes since endogenously formed $PGF_{2\alpha}$ rapidly diffuses out of brain slices.

2.5. Cerebrospinal Fluid

Prostaglandinlike activity was reported by Ramwell (1964) in cerebrospinal fluid soon after these compounds were chemically characterized. The possible implication of prostaglandins in the genesis of pyrogen fever (see section 2.6.4a) stimulated comparison of prostaglandin activity by bioassay methods in third ventricle and cisterna magna cerebrospinal fluid of cats nonfebrile and febrile following the administration of bacterial pyrogen (Feldberg et al., 1972; Feldberg and Gupta, 1973). Prostaglandin levels were significantly elevated in febrile animals and decreased when the fever subsided or the animals were treated with antipyretic drugs known to inhibit prostaglandin synthesis. Based on chromatographic properties, prostaglandin E_2 was thought to be the active type.

In a more systematic study using precise mass-spectrometric methods, Wolfe and Mamer (1974) measured $PGF_{2\alpha}$ concentration in human cell-free

TABLE 5.   Prostaglandin $F_{2\alpha}$ in Human
Cerebrospinal Fluid[a]

Group	$PGF_{2\alpha}$ (pg/ml),[b] Mean $\pm$ SEM
"Normals"[c]	92 ± 10 (10)
Epilepsy, before surgery	559 ± 124 (11)
Epilepsy, 1–9 days after surgery	1221 ± 444 (10)
Meningitis–encephalitis	1081 ± 414 (5)

[a] CSF was obtained during pneumoencephalography, immediately centrifuged, and supernatant frozen until analyzed.
[b] $PGF_{2\alpha}$ was measured by gas chromatography–mass fragmentography following purification. $3,3,4,4\text{-}^2H_4\text{-}PGF_{2\alpha}$ was added as a carrier and internal standard. m/e 423 and 427 of the methyl ester trimethylsilyl ether derivatives were monitored.
[c] Patients with no organic neurological disease and normal pneumograms.

cerebrospinal fluid obtained during routine diagnostic pneumoencephalography. Summaries of the results obtained so far are given in Table 5. In the normal group, low but measurable levels were obtained. The result is in contrast to that for plasma, where the natural prostaglandins could not be detected because of the rapid metabolism, and is in agreement with the very low activities of the catabolizing enzymes in brain. Patients with seizures not surprisingly show increased levels of $PGF_{2\alpha}$, in line with the frequently demonstrated increases in formation and release after stimulation. The greatly increased levels in seizure patients following surgery is probably due to the stimulated synthesis by the surgical tissue trauma. Higher amounts are also found in acute inflammatory conditions. $PGF_{2\alpha}$ is greatly increased (38 pg/ml in normal to 655 pg/ml) in cerebrospinal fluid in patients with subarachnoid hemorrhage and following brain damage (Patrono and La Torre, 1974). No correlation was found with the degree of vasospasm. It is important to extend these studies to the measurement of PGE_2 and also to include a brain-tumor group. Hammarström et al. (1973) have reported rather dramatic increases in PGE_2 levels in cells and culture media of fibroblast transformed by oncogenic viruses. A similar stimulation of PGE_2 synthesis may occur in glioblastoma multiforme and be reflected in the cerebrospinal fluid levels.

A migraine-like headache is a side effect following intravenous administration of PGE_1 (Bergström et al., 1965). An unknown vasoactive principle that could be an acidic lipid has been reported in the CSF of a patient with migraine (Barrie and Jowett, 1967). Elevation of cerebrospinal fluid PG's during a migraine attack has not been found so far (Sandler, 1972). However, the data are quite inadequate and a more careful study is needed before prostaglandins can be excluded from a role in the intracerebral vascular changes during a migraine attack.

2.6.   Effects on Brain Function

2.6.1.   *Behavior*

The extensive investigations of Horton and his group showed that the E prostaglandins have a sedative–tranquilizer action on several animal species (see review by Horton, 1972). The most intense and prolonged effects were obtained by direct intraventricular injections of PGE_1 (3–20 μg/kg in the cat), which after a 5–20 min latent period produced a stuporous state progressing to catatonia (Horton, 1964). Parenteral administrations of PGE_1 were also effective but at much higher nonphysiological doses because of the substantial enzymatic inactivation before the compound reaches the brain. Furthermore, PGE_1 was found to potentiate the action of barbiturates and protected animals against convulsions produced by pentylenetetrazol, strychnine, or electroshock (Horton, 1972; Duru and Türker, 1969). Prostaglandins of the F type were completely inactive. PGF_2 injected intraperitoneally or subcutaneously into rodents and primates causes a marked depression of conditioned avoidance and escape responses in both naïve and trained animals (Potts and East, 1971a,b; Potts *et al.*, 1973).

The mechanism of the sedative effects is unknown, but action on brain-stem neurons or pathways is most likely. The effects are prolonged—existing long after the prostaglandins have been removed. Studies with tritiated PGE_1 by Holmes and Horton (1968c) showed that, within minutes after injection into the ventricular system, the prostaglandin had been removed and only very small amounts were taken up by brain tissue. This clearance is very likely an active process through the choroid plexus in view of the findings of Bito (1972a) that the choroid plexus *in vitro* is highly active in accumulating prostaglandins. The prolonged effects thus must arise through a slowly reversible alteration of chemical neurotransmission in brain-stem pathways (see Daugherty *et al.*, 1974). Alterations of blood supply through arteriolar vasoconstriction (Gilmore and Shaikh, 1972; Yamamoto *et al.*, 1973a,b; White *et al.*, 1974) may contribute to these effects, but probably of greater significance is a reduction of neurotransmitter release. Bergström *et al.* (1973) found that PGE_2 reduces stimulated release of norepinephrine and dopamine from rat cerebral cortex and neostriatum *in vitro* and also decreases the disappearance time *in vivo* of dopamine histofluorescence in the neostriatum of rats pretreated with a tyrosine hydroxylase inhibitor. Similar reduction of acetylcholine release from neurons in the ascending reticular-activating arousal pathways to the cerebral cortex may well account for the behavioral depression produced by the E prostaglandins.

2.6.2.   *Spinal Cord and Motor Pathways*

The effects of prostaglandins on spinal reflexes are complex, results varying with animal species, the type of experiment, and the prostaglandin used (for comprehensive reviews, see Horton, 1972; Coceani, 1974). $PGF_{1\alpha}$ and $PGF_{2\alpha}$ given intravenously cause immediate and extreme extension in the chick but not in the cat unless a decerebrate preparation is used. PGE_1 gives inconsistent results in the cat—facilitation, inhibition, or biphasic responses, depending upon the type of preparation. It is exceedingly difficult to separate actions of prostaglandins on blood supply to the spinal cord from direct actions on monosynaptic and polysynaptic reflexes. The inhibitory effects of PGE_1 could be related to a vasoconstrictor action or to actions at a number of sites, spinal as well as supraspinal. The general conclusion is that the main effect of both E and F prostaglandins on spinal reflexes is at the spinal cord level and is primarily an excitation of α-motoneurons (Horton and Main, 1967b, 1969; Duda *et al.*, 1968). The studies of Coceani *et al.*(1971), Coceani and Viti (1973), Phillis and Tebécis (1968) in the isolated superfused frog spinal cord are in accord with this view. Again it is apparent that the spinal cord effects are prolonged, greatly exceeding the time the compounds are actually in contact with or present in the tissue. Such prolonged changes are inconsistent with a transmitter-like role of the prostaglandins. As more information becomes available on the specific effects of prostaglandins on neurotransmitter release in the spinal cord, clearer explanations of these diverse effects should be possible.

2.6.3.   *Brain Stem*

Several lines of investigation indicate that both E- and F-type prosta-glandins have actions on brain stem neurons. Kaplan *et al.* (1969) present convincing evidence that PGE_1 stimulates brain-stem cardioregulatory centers. Injected through the carotid arteries into the vascularly isolated, neurally intact head of a dog perfused by a donor dog, PGE_1 raised the systemic blood pressure. Intravertebral infusion of $PGF_{2\alpha}$ also produces a dose-dependent rise in systemic blood pressure owing to an increase in cardiac output, but PGE_1 by this route only causes tachycardia (Lavery *et al.*, 1970, 1971). Again these effects are attributed to activation of cardiovascular brain-stem centers. Not all researchers agree on this point. Sweet *et al.* (1971) conclude that the hypertensive response to intravertebral infusion of $PGF_{2\alpha}$

is due to stimulation of the sympathetic nervous system. The quick reduction of sinus arrhythmia in dogs by intracarotid PGE_1 is also attributed to alteration of the interactions between the respiratory and cardio-inhibitory centers (McQueen and Ungar, 1969). The effect is prolonged and unaffected by denervation of the carotid sinus. Carlson *et al.* (1969) in their study of PGE_1 infusion in normal human subjects reported marked changes in ventilation leading to a fall in arterial pCO_2 and respiratory alkalosis. These increases in lung ventilation could arise by direct stimulation of the brainstem respiratory centers. The findings highlight the importance of monitoring blood pCO_2 during studies on the effect of prostaglandins *in vivo*. Since hypocapnea will vasoconstrict cerebral blood vessels, stimulation of brainstem centers particularly following intracisternal infusions can markedly modify cerebral blood flow indirectly through changes in ventilation. Local application of $PGF_{2\alpha}$ (10 μg/ml) to the dorsal medulla oblongata depresses synaptic transmission through the cuneate nucleus (Coceani *et al.*, 1969). In this system PGE_1 was inactive. Orthodromically evoked responses in the lemniscal fibers by direct stimulation of cuneate neurons or peripheral nerves were also reduced by $PGF_{2\alpha}$ (Coceani *et al.*, 1971). In conclusion, it is evident that prostaglandins stimulate or depress synaptic events in the brain stem depending on the specificity of particular neurons and pathways for individual prostaglandins.

2.6.4. *Hypothalamus*

2.6.4a. Fever and Thermoregulation. The implication of prostaglandins in fever production and thermoregulation was due to the discovery by Milton and Wendlandt (1970, 1971*a,b*) that single intraventricular injections of pyrogen-free solutions of PGE_1 or PGE_2 into unanesthetized cats in doses down to 10 ng produced a prompt elevation of body temperature associated with skin vasoconstriction, shivering, and piloerection. The temperature response was dose-related and lasted up to 5 hr. The responses to $PGF_{1\alpha}$, $PGF_{2\alpha}$, and PGA_1 in doses of 1–10 μg were variable—no effect, small temperature increases, or delayed effects. These experiments triggered a new approach in the complex field of thermoregulation, and the evidence is now very convincing that the E-type prostaglandins are natural mediators for pyrogen-induced hyperthermia. A brief summary of recent developments follows.

The E prostaglandins raise the temperature in all animal species examined so far: cat, mouse, rat, and rabbit (Milton and Wendlandt, 1971*a,b*; Feldberg and Saxena, 1971*a,b*; Feldberg, 1971; Potts and East, 1972; Willis *et al.*, 1972; Stitt, 1973). Recently, using surgically implanted telemeters, the core temperature of hamsters was monitored in the unrestrained state

(Miller and Sutton, 1974). Both PGE_2 and $PGF_{2\alpha}$ given subcutaneously caused a pyrexia that was unaffected by pretreatment with aspirin. In women, pyrexia associated with chills and shivering is a fairly frequent side effect when the prostaglandins are administered by intravenous, intrauterine, intravaginal, or intramuscular routes for the termination of second trimester pregnancies (Hendricks et al., 1971; Gillett et al., 1972; Embrey and Hillier, 1972). It is interesting that this occurs not only with PGE_2 but also with $PGF_{2\alpha}$, particularly with high doses and intravenous administration. Furthermore, early clinical trials with the synthetic prostaglandin analogues 15(S),15-methyl prostaglandin E_2 and $F_{2\alpha}$ methylesters, which are resistant to metabolism, have shown that sometimes quite severe pyrexia is a frequent side effect (Karim et al., 1973).

The site of action of the prostaglandins has been localized to the anterior hypothalamus, particularly the rostral part. Microinjections through stereotaxically placed cannulas in unanesthetized cats of as little as 2 ng PGE_1 produced significant hyperthermia. It was also shown that, during barbiturate anesthesia known to produce hypothermia by an action on the hypothalamus, the sensitivity to prostaglandins was greatly diminished (Feldberg, 1971; Stitt, 1973).

Earlier studies by Milton and Wendlandt (1968) showed that the normal temperature of unanesthetized cats was not affected by intraperitoneal injections of the antipyretic drug 4-acetamidophenol (paracetamol) but that the pyrexia produced by intracerebral injections of 5-hydroxytryptamine and pyrogen (TAB vaccine) was. In later experiments with prostaglandin fever, they found that is was also resistant to paracetamol and concluded that this drug might interfere with the release of prostaglandins (Milton and Wendlandt, 1971c). Vane's (1971) important discovery that certain anti-inflammatory and antipyretic drugs (aspirin and indomethacin) were potent inhibitors of prostaglandin biosynthesis added further weight to the idea that prostaglandins were mediating the pyrogen fever responses. Flower and Vane (1972) subsequently showed that brain prostaglandin synthetase was more sensitive to inhibition by paracetamol than were other tissues. These results suggest that prostaglandin synthesis is involved in the fever production and that the therapeutic action of these drugs is related to inhibition of its synthesis (Vane, 1973). Indeed, prostaglandin-like activity was found in cerebrospinal fluid during fever produced by bacterial pyrogens and endotoxins (Feldberg et al., 1972; Feldberg and Gupta, 1973; Milton, 1973).

Recently, more detailed investigations have been made on prostaglandin release in fever produced in cats by the pyrogen of Shigella dysenteriae (Feldberg et al., 1973). In cats without fever, prostaglandin-like activity of cisternal cerebrospinal fluid bioassayed on the rat stomach fundus strip was less than 1 ng/ml (below the threshold sensitivity of the method). Addition of pyrogen into the third ventricle into the cisternal magna, or intravenously increased the prostaglandin-like activity to as high as 100 ng, but there was considerable variability among animals. Antipyretic drugs decreased the fever and the release of prostaglandins. The bacterial pyrogens increased prostaglandin synthesis not only in the preoptic anterior hypothalamic area but also in other parts of the brain. Thin-layer chromatography showed that the activity was concentrated in the E zone and probably was due to PGE_2. Thus these studies strongly support a role of prostaglandins in fever production. Incubated slices from the cat anterior hypothalamus show considerable endogenous synthesis of both PGE_2 and $PGF_{2\alpha}$ determined by gas chromatography–mass fragmentography (see Table 4).

The current hypothesis is that pyrogens (bacterial or leukocytic) and endotoxins accelerate the biosynthesis of prostaglandins in brain and specifically in the anterior hypothalamus through stimulation of the rate-controlling step releasing the precursor fatty acids. The prostaglandins formed or the endoperoxide intermediates act locally on neurons, a process that leads to fever responses, and are liberated into the cerebrospinal fluid where they may affect behavior through actions on other brain centers. Ultimately the prostaglandins are cleared in the venous circulation and inactivated by metabolism in the lung and liver. The presence of prostaglandins probably also explains the pyrexia produced in cross-perfusion experiments of cerebrospinal fluid from cooled, shivering monkeys to other animals (Myers, 1967). Furthermore, perfusion of cerebral ventricles of unanesthetized cats with a calcium-free saline solution causes an immediate intense hyperthermia (Feldberg et al., 1970). However, a long-lasting rise in temperature was observed independent of the composition of the perfusion fluid. This response may well be due to prostaglandins released through damage to cerebral tissues by the cannulation procedure.

The action of the E prostaglandins differs in a number of respects from the effects of monoamines (norepinephrin, dopamine, 5-hydroxytryptamine), which are widely thought to be the effectors of temperature regulation in mammals (Feldberg and Myers, 1964; Lomax, 1970; Veale and Cooper, 1973). The prostaglandins are about 1000 times more potent and always produce a temperature increase which is little affected by the ambient temperature in all species studied. The sign of response for each monoamine, on the other hand, is species dependent and conditioned by a high or low ambient temperature. A current theory explains temperature regulation in terms of an antagonistic relationship (thermogenic or thermolytic) between the catecholamines and 5-hydroxytryptamine (Veale and Cooper, 1973). However, the evidence is inconclusive that biogenic amines are directly involved in the production of pyrogen fever (Cooper et al., 1967; Feldberg, 1971), and the E prostaglandins appear much more likely candidates.

However, prostaglandin release by pyrogens may alter the balance between catecholamines and serotonin through their known inhibitory actions on the release of norepinephrin from nerve terminals (Hedqvist, 1972), which would reduce the thermolytic action of the catecholamine. Another action of prostaglandins must also be considered in this regard, namely, their vasoconstrictive action on small cerebral arterioles, which could also affect the balance of neurotransmitter release by production of a local ischemia.

Although there is much evidence to implicate prostaglandins in the genesis of pyrogen fever, there is little evidence that normal body temperature is maintained by a continuous release of prostaglandins. Antipyretic drugs that inhibit prostaglandin synthesis do not generally affect normal body temperature. On the other hand, a recent report (Satinoff, 1973) demonstrated in rats that sodium salicylate lowered the rectal temperature by up to 5.5°C when the animals were placed in a 5°C environment but that at 23°C the hypothermia was less marked. This suggests that prostaglandins may be involved after all in normal temperature control and that cold stress may accelerate the local release of prostaglandins. If synthesis and release are inhibited, body temperature would fall. Intraventricular infusion in the dog of 5-hydroxytryptamine (thermogenic in this species) stimulates the release of E-type prostaglandins (Holmes, 1970). It is possible that stimulation of the release of serotonin from neurons in the anterior hypothalamus accelerates prostaglandin-E synthesis, which would initiate the thermogenic response. Clearly, more research is needed before prostaglandins can be implicated in the normal physiological control of temperature or in all pharmacological or pathological thermogenic responses. For example, exercise pyrexia, etiocholanolone fever, familial Mediterranean fever, and anesthetic malignant hyperpyrexia are unaffected by antiinflammatory and antipyretic drugs and thus are probably not mediated by prostaglandin release.

2.6.4b. Pituitary Hormone Release. Hormonal secretions by the anterior pituitary are regulated by peptide hormones released by the hypothalamus into the hypophyseal portal blood vessels (McCann and Porter, 1969). There is ever-increasing evidence that prostaglandins of the E and F types have pharmacological actions suggesting their implication in the physiological control of hormone-release processes at the hypothalamus–pituitary axis. Stimulation of ACTH release by intravenous injection of low doses of PGE_1 has been observed in several laboratories (deWied et al., 1969; Peng et al., 1970; Hedge and Hanson, 1972) and is regarded as a hypothalamic stimulation of the release of the corticotropin-releasing hormone (CRH). PGE_1 did not increase significantly the release of ACTH from anterior pituitary tissue *in vitro*, whereas even impure preparations of CRH are exceedingly active (deWied et al., 1969). On the other hand, Vale et al. (1971) report increases in ACTH and TSH secretion *in vitro* by PGE_1 in the high

μg/ml dose range which are diminished by the antagonist 7-oxa-13-prosty-noic acid. This is probably due to a direct action resulting in an increase in intracellular cAMP, which is also elevated by CRH (Zor et al., 1970; Kuehl et al., 1973). Microinjections of prostaglandins of both the E and F series (0.5–1 μg) directly into the basal hypothalamic region were very effective in causing ACTH secretion (Hedge and Hanson, 1972). The effect was diminished by dexamethasone and abolished by morphine. Microinjections into the pituitary have absolutely no effect. It is unclear why only the E series is active intravenously but both E and F are active when applied directly to the hypothalamus. This difference is also apparent with the release of other pituitary hormones. Differences in rate of inactivation of the E and F types or differences in penetrability into brain have been postulated, but there really is no evidence to support either of these views. Direct injections of PGE_2 into the third ventricle of ovariectomized rats greatly increased plasma levels of luteinizing hormone (LH) and follicle-stimulating hormone (FSH) but was ineffective when injected into the anterior pituitary (Harms et al., 1973). $PGF_{1\alpha}$ and $PGF_{2\alpha}$ were ineffective. Again this gives support for the indirect evidence that prostaglandins can affect ovulation at the hypothalamic level (Labhsetwar, 1970; Orczyke and Behrman, 1972; Carlson et al., 1973).

Prostaglandin E_1 at low concentrations does not stimulate the release of LH from pituitary tissue in vitro, but high doses (10^{-4} M) do increase release and elevate the tissue cyclic AMP (Ratner et al., 1974). Several laboratories have reported an increase in growth hormone (GH) release by PGE_1 from anterior pituitary tissue in vitro (Zor et al., 1970; Schofield, 1970; McLeod and Lehmeyer 1970; Hertelendy, 1971) and also have reported that the release is independent of protein synthesis. Intravenous PGE_1 (50–140 μg/kg/min) does increase plasma GH in man, and it is thought that the effect is at the hypothalamic level (Ito et al., 1971). Intracarotid injections of PGE_2 (1–20 μg) markedly increase urine osmolarity and decrease urine flow in rats (Vilhardt and Hedqvist, 1970), and again this effect on vasopressin secretion could be via the hypothalamus. Intravenous $PGF_{2\alpha}$ (single 5-mg dose or infusion at 0.5 mg/min) to heifers increased plasma prolactin, GH, glucocorticoids, and LH (Louis et al., 1974). Administration of single doses of 10–20 μg $PGF_{2\alpha}$ to breast-feeding women brought about milk ejection of variable latency (Cobo et al., 1974). It was concluded that the effect was due to a central stimulation of oxytocin release. In a series of interesting experiments, Labhsetwar and Zolovick (1973) found that microinjections of aspirin directly into the hypothalamus inhibited markedly the progesterone-induced ovulation in immature rats primed with pregnant mare serum gonadotrophin. Injections of $PGF_{2\alpha}$ or dopamine simultaneously with aspirin restored ovulation, but dopamine alone had no effect. It was suggested that $PGF_{2\alpha}$ modulates the neurotransmitter role of catecholamines and thus potentiates adrenergic neurotransmission and the release of gonadotrophin-releasing hormones.

It is much too early to make any generalizations on a physiological role of prostaglandins in the regulation of release of hypothalamic-releasing hormones. It is clear, though, that prostaglandins are not releasing hormones. Many of the effects of prostaglandins reported, particularly those on cAMP levels, may be straight pharmacological responses and bear little relationship to the *in vivo* situation. There is clear divergence of results with the E- and F-type prostaglandins when they are injected directly into the hypothalamus or given intravenously. It is quite possible that the specific neuronal pathways for the release of each specific releasing hormone may respond differently to the E or F prostaglandins and that one or the other type might be preferentially synthesized. The most reasonable position at present is that prostaglandins formed locally might interact with catecholamine release mechanisms thereby effecting release of the hypothalamic hormones.

    2.6.2c.   Control of Food Intake. Prostaglandins E_1 (0.1 mg/kg) and A_1, $F_{1\alpha}$, and $F_{2\alpha}$ (1 mg/kg) administered subcutaneously to fasted rats reduced their feeding behavior for at least 45 min (Scaramuzzi *et al.*, 1971). Microinjections of PGE_1 into the medial and lateral hypothalamus of rats and sheep also decreased food intake (Baile *et al.*, 1973; Martin and Baile, 1973; see review by Baile and Forbes, 1974). The prostaglandin inhibitor polyphloretin phosphate blocked the PGE_1 effect, but this action could be nonspecific. In sheep, feeding is increased if the injections are made into the anterior hypothalamus. As in other hypothalamic regions, the satiety and hunger centers and the control of energy balance might involve endogenously synthesized prostaglandins modulating noradrenergic neurotransmission.

2.7. Direct Applications to Neurons

Prostaglandins have variable effects when applied by microiontophoresis to central neurons. Avanzino *et al.* (1966a,b) reported predominantly excitatory responses of brain-stem neurons to PGE_1, PGE_2, and $PGF_{2\alpha}$, but over 50% of the neurons tested were unresponsive and the excitatory action showed rapid desensitization. Neurons in the cerebral cortex and cuneate nucleus are unresponsive (Krnjević, 1965; Coceani *et al.*, 1971). Bloom's group (Siggins *et al.*, 1971a,b; Hoffer *et al.*, 1971, 1972) found excitation predominantly of neurons in the cerebellar cortex, hippocampus, and brain system of the rat by PGE_1 and PGE_2. Furthermore, there was a consistent antagonism of the inhibitory action of norepinephrine applied concurrently. Their hypothesis was that an intracellular cAMP increase mediates the inhibitory effects of norepinephrine and PGE's block this through effects on adenyl cyclase. Iontophoretically applied cAMP also inhibited Purkinje cells, but this was not antagonized by PGE_1. These results have been widely quoted, perhaps because they were consistent with the early negative feedback hypothesis of Bergström (1967) and the inhibitory effects of PGE_1 on dopamine action in the sympathetic ganglia (McAfee and Greengard, 1972). Caution is needed in these interpretations: First, they run counter to the Hedqvist hypothesis that PGE's act on presynaptic terminals to reduce transmitter release; second, the most common response of many cells including nerve cells to the PGE's is an increase in cAMP; and, third, cAMP can penetrate nerve cell membranes in only one direction, namely from inside to outside, and extracellular cAMP cannot enter cells (Lindl and Cramer, 1974). In addition, the experiments of Siggins et al. (1971) could not be reproduced by others nor have similar results been obtained in cerebral cortex or brain stem (Anderson et al., 1973; Lake et al., 1972, 1973; Godfraind and Pumain, 1971, 1972).

2.8.   Adenylate and Guanylate Cyclase Systems

There is now much evidence that the E prostaglandins stimulate cAMP formation and increase intracellular cAMP contents in many tissues (Butcher, 1970; Robinson et al., 1971; Hittelman and Butcher, 1973). The adipocyte is an exception in that PGE's decrease hormonally stimulated cAMP levels but have no effect on unstimulated cells. Several laboratories have shown stimulation by PGE_1 of cAMP formation in cultured neural tissues and in slices of cerebral cortex in vitro (Gilman and Nirenberg, 1971; Asakawa and Yoshida, 1971; Gilman, 1972; Gilman and Schrier, 1972; Berti et al., 1973). The responses vary with the species studied. For example, the cAMP levels in slices of rabbit and human brain are unaffected by PGE_1 but are stimulated when rat tissues are used. Intravenous administration of PGE_1 and PGE_2 at doses of 1 mg/kg (threshold 0.5 mg/kg) to rats and mice caused an increase in the first minute in the cAMP levels in seven discrete brain regions followed by a rapid decrease (Wellmann and Schwabe, 1973). PGE_2 was the most effective and $PGF_{2\alpha}$ at the same dose level produced only a slight increase in the first 30 sec after injection. The sedation and stupor produced correlated fairly well with the increase in cAMP.

Which brain-cell types, neurons or glia, are specifically affected by the prostaglandins is not certain. Gilman and Nirenberg (1971) found no stimulatory effects of PGE_1 on cAMP in clones of rat glial tumor cells but did find such effects with norepinephrine. In contrast, several clones of human astrocytoma cell lines originally obtained from a cerebral glioma responded with a rise in cAMP content to norepinephrine, histamine, adenosine, and PGE_1 (Perkins, 1973). The effects of the four agonists are not additive, and it appears that there are receptors distinct for each stimulator. Propranolol inhibited only the response to norepinephrine, and theophylline blocked only the effect of adenosine. Interpretation of the effects of the variety of stimulators of adenyl cyclase in slices of brain cortex is complex to say the least. Synergism of action occurs at maximally effective concentrations, e.g., histamine plus norepinephrine, adenosine plus norepinephrine, PGE_1 plus norepinephrine, histamine, or adenosine (Schimizu *et al.*, 1970; Huang *et al.*, 1971; Berti *et al.*, 1973). Homogenization of the tissue destroys the hormonal responsiveness of the brain adenyl cyclase. The synergistic effects of combinations of hormones and PGE_1 observed in slices of brain in contrast to tumor glial cells could be the result of interactions on different cell types, but it is also possible that in the transformed tumor cells there is masking of hormonal receptors.

There is a growing appreciation that intracellular cAMP concentrations undergo cyclic changes during the growth cycle in cell cultures (Otten *et al.*, 1971; Sheppard, 1972; Burger *et al.*, 1972). High intracellular levels of cAMP are associated with inhibited cell growth (confluent, contact-inhibited cell lines), whereas during active mitosis (virus transformation of cell lines) the cAMP levels are lowest. These changes are also associated with morphological alterations and cell surface changes and are affected by prostaglandins (Johnson and Pastan, 1971). Mouse neuroblastoma cells in culture respond to dibutyryl cyclic AMP and to PGE_1 and PGE_2 by a striking morphological differentiation with the development of axon-like processes (Prasad, 1972). This result is in accord with the known effects of prostaglandins, which increase intracellular cAMP. However, a paradoxical situation exists which is unresolved at the present time: Specific measurements of PGE_2 biosynthesis in virus-transformed fibroblast cell cultures show marked increases in PGE_2 production compared with normal cells (Hammarström *et al.*, 1973). Thus, increased endogenous prostaglandin production occurs during transformation when levels of cAMP are low, not what would be expected from the pharmacological studies.

Another aspect of relationships between cAMP and the E prostaglandins is the recent report by Collier and Roy (1974) that morphine and related drugs inhibit the stimulation by PGE_1 of cAMP formation in homogenates of rat brain. The authors go on to correlate the pharmacological effects of opiates to the inhibition of the action of PGE_1 on intracellular cAMP. It is unfortunate that homogenates of brain rather than slices of brain were used since the stimulation of cAMP required very high doses of prostaglandins.

Guanylate cyclase has been found in particulate and high-speed supernatant fractions of many tissues, and cGMP levels like cAMP levels

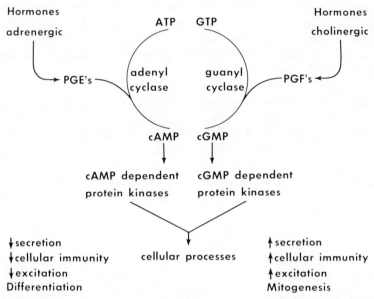

FIGURE 3. Diagrammatic representation of the dualistic hypothesis of Goldberg on the opposing actions of adrenergic and cholinergic hormones and agonists on adenylate and guanylate cyclases.

are high in brain. A surprising finding is that acetylcholine and cholinergic agonists elevate cGMP levels in many tissues including the perfused rat heart, cerebellum, and cerebral cortex (see review by Goldberg *et al.*, 1973). It is of great interest that $PGF_{2\alpha}$, oxytocin, and serotonin, like cholinergic agents, also promote cyclic GMP accumulation in the rat uterus *in vitro*. These findings and others have led to speculation that cGMP is involved in promoting cellular processes that are antagonistic to those mediated by cAMP, and Goldberg has formulated a "dualism" theory of biological control by opposing actions of the two nucleotides (Figure 3). It is premature to invoke, especially for brain, a role for $PGF_{2\alpha}$ in facilitating excitation of acetylcholine and serotonin pathways through activation of guanylcyclase, but the possibility is so interesting that it should not be long before solid data one way or the other are forthcoming.

2.9. Cerebral Blood Flow, Cerebral Vasospasm, and Cerebral Ischemia

Arterial and arteriolar spasm of cerebral blood vessels, which is a frequent occurrence in patients following subarachnoid hemorrhage, is of great clinical importance since it is implicated as one of the major causes of mortality following rupture of an intracranial aneurysm (Allcock and Drake, 1965; Brawley *et al.*, 1968). An extensive literature over the past 10 years implicates mechanical, chemical, and neurogenic factors in the genesis of clinical cerebral vasospasm (see the *Journal of Neurosurgery*, 1965–1974, and *Stroke*, 1970–1974, for many articles). There is still considerable controversy on the main causal factor, and the problem is unresolved. Evidence is mounting that vasoconstricting agents particularly associated with platelets are present in blood (Echlin, 1968; Kapp *et al.*, 1968). Serotonin released from platelets can produce vasospasm and constrict cerebral arterial smooth muscle *in vitro* (Raynor *et al.*, 1961; Echlin, 1968; Allen *et al.*, 1974). However, substances other than serotonin appear responsible for the prolonged vaso-spasm seen in the clinical situations (Buckell, 1964; Kapp *et al.*, 1970). It is well recognized that platelets form and release E- and F-type prostaglandins and endoperoxide intermediates during aggregation (Clausen and Srivastava, 1972; Smith *et al.*, 1973; Willis, 1974). Arachidonic acid causes rapid platelet aggregation and death following injection in rabbits (Silver *et al.*, 1974). Thus it is not surprising that recent interest has centered on the contribution prostaglandins might make to the normal and pathophysiological responses of cerebral blood vessels.

Studies using isolated aortic strips (Wilkins *et al.*, 1967) demonstrated a spasmogenic substance in cerebrospinal fluid from patients with sub-arachnoid hemorrhage which was not serotonin. Recent studies (White *et al.*, 1971; Denton *et al.*, 1972; Pennick *et al.*, 1972; Yamamoto *et al.*, 1973a,b) all show that $PGF_{2\alpha}$ vasoconstricts cerebral blood vessels in the dog and monkey and decreases blood flow when administered directly into the caro-tid circulation. The effect is prolonged and independent of the actions of serotonin and norepinephrine, indeed, very similar to what occurs in clinical vasospasm. Pennick *et al.* (1972), in an angiographic study in dogs, injected directly into the chiasmatic cistern $PGF_{2\alpha}$ mixed either with blood or with saline in 20 μg/kg doses. A marked spasmogenic effect was observed. Dose–response curves of segments of canine basilar and middle cerebral arteries *in vitro* to a number of vasoactive agents indicated that the KED50 (con-centration of agent to give 50% of the maximal contraction) for serotonin, PGE_1, and $PGF_{2\alpha}$ was $7 \times 10^{-9} M$, $2 \times 10^{-10} M$, and $3 \times 10^{-7} M$, respectively. It was concluded, based on the comparison of molar concentra-tions of these agents in platelets with the dose–response curves, that sero-tonin is probably the agent responsible for cerebral vasospasm. However, measurement of prostaglandin contents in platelets is subject to many errors. Furthermore, serotonin is released immediately on aggregation, whereas prostaglandins are formed and released over a much longer time course.

While it is clear that low concentrations of $PGF_{2\alpha}$ can cause cerebral vasoconstriction *in vivo* and *in vitro*, the results obtained by different groups for the E-type prostaglandins are contradictory (Denton *et al.*, 1972; Yamamoto *et al.*, 1973*a*). The reasons for the discrepancies may be related to the techniques used to measure cerebral blood flow and the size of the arterial vessels studied. The dog is not the ideal experimental animal because of the variable anastomotic vessels connecting the extracranial and intracranial circulations, unless direct measurements of cerebral flow are made (Yamamoto *et al.*, 1973*a*). It is also a frequent practice of researchers to use ethanol to dissolve PGE_1 in saline solutions, and this can reverse the prostaglandin vasoconstriction. The use of ^{133}Xe to measure microregional cerebral blood flow in epicerebral blood vessels of the dog and monkey cerebral hemispheres clearly showed that intracarotid infusions of PGE_1, PGE_2, and $PGF_{2\alpha}$ reduce blood flow up to 42%. The effect was prolonged (more than 6 hr) and was reversed by 0.1% ethanol infusions (Yamamoto *et al.*, 1973*b*). A corresponding constriction in small-diameter cerebral arterioles was found by direct measurements made from color photographs. Thus, in summary, both E- and F-type prostaglandins can vasoconstrict cerebral blood vessels in low concentrations and must be seriously considered as vasoactive agents in the genesis of clinical vasospasm, particularly since their effects are long-lasting. However, much more definitive work is needed to prove they are the key factors released from platelets following subarachnoid hemorrhage. In this regard, Wilson and Field (1974) implicate spasmogenic substances released from locally damaged brain tissue, particularly the hypothalamus, as contributing to cerebrovascular spasm, and they consider $PGF_{2\alpha}$ as the most likely substance. Their view is consistent with the considerable capacity of brain tissue to synthesize this prostaglandin.

Cerebral thromboembolism stands among the three major causes of death and one of the most common causes of neurological disability. Clearly, vasoactive factors released from platelet emboli and the damaged and necrosing ischemic brain tissue will greatly modify the blood supply surrounding an ischemic lesion and lead to the expansion of the brain damage. Prostaglandins are among the substances formed and released during ischemic brain damage. Accumulating evidence indicates that aspirin, a potent prostaglandin synthesis inhibitor as well as an inhibitor of platelet aggregation, is of real therapeutic value in focal cerebral ischemia. Whether the decrease of platelet aggregation or the inhibition of prostaglandin synthesis by platelets or brain tissue is the important factor in the therapeutic effectiveness—indeed, it may be both—is yet to be resolved. The issue has such obvious clinical importance that, with the advances in the techniques of prostaglandin measurement and collaboration between neurosurgeons, neurologists, and neurochemists, an answer to the role of prostaglandins in vascular pathophysiology should not be far away.

3. PERIPHERAL NERVOUS SYSTEM

3.1. Release Following Nerve Stimulation

Stimulation of sympathetic or parasympathetic nerves is associated with the release of prostaglandins, principally PGE_2 and $PGF_{2\alpha}$ (rat stomach, Coceani et al., 1967; Bennett et al., 1967; adipose tissue, Shaw and Ramwell, 1968, Lewis and Matthews, 1969, Fredholm et al., 1970; spleen, Davies et al., 1968, Gilmore et al., 1968; rabbit heart, Wennmalm 1971; dog kidney, Dunham and Zimmerman, 1970; seminal vesicles, Hedqvist, 1972; vas deferens, Hedqvist and von Euler, 1972; cat superior cervical ganglion, Davis et al., 1971; Auerbach's plexus, Ambache et al., 1970). The prostaglandins are not released from preformed stores, rather, de novo biosynthesis is accelerated during the stimulation period. Although unproved, the accelerated synthesis is thought to result from stimulation of acyl hydrolases that liberate the free substrate fatty acids from precursor membrane lipids to the site of the membrane-bound cyclo-oxygenases. The rate of prostaglandin release is in general related to the stimulus frequency and decreases to spontaneous levels on cessation of stimulation. There is good evidence that the postsynaptic effector cell membrane is the site of synthesis and release, since receptor blockade by drugs (hyoscine, atropine, phenoxybenzamine, dibenzyline) inhibits prostaglandin release without affecting neurotransmitter release and the addition of the neurotransmitter hormones stimulates release.

3.2. Regulation of Autonomic Neurotransmission—The Hedqvist Hypothesis

3.2.1. Sympathetic Neurotransmission

Sympathetic nerve stimulation to various organs (heart, oviduct, spleen, vas deferens) induces release of both norepinephrine and prostaglandin (principally PGE_2). Effector responses to nerve stimulation are inhibited by exogenously added PGE_1 and PGE_2 but not by the PGF series of prostaglandins (Brundin, 1968; Hedqvist and Brundin, 1969; von Euler and Hedqvist, 1969). The inhibition can be produced by exceedingly low concentrations in the picogram and nanogram range well within possible physiological concentrations (Ambache and Zar, 1970; Baum and Shropshire, 1971; Hedqvist et al., 1970). These findings led Hedqvist to speculate that endogenous PGE_2 formed and released from the postsynaptic effector

Sympathetic
Nerve Terminal   Synaptic Gap   Effector Cell

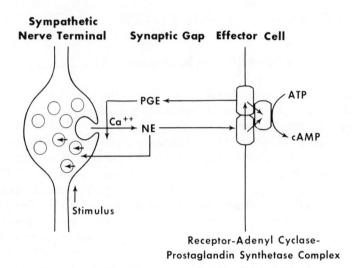

Receptor-Adenyl Cyclase-
Prostaglandin Synthetase Complex

FIGURE 4. Diagrammatic representation of the Hedqvist hypothesis of feedback control of the release of norepinephrine by the E-prostaglandins at sympathetic nerve terminals.

membrane during stimulation inhibits the release of norepinephrine from the presynaptic terminals (see reviews by Hedqvist, 1973a,b, and references therein). Good evidence for the existence of the negative feedback control hypothesis was obtained using a specific inhibitor of endogenous prostaglandin synthesis, namely 5,8,11,14-eicosatetraynoic acid (ETA). This carboxylic acid does not affect norepinephrine release at rest in the rabbit heart preparation nor interfere with uptake, but it blocks the release of prostaglandins and markedly increases, within minutes after application, the outflow of norepinephrine (Samuelsson and Wennmalm, 1971). Similar results were found for the cat spleen and guinea pig vas deferens preparations (see Hedqvist, 1973a). Furthermore, antiinflammatory drugs (aspirin, indomethacin) which are also powerful inhibitors of prostaglandin synthesis also increase the effector responses of the isolated dog spleen preparation to epinephrine (Ferreira *et al.*, 1971). Many other studies, principally by Hedqvist, Wennmalm, von Euler, Stjärne *et al.* at the Karolinska Institute, are consistent with the negative feedback hypothesis of control of neurotransmitter release. These studies have been reviewed in excellent articles by Smith (1972), Hedqvist (1973a), and Brody and Kadowitz (1974). Inconsistent observations are discussed by Weeks (1972). It is still too early to make generalizations that the physiological role in the sympathetic nervous system of stimulated biosynthesis of PGE prostaglandins is solely to "police" the release of transmitter rather than to modify the action of the mediator on its target cell. The hypothesis of a presynaptic action of prostaglandins inhibiting stimulus-coupled exocytosis of sympathetic neurotransmitter was greatly strengthened by the work of Johnson *et al.* (1971), who found that, in the innervated guinea pig vas deferens, PGE_2 inhibited the augmented release of dopamine-β-hydroxylase produced by stimulation of the presence of increased calcium concentration or phenoxybenzamine. The influx of calcium into nerve terminals is an essential component of the stimulus-coupled exocytosis of neurotransmitter, along with adenine nucleotides and dopamine-β-hydroxylase. The mechanism by which the PGE's interfere with calcium influx is unknown. That PGE_1 in nanogram quantities markedly facilitates the nonenergized binding of calcium to the mitochondrial inner membrane suggests that they might act similarly on the presynaptic terminals (Kirtland and Baum, 1972).

While the research mentioned above greatly favors the hypothesis that the E-type prostaglandins control autonomic neurotransmission by feedback inhibition, there is now growing evidence that the F-type prostaglandins have a facilitating action. For example, in studies with the perfused saphenous vein preparation and the perfused hind paw of the dog, $PGF_{1\alpha}$ and $PGF_{2\alpha}$ significantly increase the responses to norepinephrine (Kadowitz *et al.*, 1971*a,b*). $PGF_{2\alpha}$ also potentiates the action of norepinephrine on uterine blood vessels at concentrations which have no effect on uterine vascular resistance (Clark *et al.*, 1973). The vasoconstrictor effects of norepinephrine on pulmonary vessels are sensitized by $PGF_{2\alpha}$ (Kadowitz *et al.*, 1973). Neurogenically evoked vasoconstriction to cutaneous vessels is also facilitated by $PGF_{2\alpha}$ in quantities of less than a nanogram (Sweet *et al.*, 1971; Kadowitz *et al.*, 1972). All the evidence for the facilitating effects of the F-type prostaglandins cannot be reported here, and the interested reader should consult the recent reviews (Kadowitz *et al.*, 1972; Brody and Kadowitz, 1974). The evidence is quite impressive that the E- and F-type prostaglandins have competitive interactions at adrenergic nerve terminals. One hopes that future research will clarify whether the prejunctional or postjunctional interactions of the prostaglandins are the physiologically important ones.

3.2.2. *Parasympathetic Neurotransmission*

Both the E- and the F-type prostaglandins contract longitudinal smooth muscles of the gastrointestinal tract. Indeed, the most sensitive preparations from particular animal species (gerbil colon, rat stomach fundus strip) are used for bioassay. The prostaglandin action appears to be directly on the smooth muscle and not mediated by the innervation (Coceani and Wolfe, 1966). However, parasympathetic neurotransmission to the rabbit heart seems to be different. Here PGE_1 at very low concentrations inhibits the decrease in heart rate produced by stimulation of the cholinergic nerves (Wennmalm and Hedqvist, 1971) but has no effect on the response to infused acetylcholine. Thus a prejunctional effect is suspected similar to the much more extensive evidence for the sympathetic nervous system. Whether the E prostaglandins have a similar action on other cholinergic pathways is uncertain. For example, the inhibition by PGE_1 of the bronchoconstriction caused by vagus nerve stimulation (Main, 1964) in several animal species could also be due to inhibition of release of acetylcholine. Hahn and Patil (1972, 1974) have reported that $PGF_{2\alpha}$ given intravenously in dogs produced copious salivation which was augmented by physostigmine and abolished by atropine. This prostaglandin effect is interpreted as a stimulation of the release of endogenous acetylcholine. Taira and Satoh (1973) injected $PGF_{2\alpha}$ directly into the arterial supply to the submaxillary gland. Salivation and increased blood flow developed slowly and the effect was prolonged quite in contrast to the action of acetylcholine. The response could be elicited by very small amounts of $PGF_{2\alpha}$ (1–100 ng), which was many times more potent than acetylcholine. The effect on both secretion and blood vessels was abolished by tetrodotoxin. The parasympathetic postganglionic neurons, not the ganglionic neurons, appeared to be the site of action, since the salivation was unaffected by hexamethonium.

3.3. Ganglionic Neurotransmission

The fast excitatory postsynaptic action potentials produced by preganglionic stimulation of the cervical sympathetic trunk are not affected by PGE_1 or PGE_2 (Kayaalp and McIsaac, 1968). There is no evidence to support an action of prostaglandins on the release of acetylcholine or its action at the nicotinic cholinoreceptors in the superior cervical ganglion. This may not be the case for excitation through the muscarinic cholinergic receptors responsible for slow excitatory postsynaptic potentials or the slow inhibitory postsynaptic potentials mediated by dopamine release from small, intensely fluorescent interneurons (S.I.F. cells). Greengard and his group have mounted impressive evidence that the slow inhibitory postsynaptic potentials and the dopamine-induced hyperpolarization of postganglionic neurons in sympathetic ganglia are generated by an increase in cAMP (McAfee and Greengard, 1972; Greengard and Kebabian, 1974). PGE_1 virtually abolishes the slow inhibitory potentials and the hyperpolarization caused by dopamine. These results are interpreted as due to a prostaglandin inhibition of adenyl cyclase in the postsynaptic membrane rather than an inhibition of presynaptic transmitter release. A role for cGMP in the generation of the slow excitatory postsynaptic potentials at the cholinergic muscarinic receptors is also postulated. The F-type prostaglandins could act through stimulation of guanyl cyclase, as has been suggested by Goldberg *et al.* (1973).

3.4. Neuromuscular Junctions

Ramwell *et al.* (1965) and Laity (1969) have reported that PGE_1 determined by bioassay methods was released from the rat nerve diaphragm on stimulation of the phrenic nerve. However, subsequent studies (Ginsborg and Hirst, 1971; Marco and Coceani, 1973) indicate that prostaglandins are inactive at all concentrations on neurotransmission at neuromuscular junctions. Spontaneous miniature end-plate potentials and evoked end-plate potentials are unaffected by PGE_1. Prostaglandins do not appear to play any role in effector responses at nicotinic cholinoreceptors.

Acknowledgments

This review and the work of the author and associates reported in it were supported by grants from the Medical Research Council of Canada. Dr. J. E. Pike of The Upjohn Company, Kalamazoo, Michigan, generously provided the prostaglandins and deuterated standards.

4. GENERAL BIBLIOGRAPHY

Anderson, G. G., Caldwell, B. V., and Speroff, L., eds., 1972, *Prostaglandins*, Geron-X, New Haven, Conn.
Bentley, P. H., 1973, Total syntheses of prostanoids, *Chem. Soc. Rev.* **2**:29–48.
Bergström, S., ed., 1973, *International Conference on Prostaglandins, Advances in the Biosciences*, Pergamon, New York.
Bergström, S., and Samuelsson, B., eds., 1967, *Prostaglandin*, Nobel Symposium 2, Almqvist and Wiksell, Stockholm.
Bergström, S., Carlson, L. A., and Weeks, J. R., 1968, *Pharmac. Rev.* **20**:2–48.
Cuthbert, M. F., ed., 1973, *The Prostaglandins*, Pharmacological and Therapeutic Advances, Lippincott, Philadelphia.
Euler, U. S., von, and Eliasson, R., 1967, *Prostaglandins*, Academic Press, New York.
Horton, E. W., 1972, *Prostaglandins, Monographs on Endocrinology 7*, Springer–Verlag, New York.
Kahn, R. H., and Lands, W. E. M., eds., 1973, *Prostaglandins and Cyclic AMP*, Academic Press, New York.
Karim, S. M. M., ed., 1972, *The Prostaglandins*, Medical and Technical Publishing Co., Oxford, England.
Lobotsky, J., ed., 1972, *Research in Prostaglandins*, Prostaglandin Information Center of the Worcester Foundation.

Oesterling, T. O., Morozowich, W., and Roseman, T. J., Prostaglandins, *J. Pharmacol. Sci.* **61**:1862–1895.
Pickles, V. R., 1967, The prostaglandins, *Biol. Rev.* **42**:614–652.
Pike, J. E., and Weeks, J. R., eds., *The Prostaglandins*, Bibliography, The Upjohn Company, Kalamazoo, Michigan.
Prostaglandines, 1973, INSERM, Paris.
Ramwell, P. W., 1973, *The Prostaglandins, Vol. 1*, Plenum, New York.
Ramwell, P. W., and Shaw, J. E., eds., 1967, *Prostaglandin Symposium of the Worcester Foundation for Experimental Biology*, Interscience, New York.
Ramwell, P. W., and Pharris, B. B., eds., 1972, *Prostaglandins in Cellular Biology*, Plenum Press, New York.
Ramwell, P. W., and Shaw, J. E., eds., 1971, Prostaglandins, *Ann. N.Y. Acad. Sci.*, Volume 180.
Ramwell, P. W., Shaw, J. E., Clarke, G. B., Grostic, M. F., Kaiser, D. G., and Pike, J. E., 1968, in: *Progress in the Chemistry of Fats and Other Lipids*, Vol. 9 (Holman, R. T., ed.), pp. 233–273, Pergamon, New York.
Shaw, J. E., and Ramwell, P. W., 1969, in *Methods of Biochemical Analysis* (D. Glick, ed.), Interscience, New York.
Southern, E. M., ed., 1972, *The Prostaglandins. Clinical applications in human reproduction*, Futura Publishing Co., Mount Kisco, New York.

5. REFERENCES

Ahern, D. G., and Downing, D. T., 1970, Inhibition of prostaglandin biosynthesis in sheep seminal vesicular tissue by eicosa-5:8:11:14-tetraynoic acid, *Biochim. Biophys. Acta* **210**:456–461.
Allcock, J. M., and Drake, C. G., 1965, Ruptured intracranial aneurysms—the role of arterial spasm, *J. Neurosurg.* **22**:21–29.
Allen, G. S., Henderson, L. M., Chou, S. N., and French, L., 1974, Cerebral arterial spasm. Part I: *In vitro* contractile activity of vasoactive agents on canine basilar and middle cerebral arteries, *J. Neurosurg.* **40**:433–441.
Ambache, N., 1957, Properties of irin, a physiological constituent of the rabbit's iris, *J. Physiol. (London)* **135**:114–132.
Ambache, N., 1966, Biological characterization of and structure–action studies on smooth-muscle contracting fatty acids, *Mem. Soc. Endocrinol.* **14**:19–28.
Ambache, N., and Zar, M. A., 1970, An inhibitory effect of prostaglandin E_2 on neuromuscular transmission in guinea pig vas deferens, *J. Physiol. (London)* **208**:30–32P.
Ambache, N., Reynolds, M., and Whiting, J., 1963, Investigation of an active lipid in aqueous extracts of rabbit brain, and some further hydroxy-acids, *J. Physiol. (London)* **166**:251–283.
Ambache, N., Verney, J., and Zar, M. A., 1970, Evidence for the release of two atropine-resistant spasmogens from Auerbach's plexus, *J. Physiol. (London)* **207**:761–782.
Andersen, N. H., and Ramwell, P. W., 1974, Biological aspects of prostaglandins, *Arch. Intern. Med.* **133**:30–50.
Anderson, E. G., Hoas, H. L., and Hösli, L., 1973, Comparison of effects of noradrenaline and histamine with cyclic AMP on brain stem neurones, *Brain Res.* **49**:471–475.
Änggård, E., and Samuelsson, B., 1964, Smooth muscle stimulating lipids in sheep iris. The identification of prostaglandin $F_{2\alpha}$, *Biochem. Pharmacol.* **13**:281–283.

Änggård, E., Larsson, C., and Samuelsson, B., 1971, The distribution of 15-hydroxy prostaglandin dehydrogenase and prostaglandin Δ^{13}-reductase in tissues of the swine. *Acta Physiol. Scand.* **81**:396–404.

Änggård, E., Bohman, S. O., Griffin, J. E., III, Larsson, C., and Maunsbach, A. B., 1972, Subcellular localization of the prostaglandin system in the rabbit renal papilla, *Acta Physiol. Scand.* **84**:231–246.

Asakawa, T., and Yoshida, H., 1971, Studies on the functional role of adenosine 3',5'-monophosphate, histamine and prostaglandin E_1 in the central nervous system, *Japan. J. Pharmacol.* **21**:569–583.

Avazino, G. L., Bradley, P. B., and Wolstencroft, J. H., 1966a, Actions of prostaglandins E_1, E_2 and $F_{2\alpha}$ on brain stem neurones, *Brit. J. Pharmacol.* **27**:157–163.

Avazino, G. L., Bradley, P. B., and Wolstencroft, J. H., 1966b, Excitatory action of prostaglandin E_1 on brain-stem neurones, *Nature (London)* **209**:87–88.

Axen, U., Gréen, K., Hörlin, D., and Samuelsson, B., 1971, Mass spectrometric determination of picomole amounts of prostaglandins E_2 and $F_{2\alpha}$ using synthetic deuterium labeled carriers, *Biochem. Biophys. Res. Comm.* **45**:519–525.

Baile, C. A., and Forbes, J. M., 1974, Control of feed intake and regulation of energy balance in ruminants, *Physiol. Rev.* **54**:161–214.

Baile, C. A., Simpson, C. W., Bean, S. M., McLaughlin, C. L., and Jacobs, H. L., 1973, Prostaglandins and food intake in the rat, *Physiol. Behav.* **10**:1077–1086.

Baker, R. R., and Thompson, E., 1972, Positional distribution and turnover of fatty acids in phosphatidic acid, phosphoinositides, phosphatidyl choline and phosphatidyl ethanolamine in rat brain *in vivo*, *Biochim. Biophys. Acta* **270**:489–503.

Barrie, M., and Jowett, A., 1967, A pharmacological investigation of cerebrospinal fluid from patients with migraine, *Brain* **90**:785–794.

Bartels, J., Kunze, H., Vogt, W., and Wille, G., 1970, Prostaglandin: Liberation from and formation in perfused frog intestine, *Naunyn-Schmied. Arch. Pharmakol.* **266**:199–207.

Baum, T., and Shropshire, A. T., 1971, Influence of prostaglandins on autonomic responses, *Amer. J. Physiol.* **221**:1470–1475.

Bazan, N. G., 1970, Effects of ischemia and electroconvulsive shock on free fatty acid pool in the brain, *Biochim. Biophys. Acta* **218**:1–10.

Beleslin, D. B., and Myers, R. D., 1971, Release of an unknown substance from brain structures of unanaesthetized monkeys and cats, *Neuropharmacol.* **10**:121–124.

Beleslin, D. B., Radmanović, B. Z., and Rakić, M. M., 1971, Release during convulsions of an unknown substance into the cerebral ventricles of the cat's brain, *Brain Res.* **35**:625–627.

Bennett, A., Friedmann, C. A., and Vane, J. R., 1967, Release of prostaglandin E_1 from the rat stomach, *Nature (London)* **216**:873–876.

Bergström, S., 1967, Prostaglandins: Members of a new hormonal system, *Science* **157**:1–10.

Bergström, S., Ryhage, R., Samuelsson, B., and Sjövall, J., 1962, The structure of prostaglandin E_1, F_1 and F_2, *Acta Chim. Scand.* **16**:501–502.

Bergström, S., Ryhage, R., Samuelsson, B., and Sjövall, J., 1963, The structures of prostaglandin E_1, $F_{1\alpha}$ and $F_{1\beta}$, *J. Biol. Chem.* **238**:3555–3564.

Bergström, S., Danielsson, H., and Samuelsson, B., 1964a, The enzymatic formation of prostaglandin E_2 from arachidonic acid, *Biochim. Biophys. Acta* **90**:207–210.

Bergström, S., Danielsson, H., Klenberg, D., and Samuelsson, B., 1964b, The enzymatic conversion of essential fatty acids into prostaglandins, *J. Biol. Chem.* **239**:PC4006–4008.

Bergström, S., Carlson, L. A., Ekelund, L. G., and Orö, L., 1965, Cardiovascular and metabolic response to infusions of prostaglandin E_1 and to simultaneous infusions of noradrenaline and prostaglandin E_1 in man, *Acta Physiol. Scand.* **64**:332–339.

Bergström, S., Carlson, L. A., and Weeks, J. R., 1968, The prostaglandins: A family of biologically active lipids, *Pharmacol. Rev.* **20**:1–48.

Bergström, S., Farnebo, L. A., and Fuxe, K., 1973, Effect of prostaglandin E_2 on central and peripheral catecholamine neurons, *Eur. J. Pharmacol.* **21**:362–368.

Berti, F., Trabucchi, M., Bernareggi, V., and Fumagalli, R., 1973, Prostaglandins on cyclic-AMP formation in cerebral cortex of different mammalian species, *Adv. Biosci.* **9**:475–480.

Bito, L. Z., 1972a, Accumulation and apparent active transport of prostaglandins by some rabbit tissues *in vitro*, *J. Physiol. (London)* **221**:371–387.

Bito, L. Z., 1972b, Comparative study of concentrative prostaglandin accumulation by various tissues of mammals and marine vertebrates and invertebrates, *Comp. Biochem. Physiol.* **43A**:65–82.

Bradley, P. B., Samuels, G. M. R., and Shaw, J. E., 1969, Correlation of prostaglandin release from the cerebral cortex of cats with electro-corticogram following stimulation of the reticular formation, *Brit. J. Pharmacol.* **37**:151–157.

Brawley, B. W., Strandness, D. E., Jr., and Kelly, W. A., 1968, The biphasic response of cerebral vasospasm in experimental subarachnoid hemorrhage, *J. Neurosurg.* **28**:1–8.

Brody, M. J., and Kadowitz, P. J., 1974, Prostaglandins as modulators of the autonomic nervous system, *Fed. Proc.* **33**:48–60.

Brundin, J., 1968, The effect of prostaglandin E_1 on the response of the rabbit oviduct to hypogastric stimulation, *Acta Physiol. Scand.* **73**:54–57.

Buckell, M., 1964, Demonstration of substances capable of contracting smooth muscle in the haematoma fluid from certain cases of ruptured cerebral aneurysm, *J. Neurol. Neurosurg. Psychiat.* **27**:198–199.

Burger, M. M., Bombik, B. M., Breckenridge, B. McL., and Sheppard, J. R., 1972, Growth control and cyclic alterations of cyclic AMP in the cell cycle, *Nature New Biol.* **239**:161–163.

Butcher, R. W., 1970, Prostaglandins and cyclic AMP, *Adv. Biochem. Psychopharmac.* **3**:173–183.

Carlson, J. C., Barcikowski, B., and McCracken, J. A., 1973, Prostaglandin $F_{2\alpha}$ and the release of LH in sheep, *J. Reprod. Fert.* **34**:357–361.

Carlson, L. A., Ekelund, L.-G., and Orö, L., 1969, Circulatory and respiratory effects of different doses of prostaglandin E_1 in man, *Acta Physiol. Scand.* **75**:161–169.

Christ, E. J., and Dorp, D. A. van, 1972, Comparative aspects of prostaglandin biosynthesis in tissues, *Biochim. Biophys. Acta* **270**:537–545.

Christ, E. J., and Dorp, D. A. van, 1973, Comparative aspects of prostaglandin biosynthesis in animal tissues, *Adv. Biosci.* **9**:35–38.

Clark, K. E., Ryan, M. J., and Brody, M. J., 1973, Effects of prostaglandins E_1 and $F_{2\alpha}$ on uterine hemodynamics and motility, *Adv. Biosci.* **9**:779–782.

Clausen, J., and Srivastava, K. C., 1972, The synthesis of prostaglandins in human platelets, *Lipids* **7**:246–250.

Clithroe, H. J., and Pickles, V. R., 1961, The separation of the smooth-muscle stimulants in menstrual fluid, *J. Physiol. (London)* **156**:225–237.

Cobo, E. C., Rodriguez, A., and Villamizar, M. de, 1974, Milk-ejecting activity induced by prostaglandin $F_{2\alpha}$, *Amer. J. Obst. Gynecol.* **118**:831–836.

Coceani, F., 1974, Prostaglandins and the central nervous system, *Arch. Intern. Med.* **133**:119–129.

Coceani, F., and Viti, A., 1973, Actions of prostaglandin E_1 on spinal neurones in the frog, *Adv. Biosci.* **9**:481–487.

Coceani, F., and Wolfe, L. S., 1965, Prostaglandins in brain and the release of prostaglandin-like compounds from the cat cerebellar cortex, *Can. J. Physiol. Pharmacol.* **43**:445–450.

Coceani, F., and Wolfe, L. S., 1966, On the action of prostaglandin E_1 and prostaglandins from brain on the isolated rat stomach, *Can. J. Physiol. Pharmacol.* **44**:933–950.

Coceani, F., Pace-Asciak, C., Volta, F., and Wolfe, L. S., 1967, Effect of nerve stimulation on prostaglandin formation and release from the rat stomach, *Amer. J. Physiol.* **213**:1056–1064.

Coceani, F., Dreifuss, J. J., Puglisi, L., and Wolfe, L. S., 1969, Prostaglandins and membrane function, *in Prostaglandins, Peptides and Amines* (P. Mantegazza and E. W. Horton, eds.), pp. 73–84, Academic Press, New York.

Coceani, F., Puglisi, L., and Lavers, B., 1971, Prostaglandins and neuronal activity in spinal cord and cuneate nucleus, *Ann. N.Y. Acad. Sci.* **180**:289–301.

Collier, H. O. J., and Roy, A. C., 1974, Morphine-like drugs inhibit the stimulation by E prostaglandins of cyclic AMP formation by rat brain homogenate, *Nature* **248**:24–27.

Cooper, K. E., Cranston, W. I., and Honour, A. J., 1967, Observations on the site and mode of action of pyrogens in the rabbit brain, *J. Physiol. (London)* **191**:325–337.

Daniels, E. G., Hinman, J. W., Leach, B. E., and Muirhead, E. E., 1967, Identification of prostaglandin E_2 as the principal vasodepressor lipid of rabbit renal medulla, *Nature (London)* **215**:1298–1299.

Daugherty, J. H., Marrazzi, M. A., Marrazzi, A. S., 1974, The effects of prostaglandin on cerebral cortical evoked potentials, *Fed. Proc.* **33**:286.

Davies, B. N., Horton, E. W., and Withrington, P. G., 1968, The occurrence of prostaglandin E_2 in spenic venous blood of the dog following splenic nerve stimulation, *Brit. J. Pharmacol.* **32**:127–135.

Davis, H. A., Horton, E. W., Jones, K. B., and Quilliam, J. P., 1971, Identification of prostaglandins in prevertebral venous blood after preganglionic stimulation of the cat superior cervical ganglion, *Brit. J. Pharmacol.* **42**:569–583.

Denton, I. E., White, R. P., and Robertson, J. T., 1972, The effects of prostaglandins E_1, A_1 and F_{2x} on the cerebral circulation in dogs and monkeys, *J. Neurosurg.* **36**:34–42.

Destephano, D. B., Brady, U. E., and Lovins, R. E., 1974, Synthesis of prostaglandin by reproductive tissue of the male house cricket, *Acheta domesticus*, *Prostaglandins* **6**:71–79.

Dorp, D. A. van, 1966, The biosynthesis of prostaglandins, *Mem. Soc. Endocrinol.* **14**:39–47.

Dorp, D. A. van, Beerthuis, R. K., Nugteren, D. H., and Vonkeman, H., 1964a, The biosynthesis of prostaglandins, *Biochim. Biophys. Acta* **90**:204–207.

Dorp, D. A. van, Beerthuis, R. K., Nugteren, D. H., and Vonkeman, H., 1964b, Enzymatic conversion of all-*cis*-polyunsaturated fatty acids into prostaglandins, *Nature (London)* **203**:839–841.

Downing, D. T., Ahern, D. G., and Bachta, M., 1970, Enzyme inhibition by acetylenic compounds, *Biochem. Biophys. Res. Comm.* **40**:218–223.

Duda, P., Horton, E. W., and McPherson, A., 1968, The effects of prostaglandins E_1, F_{1x} and F_{2x} on monosynaptic reflexes, *J. Physiol. (London)* **196**:151–162.

Dunham, E. W., and Zimmerman, B. G., 1970, Release of prostaglandin-like material from dog kidney during nerve stimulation, *Amer. J. Physiol.* **219**:1279–1285.

Duru, S., and Türker, R. K., 1969, Effect of prostaglandin E_1 on the strychnine-induced convulsion in the mouse, *Experientia* **25**:275.

Echlin, R. A., 1968, Current concepts in the etiology and treatment of vasospasm, *Clin. Neurosurg.* **15**:133–160.

Eglington, G., Raphael, R. A., Smith, G. N., Hall, W. J., and Pickles, V. R., 1963, The isolation and identification of two smooth muscle stimulants from menstrual fluid, *Nature (London)* **200**:993–995.

Embrey, M. P., and Hillier, K., 1972, Therapeutic abortion by extraamniotic administration of prostaglandins, *in The Prostaglandins* (E. M. Southern, ed.), pp. 381–390, Brook Lodge Symposium, Futura, Mount Kisco, New York.

Euler, U. S. von, 1934, Zur Keuntnis der pharmakologischen Wirkungen von Nativsecreten und Extrackten männlicher accessorischer Geschlectsdrüsen, *Arch. Exptl. Pathol. Pharmakol.* **175**:78–84.

Euler, U. S. von, 1935*a*, A depressor substance in vesicular gland, *J. Physiol. (London)* **84**:21P.

Euler, U. S. von, 1935*b*, Über die spezifische blutdrucksenkende Substanz des menschlichen Prostata- und Samenblasensekretes, *Klin. Wochensch.* **14**:1182–1183.

Euler, U. S. von, and Hedqvist, P., 1969, Inhibitory action of prostaglandins E_1 and E_2 on the neurotransmission in the guines-pig vas deferens, *Acta Physiol. Scand.* **77**:510–512.

Feldberg, W., 1971, On the mechanism of action of pyrogens, *in Pyrogens and Fever* (G. E. W. Wolstenholm and J. Birch, eds.), pp. 115–129, Ciba Foundation Symposium, Livingstone, London.

Feldberg, W., and Gupta, K. P., 1973, Pyrogen fever and prostaglandin-like activity in cerebrospinal fluid, *J. Physiol. (London)* **228**:41–53.

Feldberg, W., and Myers, R. D., 1964, Effects of amines injected into the cerebral ventricles. A new concept of temperature regulation, *J. Physiol. (London)* **173**:226–237.

Feldberg, W., and Myers, R. D., 1966, Appearance of 5-hydroxytryptamine and an unidentified pharmacologically active lipid acid in effluents from perfused cerebral ventricles, *J. Physiol. (London)* **184**:837–855.

Feldberg, W., and Saxena, P. N., 1971*a*, Fever produced by prostaglandin E_1, *J. Physiol. (London)* **217**:547–556.

Feldberg, W., and Saxena, P. N., 1971*b*, Further studies on prostaglandin E_1 fever in cats, *J. Physiol. (London)* **219**:739–745.

Feldberg, W., Myers, R. D., and Veale, W. L., 1970, Perfusion from cerebral ventricle to cisterna magna in the unanaesthetized cat. Effect of calcium on body temperature, *J. Physiol. (London)* **207**:403–416.

Feldberg, W., Gupta, K. P., Milton, A. S., and Wendlandt, S., 1972, Effect of bacterial pyrogen and antipyretics on prostaglandin activity in cerebrospinal fluid of unanaesthetized cats, *Brit. J. Pharmacol.* **46**:550–551P.

Feldberg, W., Gupta, K. P., Milton, A. S., and Wendlandt, S., 1973, Effect of pyrogen and antipyretics on prostaglandin activity in cisternal C.S.F. of unanaesthetized cats, *J. Physiol. (London)* **234**:279–303.

Ferreira, S. H., Moncada, S., and Vane, J. R., 1971, Indomethacin and aspirin abolish prostaglandin release from the spleen, *Nature New Biol.* **231**:237–239.

Flower, R. J., and Vane, J. R., 1972, Inhibition of prostaglandin synthetase in brain explains the anti-pyretic activity of paracetamol (4-acetamidophenol), *Nature (London)* **240**:410–411.

Fredholm, B. B., Rosell, S., and Strandberg, K., 1970, Release of prostaglandin-like material from canine subcutaneous adipose tissue by nerve stimulation, *Acta Phyiol. Scand.* **79**:18–19A.

Gillett, P. G., Kinch, R. A. H., Wolfe, L. S., and Pace-Asciak, C., 1972, Therapeutic abortion with the use of prostaglandin F_{2}, *Amer. J. Obstet. Gynecol.* **112**:330–338.

Gilman, A. G., 1972, Regulation of cyclic AMP metabolism in cultured cells of the nervous system, *Adv. Cyclic Nucl. Res.* **1**:389–410.

Gilman, A. G., and Nirenberg, M., 1971, Regulation of adenosine 3′,5′-cyclic monophosphate metabolism in cultured neuroblastoma cells, *Nature* **234**:356–358.

Gilman, A. G., and Schrier, B. K., 1972, Adenosine cyclic 3′,5′-monophosphate in fetal rat brain cell culture, *Mol. Pharmacol.* **8**:410–416.

Gilmore, D. P., and Shaikh, A. A., 1972, The effect of prostaglandin E_2 in producing sedation in the rat, *Prostaglandins* 2:143–151.

Gilmore, N., Vane, J. R., and Wyllie, J. H., 1968, Prostaglandin released by the spleen, *Nature* (London) 218:1135–1140.

Ginsborg, B. L., and Hirst, G. D. S., 1971, Prostaglandin E_1 and noradrenaline at the neuromuscular junction, *Brit. J. Pharmacol.* 42:153–154.

Godfraind, J. M., and Pumain, R., 1971, Cyclic adenosine monophosphate and norepinephrine effect on Purkinje cells in the rat cerebellar cortex, *Science* 174:1257–1258.

Godfraind, J. M., and Pumain, R., 1972, Cyclic AMP and noradrenalin iontophoretic release on rat cerebellar Purkinje neurones, *Arch. Intern. Pharmacodyn.* 196:131–132.

Goldberg, N. D., O'Dea, R. F., and Haddox, M. K., 1973, Cyclic GMP, *Adv. Cyclic Nucl. Res.* 3:156–223.

Goldblatt, M. W., 1933, A depressor substance in seminal fluid, *J. Soc. Chem. Ind.* (*London*) 52:1056–1057.

Goldblatt, M. W., 1935, Properties of human seminal plasma, *J. Physiol.* (*London*) 84:208–218.

Granström, E., 1973, Structures of C14 metabolites of prostaglandin $F_{2\alpha}$, *Adv. Biosci.* 9:49–60.

Granström, E., Lands, W. E. M., and Samuelsson, B., 1968, Biosynthesis of 9α,15-dihydroxy-11-ketoprost-13-enoic acid, *J. Biol. Chem.* 243:4104–4108.

Gray, G. W., 1962, Intestinal levels of stimulant lipids in experimental obstructive ileus, *Gastroenterology* 43:51–59.

Gray, G. W., 1964, Effect of drugs on intestinal release of stimulant lipids, *J. Pharmacol. Exptl. Therap.* 146:215–224.

Gréen, K., 1973, Methods for quantitative determination of prostaglandins using gaschromatography–mass spectrometry, *in Prostaglandines 1973*, pp. 113–132, INSERM, Paris.

Gréen, K., Granström, E., Samuelsson, B., and Axen, U., 1973, Methods for quantitative analysis of $PGF_{2\alpha}$, PGE_2, 9α,11α-dihydroxy-15-keto-5-enoic acid and 9α,11α,15-trihydroxyprost-5-enoic acid from body fluids using deuterated carriers and gas chromatography–mass spectrometry, *Anal. Biochem.* 54:434–453.

Greengard, P., and Kebabian, J. W., 1974, Role of cyclic AMP in synaptic neurotransmission in the mammalian peripheral nervous system, *Fed. Proc.* 33:1059–1067.

Gryglewski, R., and Vane, J. R., 1972, The generation from arachidonic acid of rabbit aorta contracting substance (RCS) by a microsomal enzyme preparation which also generates prostaglandins, *Brit. J. Pharmacol.* 46:449–457.

Hahn, R. A., and Patil, P. N., 1972, Salivation induced by prostaglandin $F_{2\alpha}$ and modification of the response by atropine and physostigmine, *Brit. J. Pharmacol.* 44:527–533.

Hahn, R. A., and Patil, P. N., 1974, Further observations on the interaction of prostaglandin $F_{2\alpha}$ with cholinergic mechanisms in canine salivary glands, *Eur. J. Pharmacol.* 25:279–286.

Hamberg, M., 1968, On the absolute configuration of 19-hydroxyprostaglandin B_1, *Eur. J. Biochem.* 6:147–150.

Hamberg, M., 1972, Inhibition of prostaglandin synthesis in man, *Biochem. Biophys. Res. Comm.* 49:720–726.

Hamberg, M., 1973, Quantitative studies on prostaglandin synthesis in man, *Biochem. Biophys. Res. Comm.* 55:368–378.

Hamberg, J., and Samuelsson, B., 1967, 19-hydroxylated prostaglandins, *Prog. biochem. pharmacol.* 3:83–84.

Hamberg, M., and Samuelsson, B., 1969, The structure of a urinary metabolite of prostaglandin E_2 in the guinea pig, *Biochem. Biophys. Res. Comm.* 34:22–27.

Hamberg, M., and Wilson, M., 1973, Structures of new metabolites of prostaglandin E_2 in man, *Adv. Biosci.* 9:39–48.

Hamberg, M., Israelsson, U., and Samuelsson, B., 1971, Metabolism of prostaglandin E_2 in guinea pig liver, *Ann. N.Y. Acad. Sci.* **180**:164–180.

Hamberg, M., Svensson, J., Wakabayashi, T., and Samuelsson, B., 1974, Isolation and structure of two prostaglandin endoperoxides that cause platelet aggregation, *Proc. Nat. Acad. Sci.* **71**:345–349.

Hammarström, S., Samuelsson, B., and Bjursell, G., 1973, Prostaglandin levels in normal and transformed baby-hamster-kidney fibroblasts, *Nature New Biol.* **243**:50–51.

Harmes, P. G., Ojeda, S. R., and McCann, S. M., 1973, Prostaglandin involvement in hypothalamic control of gonadotropin and prolactin release, *Science* **181**:760–761.

Hedge, G. A., and Henson, S. D., 1972, The effects of prostaglandins on ACTH secretion, *Endocrinology* **91**:925–933.

Hedqvist, P., 1972, Prostaglandin induced inhibition of neurotransmission in the isolated guinea pig seminal vesicle, *Acta Physiol. Scand.* **84**:506–511.

Hedqvist, P., 1973a, Autonomic neurotransmission, *in The Prostaglandins* (P. W. Ramwell, ed.), Vol. 1, pp. 101–131, Plenum Press, New York.

Hedqvist, P., 1973b, Prostaglandin mediated control of sympathetic neuroeffector transmission, *Adv. Biosci.* **9**:461–473.

Hedqvist, P., and Brundin, J., 1969, Inhibition by prostaglandin E_1 of noradrenaline release and of effector responses to nerve stimulation in the cat spleen, *Life Sci.* **8**:389–395.

Hedqvist, P., and Euler, U. S. von, 1972, Prostaglandin controls neuromuscular transmission in the guinea-pig vas deferens. *Nature New Biol.* **236**:113–115.

Hedqvist, P., Stjärne, L., and Wennmalm, Å., 1970, Inhibition by prostaglandin E_2 of sympathetic neurotransmission in the rabbit heart, *Acta Physiol. Scand.* **79**:139–141.

Hendricks, C. H., Brenner, W. E., Ekblandh, L., Brotanek, V., and Fishburne, J. I., 1971, Efficacy and tolerance of intravenous prostaglandins $F_{2\alpha}$ and E_2, *Amer. J. Obstet. Gynecol.* **111**:564–579.

Hertelendy, F., 1971, Studies on growth hormone secretion. II. Stimulation by prostaglandins *in vitro*, *Acta Endocrin.* **68**:355–362.

Hittleman, K. J., and Butcher, R. W., 1973, Cyclic AMP and the mechanism of action of the prostaglandins, *in The Prostaglandins. Pharmacological and Therapeutic Advances* (M. F. Cuthbert, ed.), pp. 151–165, Heinemann, London.

Hoffer, B. J., Siggins, G. R., Oliver, A. P., and Bloom, F. E., 1971, Cyclic AMP mediation of norepinephrine inhibition in rat cerebellar cortex: a unique class of synaptic response, *Ann. N.Y. Acad. Sci.* **185**:520–530.

Hoffer, B. J., Siggins, G. R., Oliver, A. P., and Bloom, F. E., 1972, Cyclic AMP-mediated adrenergic synapses to cerebellar Purkinje cells, *in Advances in Cyclic Nucleotide Research*, (P. Greengard, R. Paoletti, and G. H. Robinson, eds.), Vol. 1, pp. 411–424, Raven Press, New York.

Holmes, S. W., 1970, The spontaneous release of prostaglandins into the cerebral ventricles of the dog and the effect of external factors on this release, *Brit. J. Pharmacol.* **37**:653–658.

Holmes, S. W., and Horton, E. W., 1968a, The identification of four prostaglandins in dog brain and their regional distribution in the central nervous system, *J. Physiol. (London)* **195**:731–741.

Holmes, S. W., and Horton, E. W., 1968b, Prostaglandins and the central nervous system, *in Prostaglandin Symposium of the Worcester Foundation* (P. W. Ramwell and J. E. Shaw, eds.), pp. 21–36, Wiley, New York.

Holmes, S. W., and Horton, E. W., 1968c, The distribution of tritium labelled prostaglandin E_1 injected in amounts sufficient to produce central nervous effects in cats and chicks, *Brit. J. Pharmacol.* **34**:32–37.

Holub, B. J., Kuksis, A., and Thompson, W., 1970, Molecular species of mono-, di-, and tri-phosphoinositides of bovine brain, *J. Lipid Res.* **11**:558–564.

Hopkin, J. M., Horton, E. W., and Whittaker, V. P., 1968, Prostaglandin content of particulate and supernatant fractions of rabbit brain homogenate, *Nature* **217**:71–72.

Horton, E. W., 1964, Actions of prostaglandins E_1, E_2 and E_3 on the central nervous system, *Brit. J. Pharmacol.* **22**:189–192.

Horton, E. W., 1972, Prostaglandins, Monographs on Endocrinology, Vol. 7, pp. 117–149, Springer-Verlag, New York.

Horton, E. W., and Main, I. H. M., 1967a, Identification of prostaglandins in central nervous tissues of the cat and chicken, *Brit. J. Pharmacol.* **30**:582–602.

Horton, E. W., and Main, I. H. M., 1967b, Further observations on the central nervous actions of prostaglandins $F_{2\alpha}$ and E_1, *Brit. J. Pharmacol.* **30**:568–581.

Horton, E. W., and Main, I. H. M., 1969, Actions of prostaglandin E_1 on spinal reflexes in the cat, *in Prostaglandins, Peptides and Amines* (P. Mantegazza and E. W. Horton, eds.), pp. 121–122, Academic Press, London.

Huang, M., Shimizu, H., and Daly, J., 1971, Regulation of adenosine cyclic 3',5'-phosphate formation in cerebral cortical slices, *Mol. Pharmacol.* **7**:155–162.

Ito, H., Momose, G., Katayama, T., Takagishi, H., Ito, L., Nakajimi, H., and Takei, Y., 1971, Effect of prostaglandin on the secretion of human growth hormone, *J. Clin. Endocrinol.* **32**:857–859.

Johnson, G. S., and Pastan, I., 1971, Change in growth and morphology of fibroblasts by pros-taglandins, *J. Natl. Cancer Inst.* **47**:1357–1364.

Johnson, D. G., Thoa, N. B., Weinshilboum, R., Axelrod, J., and Kopin, I. J., 1971, Enhanced release of dopamine-β-hydroxylase from sympathetic nerves by calcium and phenoxy-benzamine and its reversal by prostaglandins, *Proc. Natl. Acad. Sci.* **68**:2227–2230.

Jones, R. L., 1974, Preparation of prostaglandins C: chemical fixation of prostaglandin A isom-erase to a gel support and partition chromatography of prostaglandins A, B and C, *Prostaglandins* **5**:283–290.

Jones, R. L., and Cammock, S., 1973, Purification, Properties and Biological Significance of Prostaglandin A Isomerase, *Adv. Biosci.* **9**:61–70.

Jouvenaz, G. H., Nugteren, D. H., Beerthuis, R. K., and Dorp, D. A. van, 1970, A sensitive method for the determination of prostaglandins by gas chromatography with electron-capture detection, *Biochim. Biophys. Acta* **202**:231–234.

Kadowitz, P. J., Sweet, C. S., and Brody, M. J., 1971a, Potentiation of adrenergic venomotor responses by angiotensin, prostaglandin $F_{2\alpha}$ and cocain, *J. Pharmacol. Exptl. Ther.* **176**:167–173.

Kadowitz, P. J., Sweet, C. S., and Brody, M. J., 1971b, Differential effects of prostaglandins E_1, E_2, $F_{1\alpha}$ and $F_{2\alpha}$ on adrenergic vasoconstriction in the dog hindpaw, *J. Pharmacol. Exptl. Ther.* **177**:641–649.

Kadowitz, P. J., Sweet, C. S., and Brody, M. J., 1972a, Influence of prostaglandin on adrenergic transmission to vascular smooth muscle, *Circ. Res.* **31**:36–50.

Kadowitz, P. J., Sweet, C. S., and Brody, M. J., 1972b, Enhancement of sympathetic neuro-transmission by prostaglandin $F_{2\alpha}$ in the cutaneous vascular bed of the dog, *Eur. J. Phar-macol.* **18**:189–194.

Kadowitz, P. J., George, W. J., Joiner, P. D., and Hyman, A. L., 1973, Effect of prostaglandins E_1 and $F_{2\alpha}$ on adrenergic responses in the pulmonary circulation, *Adv. Biosci.* **9**:501–506.

Kaplan, H. R., Grega, G. J., Sherman, G. P., and Buckley, J. P., 1969, Central and reflexogenic cardiovascular actions of prostaglandin E_1, *Intern. J. Neuropharmacol.* **8**:15–24.

Kapp, J., Mahaley, M. S., and Odom, G. L., 1968, Cerebral arterial spasm, Part I and II, *J. Neurosurg.* **29**:331–349.

Kapp, J., Mahaley, M. S., and Odom, G. L., 1970, Experimental evaluation of potential spasmolytic drugs, *J. Neurosurg.* **32**:468–472.

Karim, S. S. M., Sharma, G. M., Filshie, G. M., Salmon, J. A., and Ganesan, P. A., 1973, Termination of pregnancy with prostaglandin analogs, *Adv. Biosci.* **9**:811–830.

Kataoka, K., Ramwell, P. W., and Jessup, S., 1967, Prostaglandins: localization in subcellular particles of rat cerebral cortex, *Science* **157**:1187–1189.

Kayaalp, S. O., and McIsaac, R. J., 1968, Absence of effects of prostaglandins E_1 and E_2 on ganglionic transmission, *Eur. J. Pharmacol.* **4**:283–288.

Kirtland, S. J., and Baum, H., 1972, Prostaglandin E_1 may act as a "Calcium Ionophore," *Nature New Biol.* **236**:47–49.

Krnjević, K., 1965, Actions of drugs on single neurones in the cerebral cortex, *Brit. Med. Bull.* **21**:10–14.

Kuehl, F. A., Cirillo, V. J., Ham, E. A., and Humes, J. L., 1973, The regulatory role of the prostaglandins on the cyclic 3′,5′-AMP system, *Adv. Biosci.* **9**:155–172.

Kurzrok, R., and Lieb, C. C., 1930, Biochemical studies of human semen, *Proc. Soc. Exptl. Biol. Med.* **28**:268–272.

Labhsetwar, A. P., 1970, Effects of prostaglandin $F_{2\alpha}$ on pituitary luteinizing hormone content of pregnant rats, *J. Reprod. Fert.* **23**:155–159.

Labhsetwar, A. P., and Zolovick, A., 1973, Hypothalamic interaction between prostaglandins and catecholamines in promoting gonadotropin secretion for ovulation, *Nature New Biol.* **246**:55–56.

Laity, J. L. H., 1969, The release of prostaglandin E_1 from rat phrenic nerve–diaphragm preparation, *Brit. J. Pharmacol.* **37**:698–704.

Lake, N., Jordan, L. M., and Phillis, J. W., 1972, Mechanism of noradrenalin action in cat cerebral cortex, *Nature* **240**:249–250.

Lake, N., Jordan, L. M., and Phillis, J. W., 1973, Evidence against cyclic adenosine 3′,5′-monophosphate (AMP) mediation of noradrenaline depression of cerebral cortical neurones, *Brain Res.* **60**:411–421.

Lands, W. E. M., and Samuelsson, B., 1968, Phospholipid precursors of prostaglandins, *Biochim. Biophys. Acta* **164**:426–429.

Lands, W. E. M., Lee, R., and Smith, W., 1971, Factors regulating the biosynthesis of various prostaglandins, *Ann. N.Y. Acad. Sci.* **180**:107–122.

Lands, W. E. M., LeTellier, P. R., Rome, L. H., and Vanderhoek, J. Y., 1973, Inhibition of prostaglandin biosynthesis, *Adv. Biosci.* **9**:15–28.

Lavery, H. A., Lowe, R. D., and Scroop, G. F., 1970, Cardiovascular effects of prostaglandins mediated by the central nervous system of the dog, *Brit. J. Pharmacol.* **39**:511–519.

Lavery, H. A., Lowe, R. D., and Scroop, G. C., 1971, Central autonomic effects of prostaglandin $F_{2\alpha}$ on the cardiovascular system of the dog, *Brit. J. Pharmacol.* **41**:454–461.

Lee, J. B., Covino, B. G., Takenan, B. H., and Smith, E. R., 1965, Renomedullary vasodepressor substance, medullin: isolation, chemical characterization and physiological properties, *Circulation Res.* **17**:57–77.

Leslie, C. A., and Levine, L., 1973, Evidence for the presence of a prostaglandin E_2-9-keto reductase in rat organs, *Biochem. Biophys. Res. Comm.* **52**:717–724.

Lewis, G. P., and Matthews, J., 1969, The cause of the vasodilatation accompanying free fatty acid release in rabbit adipose tissue, *J. Physiol. (London)* **202**:95–96P.

Lindl, T., and Cramer, H., 1974, Formation, accumulation and release of adenosine 3′,5′-monophosphate induced by histamine in the superior cervical ganglion of the rat *in vitro*, *Biochim. Biophys. Acta* **343**:182–191.

Lomax, P., 1970, Drugs and body temperature, *Int. Rev. Neurobiol.* **12**:1–43.

Louis, T. M., Stellflug, J. N., Tucker, H. A., and Hafs, H. D., 1974, Prostaglandin $F_{2\alpha}$, prolactin, and growth hormone after intravenous administration of $PGF_{2\alpha}$ in heifers, *Fed. Proc.* **33**:263.

Lunt, G. G., and Rowe, C. E., 1968, The production of unesterified fatty acid in brain, *Biochim. Biophys. Acta* **152**:681–693.

Main, I. H. M., 1964, The inhibitory action of prostaglandins on respiratory smooth muscle, *Br. J. Pharmac. Chemother.* **22**:511–519.

Marco, L. S., and Coceani, F., 1973, The action of prostaglandin E_1 on frog skeletal muscle, *Can. J. Physiol. Pharmacol.* **51**:627–634.

Marrazzi, M. A., Shaw, J. E., Tao, F. T., and Matschinsky, F. M., 1972, Reversibility of 15-OH prostaglandin dehydrogenase from swine lung, *Prostaglandins* **1**:389–395.

Martin, F. H., and Baile, C. A., 1973, Feeding elicited in sheep by intrahypothalamic injections of PGE_1, *Experientia* **29**:306–307.

Matsuura, S., Kawaguchi, S., Ichiki, M., Sorimachi, M., Kataoka, K., and Inouye, A., 1969, Perfusion of frog's spinal cord as a convenient method for neuropharmacological studies, *Eur. J. Pharmacol.* **6**:13–16.

McAfee, D. A., and Greengard, P., 1972, Adenosine 3',5'-monophosphate: electrophysiological evidence for a role in synaptic transmission, *Science* **178**:310–312.

McCann, S. M., and Porter, J. C., 1969, Hypothalamic pituitary stimulating and inhibiting hormones, *Physiol. Rev.* **49**:240–284.

McLeod, R. M., and Lehmeyer, J. E., 1970, Release of pituitary growth hormone by prostaglandins and dibutyryl adenosine cyclic 3':5'-monophosphate in the absence of protein synthesis, *Proc. Natl. Acad. Sci.* **67**:1172–1179.

McQueen, D. S., and Ungar, A., 1969, The modification by prostaglandin E_1 of central nervous interaction between respiratory and cardioinhibitor pathways, *in Prostaglandins, Peptides and Amines* (P. Mantegazza and E. W. Horton, eds.), pp. 123–124, Academic Press, New York.

Miller, W. L., and Sutton, M. J., 1974, Measurement of hamster core temperature by telemetry: effects of norepinephrine, serotonin and prostaglandins E_2 and $F_{2\alpha}$, *Fed. Proc.* **33**:589.

Milton, A. S., 1973, Prostaglandin E_1 and endotoxin fever, *Adv. Biosci.* **9**:415–500.

Milton, A. S., and Wendlandt, S., 1968, The effect of 4-acetamidophenol in reducing fever produced by the intracerebral injection of 5-hydroxytryptamine and pyrogen in the conscious cat, *Brit. J. Pharmacol.* **34**:215P.

Milton, A. S., and Wendlandt, S., 1970, A possible role for prostaglandin E_1 as a modulator for temperature regulation in the central nervous system of the cat, *J. Physiol. (London)* **20**:76–77P.

Milton, A. S., and Wendlandt, S., 1971a, The effect of different environmental temperatures on the hyperpyrexia produced by the intraventricular injection of pyrogen, 5-hydroxytryptamine and prostaglandin E_1 in the conscious cat, *J. Physiol. (Paris)* **63**:340–342.

Milton, A. S., and Wendlandt, S., 1971b, Effects on body temperature of prostaglandins of the A, E and F series on injection into the third ventricle of unanaesthetized cats and rabbits, *J. Physiol. (London)* **218**:325–336.

Milton, A. S., and Wendlandt, S., 1971c, The effects of 4-acetamidophenol (paracetamol) on the temperature of the conscious rat to the intracerebral injection of prostaglandin E_1, adrenalin and pyrogen, *J. Physiol. (London)* **217**:33–34.

Myers, R. D., 1967, Release of chemical factors from the diencephalic region of the unanaesthetized monkey during changes in body temperature, *J. Physiol. (London)* **188**:50–51P.

Nakano, J., Prancan, A. V., and Moore, S. E., 1972, Metabolism of prostaglandin E_1 in the cerebral cortex and cerebellum of the dog and rat, *Brain Res.* **39**:545–548.

Nugteren, D. H., and Hazelhof, E., 1973, Isolation and properties of intermediates in prostaglandin biosynthesis, *Biochim. Biophys. Acta* **326**:448–461.

Orczyke, G. P., and Behrman, H. R., 1972, Ovulation blockade by aspirin or indomethacin—*in vivo* evidence for a role of prostaglandin in gonadotrophin secretion, *Prostaglandins* **1**:3–20.

Otten, J., Johnson, G. S., and Pastan, I., 1971, Cyclic AMP levels in fibroblasts: relationship to growth rate and contact inhibition of growth, *Biochem. Biophys. Res. Comm.* **44**:1192–1199.

Pace-Asciak, C., and Wolfe, L. S., 1968, Inhibition of prostaglandin synthesis by oleic, linoleic and linolenic acids, *Biochim. Biophys. Acta* **152**:784–787.

Pace-Asciak, C., and Wolfe, L. S., 1970, Biosynthesis of prostaglandins E_2 and $F_{2\alpha}$ from tritium labelled arachidonic acid by rat stomach homogenates, *Biochim. Biophys. Acta* **218**:539–542.

Pace-Asciak, C., Morawska, K., Coceani, F., and Wolfe, L. S., 1968, The biosynthesis of prostaglandins E_2 and $F_{2\alpha}$ in homogenates of the rat stomach, in *Prostaglandin Symposium of the Worcester Foundation* (P. W. Ramwell and J. E. Shaw, eds.), pp. 371–378, Wiley, New York.

Pappius, H. M., Rostworowski, K., and Wolfe, L. S., 1974, Biosynthesis of prostaglandin $F_{2\alpha}$ and E_2 by brain tissue *in vitro*, *Trans. Amer. Soc. Neurochem.* **5**:119 (Abstract), and unpublished results.

Patrono, C., and La Torre, E., 1974, Prostaglandin $F_{2\alpha}$ in cerebrospinal fluid in a patient with subarachnoid hemorrhage, *Clin. Res.* **23**(3):346A.

Peng, T.-C., Six, K. M., and Munson, P. L., 1970, Effects of prostaglandin E_1 on the hypothalamo–hypophyseal–adrenocortical axis in rats, *Endocrinology* **86**:202–206.

Pennick, M., White, R. P., Crockarell, J. R., and Robertson, J. T., 1972, Role of prostaglandin $F_{2\alpha}$ in the genesis of experimental cerebral vasospasm, *J. Neurosurg.* **37**:398–406.

Perkins, J. P., 1973, Adenyl cyclase, *Adv. Cyclic Nucl. Res.* **3**:2–64.

Phillis, J. W., and Tebécis, A. K., 1968, Prostaglandins and toad spinal cord responses, *Nature* **217**:1076–1077.

Piper, P. J., and Vane, J. R., 1969, Release of additional factors in anaphylaxis and its antagonism by anti-inflammatory drugs, *Nature (London)* **223**:29–35.

Piper, P. J., and Vane, J. R., 1971, The release of prostaglandins from lung and other tissues, *Ann. N.Y. Acad. Sci.* **180**:363–385.

Potts, W. J., and East, P. F., 1971a, Effects of prostaglandins and prostaglandin precursors on the conditioned avoidance response (CAR) in rats, *Pharmacologist* **13**:392.

Potts, W. J., and East, P. F., 1971b, The effect of prostaglandin E_2 on conditioned avoidance response performance in rats, *Arch. Int. Pharmacodyn.* **191**:74–79.

Potts, W. J., and East, P. F., 1972, Effects of prostaglandin E_2 on the body temperature of conscious rats and cats, *Arch. Int. Pharmacodyn.* **197**:31–36.

Potts, W. J., East, P. F., Landry, D., and Dixon, J. P., 1973, The effects of prostaglandin E_2 on conditioned avoidance response behavior and the electroencephalogram, *Adv. Biosci.* **9**:489–494.

Prasad, E. N., 1972, Morphological differentiation induced by prostaglan in mouse neuroblastoma cells in culture, *Nature New Biol.* **236**:49–52.

Price, C. J., and Rowe, C. E., 1972, Stimulation of the production of unesterified fatty acids in nerve endings of guinea pig brain *in vitro* by noradrenalin and 5-hydroxytryptamine, *Biochem. J.* **126**:575–585.

Ramwell, P. W., 1964, The action of cerebrospinal fluid on the frog rectus abdominis muscle and other isolated tissue preparations, *J. Physiol. (London)* **170**:21–38.

Ramwell, P. W., and Shaw, J. E., 1966, Spontaneous and evoked release of prostaglandins from cerebral cortex of anesthetized cats, *Amer. J. Physiol.* **211**:125–134.

Ramwell, P. W., and Shaw, J. E., 1967, Prostaglandin release from tissues by drug, nerve and hormone stimulation, *in Prostaglandins* (S. Bergström and B. Samuelsson, eds.), pp. 283–292, Nobel Symposium 2, Almqvist and Wiksell, Stockholm.

Ramwell, P. W., Shaw, J. E., and Kucharski, J., 1965, Prostaglandin release from the rat phrenic nerve–diaphragm preparation, *Science* **149**:1390–1391.

Ramwell, P. W., Shaw, J. E., and Jessup, R., 1966, Spontaneous and evoked release of prostaglandins from frog spinal cord, *Amer. J. Physiol.* **211**:998–1004.

Ratner, A., Wilson, M. C., Srivastava, L., and Peake, G. T., 1974, Stimulatory effects of prostaglandin E_1 on rat anterior pituitary cyclic AMP and luteinizing hormone release, *Prostaglandins* **5**:165–171.

Raynor, R. B., McMurtry, J. G., and Pool, J. L., 1961, Cerebrovascular effects of topically applied serotonin in the cat, *Neurology* **11**:190–195.

Robison, G., Cole, B., Arnold, A., and Hartman, R., 1971, Effects of prostaglandins on function and cyclic AMP levels of human blood platelets, *Ann. N.Y. Acad. Sci.* **180**:324–331.

Samuelsson, B., 1964, Identification of a smooth muscle-stimulating factor in bovine brain, *Biochim. Biophys. Acta* **84**:218–219.

Samuelsson, B., 1972, Biosynthesis of prostaglandins, *Fed. Proc.* **31**:1442–1450.

Samuelsson, B., 1973a, Quantitative aspects of prostaglandin biosynthesis in man, *Adv. Biosci.* **9**:7–14.

Samuelsson, B., 1973b, Biosynthesis and metabolism of prostaglandins, *in Prostaglandines 1973*, pp. 21–41, INSERM, Paris.

Samuelsson, B., and Wennmalm, Å., 1971, Increased nerve stimulation induced release of noradrenaline from the rabbit heart after inhibition of prostaglandin synthesis, *Acta Physiol. Scand.* **83**:163–168.

Sandler, M., 1972, Migraine: a pulmonary disease? *Lancet* **1**:618–619.

Satinoff, E., 1973, Salicylate: action on normal body temperature in rats, *Science* **176**:532–533.

Scaramuzzi, O. E., Baile, C. A., and Mayer, J., 1971, Prostaglandins and food intake in rats, *Experientia* **27**:256–257.

Schimizu, H., Creveling, C. R., and Daly, J. W., 1970, The effect of histamine and other compounds on the formation of adenosine 3′,5′-monophosphate in slices from cerebral cortex, *J. Neurochem.* **17**:441–444.

Scholfield, J. G., 1970, Prostaglandin E_1 and the release of growth hormone *in vitro*, *Nature (London)* **228**:179.

Shaw, J. E., and Ramwell, P. W., 1968, Release of prostaglandin from rat epididymal fat pad on nervous and hormonal stimulation, *J. Biol. Chem.* **243**:1498–1503.

Sheppard, J. R., 1972, Difference in the cyclic adenosine 3′,5′-monophosphate levels in normal and transformed cells, *Nature New Biol.* **236**:14–16.

Siggins, G. R., Hoffer, B. J., and Bloom, F. E., 1971a, Studies of norepinephrine-containing afferents to Purkinje cells of rat cerebellum, *Brain Res.* **25**:535–553.

Siggins, G. R., Hoffer, B., and Bloom, F., 1971b, Prostaglandin–norepinephrine interactions in brain, *Ann. N.Y. Acad. Sci.* **180**:302–323.

Silver, M. J., Smith, J. B., Ingerman, C., and Kocsis, J. J., 1973, Arachidonic acid–induced human platelet aggregation and prostaglandin formation, *Prostaglandins* **4**:863–875.

Silver, M. J., Hoch, W., Kocsis, J. J., Ingerman, C. M., and Smith, J. B., 1974, Arachidonic acid causes sudden death in rabbits, *Science* **183**:1085–1087.

Smith, A. D., 1972, Cellular control of the uptake, storage and release of noradrenaline in sympathetic nerves, *in Neurotransmitters and Metabolic Regulation* (R. M. S. Smellie, ed.), pp. 103–131, Biochemical Society, London.

Smith, W. L., and Lands, W. E. M., 1972, Oxygenation of polyunsaturated fatty acids during prostaglandin biosynthesis by sheep vesicular gland, *Biochemistry* 11:3276–3285.

Smith, J. B., Ingerman, C., Kocsis, J. J., and Silver, M. J., 1973, Formation of prostaglandins during aggregation of human blood platelets, *J. Clin. Invest.* 52:965–969.

Stitt, J. T., 1973, Prostaglandin E₁ fever induced in rabbits, *J. Physiol. (London)* 232:163–180.

Strong, C. G., Boucher, R., Nowaczynski, W., and Genest, J., 1966, Renal vasodepressor lipid, *Proc. Staff Meetings Mayo Clinic* 41:433–452.

Sweet, C. S., Kadowitz, P. J., and Brody, M. J., 1971, A hypertensive response to infusion of prostaglandin $F_{2\alpha}$ into the vertebral artery of the conscious dog, *Eur. J. Pharmacol.* 16:229–232.

Taira, N., and Satoh, S., 1973, Prostaglandin $F_{2\alpha}$ as a potent excitant of the parasympathetic postganglionic neurons of the dog salivary gland, *Life Sci.* 13:501–506.

Vale, W., Rivier, C., and Guillemin, R., 1971, A "prostaglandin receptor" in the mechanisms involved in the secretion of anterior pituitary hormones, *Fed. Proc.* 30:363 (Abstract).

Vanderhoek, J. Y., and Lands, W. E. M., 1973, Acetylenic inhibitors of sheep vesicular gland oxygenase, *Biochim. Biophys. Acta* 296:374–381.

Vane, J. R., 1971, Inhibition of prostaglandin synthesis as a mechanism of action of aspirin-like drugs, *Nature New Biol.* 231:232–235.

Vane, J. R., 1973, Inhibition of prostaglandin biosynthesis on the mechanism of action of aspirin-like drugs, *Adv. Biosci.* 9:395–411.

Vargaftig, B. B., and Dao Hai, N., 1971, Release of vasoactive substances from guinea pig lung by slow reacting substance C and arachidonic acid, *Pharmacology* 6:99–108.

Vargaftig, B. B., and Dao Hai, N., 1972, Interference of some thiol derivatives with the pharmacological effects of arachidonic acid and slow reacting substance C and with the release of rabbit aorta contracting substances, *Eur. J. Pharmacol.* 18:43–55.

Veale, W. L., and Cooper, K. E., 1973, Species differences in the pharmacology of temperature regulation, *in The Pharmacology of Thermoregulation* (E. Schönbaum and P. Lomax, eds.), pp. 1–583, Karger, Basel.

Vilhardt, H., and Hedqvist, P., 1970, A possible role of prostaglandin E₂ in the regulation of vasopressin secretion in rats, *Life Sci.* 9:825–830.

Vogt, W., 1958, Naturally occurring lipid-soluble acids of pharmacological interest, *Pharmacol. Rev.* 10:407–435.

Vogt, W., Suzuki, T., and Babilli, S., 1966, Prostaglandins in SRS-C and in Darmstoff preparation from frog intestinal dialysates, *Mem. Soc. Endocrinol.* 14:137–142.

Waitzman, M. B., Bailey, W. R., and Kirby, C. G., 1967, Chromatographic analysis of biologically active lipids from rabbit irides, *Exptl. Eye Res.* 6:130–137.

Weeks, J. R., 1972, Prostaglandins, *Ann. Rev. Pharmacol.* 12:317–336.

Weinheimer, A. J., and Spraggins, R. L., 1969, The occurrence of two new prostaglandin derivatives (15-epi-PGA₂ and its acetate, methyl ester) in the gorgonian *Plexaura homomalla*, *Tetrahedron Lett.* 59:5185–5188.

Wellmann, W., and Schwabe, U., 1973, Effects of prostaglandins E₁, E₂ and $F_{2\alpha}$ on cyclic AMP levels in brain *in vivo*, *Brain Res.* 59:371–378.

Wennmalm, Å., 1971, Studies on the mechanisms controlling the secretion of neurotransmitters in the rabbit heart, *Acta Physiol. Scand.* Suppl. 365:1–36.

Wennmalm, Å., and Hedqvist, P., 1971, Inhibition by prostaglandin E₁ of parasympathetic neurotransmission in the rabbit heart, *Life Sci.* 10:465–470.

White, R. P., Heaton, J. A., and Denton, I. C., 1971, Pharmacological comparison of prostaglandin $F_{2\alpha}$, serotonin and norepinephrine on cerebrovascular tone of monkey, *Eur. J. Pharmacol.* 15:300–309.

White, R. P., Hagen, A. A., Dawson, W. N., Morgan, H., and Robertson, J. R., 1974, Arteriographic study of effects of prostaglandins, platelets and other substances on basilar arteries of dogs, *Fed. Proc.* **33**:575.

de Wied, D. A., Witter, A., Versteeg, D. H. G., and Mulder, A. H., 1969, Release of ACTH by substances of central nervous system origin, *Endocrinology* **85**:561–569.

Wilkins, R. H., Wilkins, G. K., Gunnels, J. C., and Odom, G. L., 1967, Experimental studies of intracranial arterial spasm using aortic strip assays, *J. Neurosurg.* **27**:490–500.

Willis, A. L., 1974, Isolation of a chemical trigger for thrombosis, *Prostaglandins* **5**:1–25.

Willis, A. L., Davison, P., Ramwell, P. W., Brocklehurst, W. E., and Smith, B., 1972, Release and actions of prostaglandins in inflammation and fever, in *Prostaglandins in Cellular Biology* (P. W. Ramwell and B. B. Pharriss, eds.), pp. 227–267, Plenum Press, New York.

Wilson, J. L., and Field, J. R., 1974, The production of intracranial vascular spasm by hypothalamic extract, *J. Neurosurg.* **40**:473–479.

Wlodawer, P., and Samuelsson, B., 1973, On the organization and mechanism of prostaglandin synthetase, *J. Biol. Chem.* **248**:5673–5678.

Wlodawer, P., Samuelsson, B., Albonico, S. M., and Corey, E. J., 1971, Selective inhibition of prostaglandin synthetase by a bicyclo[2.2.1] heptane derivative, *J. Am. Chem. Soc.* **93**:2815–2816.

Wolfe, L. S., and Mamer, O., 1975, Measurement of prostaglandin F_{2} levels in human cerebrospinal fluid in normal and pathological conditions, *Prostaglandins*, 9, Feb. issue.

Wolfe, L. S., Coceani, F., and Spence, M. W., 1965, Prostaglandins in brain, *Proc. 8th Intern. Congr. Neurol.* **4**:159–164.

Wolfe, L. S., Coceani, F., and Pace-Asciak, C., 1967, Brain prostaglandins and studies of the action of prostaglandins on the isolated rat stomach, in *Prostaglandins* (S. Bergström and B. Samuelsson, eds.), pp. 265–275, Nobel Symposium 2, Almqvist and Wiksell, Stockholm.

Yamamoto, Y. L., Feindel, W., Wolfe, L. S., Katoh, H. K., and Hodge, C. P., 1973a, Experimental vasoconstriction of cerebral arteries by prostaglandins, *J. Neurosurg.* **37**:385–397.

Yamamoto, Y. L., Feindel, W., Wolfe, L. S., and Hodge, C. P., 1973b, Prostaglandin induced vasoconstriction of cerebral arteries and its reversal by ethanol, *Adv. Biosci.* **9**:359–367.

Ziboh, V. A., Vanderhoek, J. Y., and Lands, W. E. M., 1974, Inhibition of sheep vesicular gland oxygenase by unsaturated fatty acids from skin of essential fatty acid deficient rats, *Prostaglandins* **5**:233–240.

Zor, U., Kaneko, H. P. G., Schneider, S., McCann, M., and Field, J. B., 1970, Further studies of stimulation of anterior pituitary cyclic adenosine 3',5'-monophosphate formation by hypothalamic extract and prostaglandins, *J. Biol. Chem.* **245**:2883–2888.

HYDROLASES OF THE SIMPLE SPHINGOLIPIDS: Ceramide, Glucocerebroside, and Galactocerebroside

NORMAN S. RADIN

Mental Health Research Institute
and
Department of Biological Chemistry, University of Michigan
Ann Arbor, Michigan

1. PREVIOUS REVIEWS ON THE SPHINGOLIPID HYDROLASES

Publications covering the sphingolipids in some depth are beginning to appear. Burton and Guerra (1974) have just edited a book on lipid chemistry which contains a detailed chapter by Burton on sphingolipids. Proceedings of a 1971 symposium contain useful informal reviews (Volk and Aronson, 1972). Another recent symposium collection by Bernsohn and Grossman (1971) contains articles on the hydrolases. A detailed review of sphingolipid metabolism by Morell and Braun (1972) covers the lipids lacking sialic acid. Gatt (1973) has one chapter on sphingolipid enzymes in a Milan symposium and one with Barenholz (1973) on enzymes of complex lipid metabolism in *Annual Reviews*. Chapters by Radin and Rosenberg (1970) on cerebrosides and sphingomyelin appeared in Volume 3 of *Handbook of Neurochemistry*. A chapter on glycolipid metabolism by Dawson (1974) has recently appeared in an edited volume.

The *Methods in Enzymology* series should also be consulted, particularly for recommended methods of assay and substrate preparation. Relevant chapters, which appear in Volumes 14 and 28, will be referred to throughout the following text. A valuable description of recent progress in the sphingolipid disorders was published by The National Foundation—March of Dimes (Bergsma, 1973).

2. RECENT DEVELOPMENTS IN SPHINGOLIPID HYDROLYSIS

The topic of sphingolipid hydrolysis has been relatively unpopular until recent years, as illustrated by the absence of chapters on the subject in books entitled *Lipid Metabolism* or *Lipid Biochemistry*. However, several new developments have made the subject somewhat more interesting.

1. *The development of improved methods for making labeled substrate and for assaying the enzymatic products.* In the case of the galactolipids, the commercial availability of galactose oxidase (*P. circinatus*) made it convenient to oxidize the 6-position of the galactose moieties and then to reduce the aldehydes with tritium-labeled sodium borohydride. Because this unusual enzyme has little specificity with respect to other moieties that might be attached to the galactose, any galactolipid can be attacked more or less rapidly. Another fortunate feature is that the oxidase works quite well in tetrahydrofuran–water 1:1, which dissolves the glycolipids (Agranoff *et al.*, 1962).

Other advances in labeling have come from improvements in sphingolipid chemistry and chromatography. Catalytic hydrogenation of the double bond present in sphingosine is a hypothetical route to the synthesis of any labeled sphingolipid, but the problem of separating enzyme product from substrate can be difficult and there are some hints in the literature that this mode of labeling produces unstable materials. Several of the sphingolipids can readily be converted to the "lyso" form by hydrolysis and then reacylated with labeled fatty acid. This method has the advantage that specific chain lengths can be used, rather than a mixture of naturally occurring fatty acid derivatives.

2. The discovery that a host of human genetic disorders are due to defects in the hydrolysis of sphingolipids. Accompanied by recent developments in amniotic fluid sampling, cell culturing, enzyme assaying, and attitudes toward abortion, this discovery has already had some spectacular successes in prevention of genetic disorders. Because the promise is strong for therapeutic treatment of affected individuals, the field is now very active. While most of the interest is in the ganglioside disorders, this review is limited to the simple sphingolipids.

3. The discovery that cultured cells undergo marked changes in glycolipid content when they are transformed by a virus. It had previously been shown by Rapport and by Hakomori that tumors could contain abnormally large amounts of certain glycolipids, and more recent work has indicated that sugar residues on the surfaces of cultured cells might be involved in malignant transformation. The field is now progressing from purely analytical evaluations to study of the changes in glycolipid synthetases and hydrolases. This development could be extremely important.

4. The discovery that "helper proteins" or "cohydrolases" exist which have the ability to stimulate greatly a number of hydrolases. From present evidence, it appears that the co-glycosidases are glycoproteins, are heat-stable, and are found in the cytosol. It is possible that all the sphingolipid hydrolases possess such proteins. Elucidating their function will be a significant research activity in the next few years.

5. The discovery that many hydrolases themselves are glycoproteins. Increasing lines of evidence support the generality of the finding, which should be very useful in purifying the enzymes since several types of carbohydrate-binding affinity columns are now commercially available. The carbohydrate chains on the hydrolase molecules may be involved in a potentially important phenomenon: the uptake of hydrolases by cells from the intercellular fluid (Hickman *et al.*, 1974).

The entire field of sphingolipid biochemistry is being retarded by the high cost of commercially available lipids and the unavailability of many sphingolipids. Purity of commercial products has sometimes been a problem too. While researchers are becoming accustomed to the high prices, their work is undoubtedly being held to an unnecessarily unsophisticated level by impurity of product. This difficulty is almost as severe in the phospholipid field. Perhaps it is time to establish a Lipid Center, like the New England Enzyme Center, to which individuals can come and prepare large batches of the sphingolipids in pilot plant scale. Permanent staff could be available to carry out the standard preparations as well as organic syntheses of labeled and unlabeled materials. The Lipid Preparations Laboratory of the Hormel Institute was a pacesetter for many years for biochemists needing high-quality fatty acids and their simple derivatives.

3. CERAMIDASE

$$
\begin{array}{c}
\text{R}-\text{CH}-\text{CH}-\text{CH}_2 \\
\;\;\;\; | \quad\;\; | \quad\;\; | \\
\;\;\;\; \text{OH} \;\;\; \text{NH} \;\; \text{OH} \\
\qquad\quad | \\
\qquad\quad \text{C}=\text{O} \\
\qquad\quad | \\
\qquad\quad \text{R}'
\end{array}
\;\; + \text{H}_2\text{O} \rightarrow \text{Sphingosine} + \text{Fatty Acid}
$$

The enzyme ceramidase was found in brain, liver, and kidney by Gatt (1966*a*), who subsequently described it for *Methods in Enzymology* (Gatt and Yavin, 1969). The enzyme from rat brain received the most attention, particularly its ability to catalyze the reverse reaction (Yavin and Gatt, 1969). More recently the enzyme entered the "clinical alert" status when it was found to be deficient in humans suffering from the disease lipogranulomatosis (Sugita *et al.*, 1972).

3.1. Substrate Preparation and Enzyme Assay

A number of syntheses have been reported for ceramide, with or without an isotopic label. Gatt (1966*a*) started with palmitoyl chloride and sphingosine-3-benzoate and removed the benzoyl group by mild saponification. It is not clear why the benzoyl group was used; there is no need to protect the hydroxyl group from acylation as long as the pH is kept just above 7 and water (not pyridine) is present. We followed the procedure described by Kopaczyk and Radin (1965) for psychosine acylation. Full details, not previously published, are as follows:

> Purchase the acid chloride or prepare it by refluxing 1 mmol of the acid with 3 ml thionyl chloride (unpurified). Of course, protect the reagents from water. After 30 min cool the solution in ice and apply an aspirator vacuum to the flask. You must shake the flask to prevent splashing. After a while remove the ice bath and complete the removal of remaining thionyl chloride. Pump for an additional 15 min after the sample has come to room temperature. Now dissolve the acid chloride in 1 ml tetrahydrofuran, freshly distilled from KOH pellets. Transfer this, with a rinse of 2 ml tetrahydrofuran, to a test tube containing 1 mmol of sphingosine (Morell *et al.*, 1970) in 3 ml sodium acetate (50 g NaOAc·3H$_2$O + 64 ml water). Stir the two phases vigorously for 2 hr and then add 24 ml chloroform, 12 ml methanol, and 6 ml water. Adjust the pH to 10–11 with NaOH, with good mixing, and discard the upper layer. Now add 10 ml water and adjust the pH to 3–4, with good mixing; discard the upper layer. Wash the lower layer twice with water, adding a little methanol if emulsions form. Evaporate off the solvent under vacuum, displacing it with benzene, and lyophilize the benzene solution. The ceramide

is fairly pure at this stage but can be purified further with a column of silica gel (Unisil) in the usual way, starting with hexane–chloroform 90 : 10 and finishing with plain chloroform.

An excess of amine or acid should be used, depending on which is the more expensive. The unused acid can be recovered from the alkaline wash liquid and the first column effluents. In the case of short-chain ceramides, a chloroform wash of the pooled upper layers will increase the recovery, which generally is about 75 % of the recovery predicted theoretically.

Several other synthetic methods have been proposed: the condensation of sphingosine and fatty acid esters of *N*-hydroxysuccinimide (Ong and Brady, 1972); the condensation of sphingosine and fatty acid by a carbodiimide (Hammarström, 1971); and the reaction of acyl chloride with amine in the presence of pyridine and dimethylformamide (Weiss and Raizman, 1958). It is my impression that these methods give lower yields or offer no advantage over the method we use.

The assay of ceramidase requires conversion of the radioactive ceramide to an emulsion. Gatt (1966a) used 45 or 80 nmol of ceramide with 0.1 mg Tween 20, dissolved in chloroform–methanol and evaporated together to dryness. The residue was taken up in aqueous Triton X-100, 1 mg/ml final mixture, together with sodium cholate. It would seem possible to utilize less detergent by drying down both the Tween and Triton together with the ceramide. Bowen and Radin (1969a) used 0.92 mg ceramide (1.63 μmol) dried with 10 mg Tween 20 and 5 mg Myrj 59, taken up subsequently in aqueous bile salt. The difference in ceramide: detergent ratios is due to the use by Gatt of the more easily dispersed oleoyl sphingosine while Bowen and Radin used stearoyl sphingosine. Nilsson (1969) has assayed the enzyme without any detergent, simply sonicating the lipid in sodium taurodeoxy-cholate solution. No systematic study seems to have been made of dispersion methods.

The most detailed description of assay methods for ceramidase appears in *Methods in Enzymology* (Gatt and Yavin, 1969). One oddity of the enzyme is its effectiveness in catalyzing the reverse reaction, in particular with oleic acid as substrate. This is like the situation with cholesterol ester hydrolase, which is often assayed through the reverse reaction.

3.2. Enzyme Purification

The only method available is from Yavin and Gatt (1969), who purified ceramidase from rat brain over 200-fold. The enzyme was first extracted with a cholate–EDTA solution, dialyzed, and then treated with a mixture of trypsin and chymotrypsin. This extraction step is probably suitable for all the sphingolipid hydrolases, and the stability against proteases may also be typical, especially if all the sphingolipid hydrolases are glycoprotein. However, proof must be furnished that the digestion-resistant enzyme is identical to the original enzyme.

3.3. Enzyme Characteristics

The rat brain enzyme in the dialyzed cholate extract was stable in the freezer for years. After proteolytic treatment, the enzyme was less stable. Heat stability also depended on the degree of purification, a point that bears attention when one wishes to compare different tissues, species, or individuals for differences in the heat denaturability of an enzyme.

Yavin and Gatt (1969) have emphasized the reversibility of the enzyme and made a considerable effort to separate and to characterize the two activities. However, there is little question about the "oneness" of the enzyme. The differences in the two types of activity are undoubtedly due to differences in dispersibility and solubility of the lipid interactants. It is true that evidence for reversibility—frequently reported for hydrolases of all sorts—raises the possibility that the hydrolases have the additional function of synthesizing, as well as hydrolyzing. However, there do exist synthetases for ceramides which utilize acyl CoA esters; thus, the need for a second synthetic mechanism does not seem strong. It should be noted that the reverse reaction catalyzed by ceramidase is very slight for fatty acids that occur most commonly in ceramides and other sphingolipids.

The synthetases show a different subcellular distribution from the hydrolase (Morell and Radin, 1970). In addition, ceramidase is absent in kidney and cerebellum of Farber's disease (Sugita et al., 1972), as is its reverse activity, yet ceramide accumulates considerably in an affected person's tissues. Evidently the synthetases in these patients are working normally, without significant feedback, as in other lipidoses.

One of the curious features of ceramidase of rat brain is that a variety of substances can stimulate the reverse reaction but not the hydrolysis (Yavin and Gatt, 1969). These include SH compounds, EDTA, and hydrazine. The importance of an enzyme SH group is indicated by the toxicity of hydroxymercuribenzoate. (Investigators have found that the more soluble mercuribenzenesulfonate is much more effective at the low pH needed by lysosomal hydrolases.) Ceramidase is inhibited fairly well by free palmitic acid and less so by sphingosine, but product inhibition does not become noticeable under the usual assay conditions.

While Bowen and Radin (1969a) assayed ceramidase in the presence of taurocholate, subsequent work in my laboratory has shown that cholate is a much better stimulator. No one seems to have compared the various bile salts in enough detail to report. Neither has a comparison been made of the relative activities of the different kinds of ceramide as substrate (fatty acid chain length, presence of an OH on the fatty acid).

There is no sign in tissues of the possible presence of an endogenous stimulator. Bowen and Radin found that doubling the concentration of brain homogenate in the incubation tube led to less than double the activity (rather than an increase) and attributed this to dilution of radioactive substrate by endogenous ceramide. However, this question could be confused by the presence of an endogenous inhibition which counteracts the endogenous stimulator, and a special search ought to be made in the heated cytosol.

The ceramidase of intestinal mucosa (Nilsson, 1969) is interesting in that its pH optimum is 7.6 while the rat brain enzyme has an optimum of 4.8. (Nilsson's text gives the figure 7.6 but his Figure 1C shows it is really 7.1.) Perhaps this is a digestive enzyme of relatively low specificity.

Assay of ceramidase in the brains of rats sacrificed at different ages revealed the presence of some activity at 4 days, a threefold rise by 15 days, and a small decrease to a steady value that held for at least 320 days (Bowen and Radin, 1969a). The peak activity was reached about the same time by sulfatase, but galactocerebrosidase peaked somewhat later. The finding that activity was retained well after "maturation" suggests that ceramidase is active throughout life and that it plays a significant role in the metabolism of the sphingolipids.

3.4. Clinical Aspects of Ceramidase

Farber's disease, or lipogranulomatosis, is a human disorder, apparently genetic in origin, found in young children. The symptoms include swollen joints, subcutaneous nodules, hoarseness, respiratory difficulty, and—generally—psychomotor retardation. Foam cells appear, and ceramide accumulation in several organs has been demonstrated. Not only ordinary ceramides (containing typical sphingolipid nonhydroxy fatty acids) but also ceramides containing hydroxy fatty acids are found (Sugita *et al.*, 1973). The latter have been hypothesized as intermediates in cerebroside biosynthesis (Morell and Radin, 1969); at least two enzymes catalyze their synthesis (Ullman and Radin, 1972), but they have not yet been isolated from fresh tissue. Presumably the accumulated ceramides arise from the degradation of cerebrosides and other sphingolipids, the latter furnishing only the nonhydroxy ceramides. It is of interest that the hydroxy ceramides were found in kidney as well as brain, despite the rather low concentration of hydroxy acid sphingolipids in that organ. This fact may signify that the hydroxy acid sphingolipids have a rather high turnover rate in kidney.

A survey of several enzymes in affected cerebellum and kidney (Sugita *et al.*, 1972) showed that ceramidase was undetectable while neuraminidase, hexosaminidase, galactosidase, and acid phosphatase were present at normal levels. Among the tissues from other individuals used for comparison, the activity of ceramidase was rather low in an infant with Gaucher's disease. Perhaps this is a sign that the level of ceramidase is controlled by the level of its substrate, which is probably derived mainly from breakdown of glucocerebroside rather than from synthesis from long-chain base and fatty acid. (Galactocerebroside hydrolysis is probably a minor source of ceramide.)

A lipid analysis of a case with Farber's disease (Moser *et al.*, 1969) disclosed not only an accumulation of ceramides but also some accumulation of gangliosides in extraneural tissues. Perhaps the rate of ganglioside synthesis in those organs is limited by the rate of ceramide production. Incidentally, this report, which stated that ceramidase was *not* deficient in the patient's tissues, is a good example of the need for lipid enzymologists to assume full responsibility for their "service" assays. Clinicians should furnish enough tissue for assay evaluation and should insist on details of method validation, even for "standard" assays.

4. GLUCOCEREBROSIDASE

Glucocerebroside → Ceramide + Glucose

Glucocerebrosidase is a β-glucosidase which was found by Brady *et al.* (1965*a,b*) in rat spleen, human spleen, and rat intestine. Gatt (1966*b*) subsequently purified the enzyme from ox brain, following the purification steps with nitrophenyl glucoside (Gatt and Rapport, 1966). The use of aryl glucoside has dominated the field of glucosidase study, unfortunately, and it is not clear how much of the activity measured by the unnatural substrate reflects glucocerebrosidase activity. Glucose is known to occur in some glycoproteins, although the nature of the linkage (α vs β) is unknown. β-Glucosides also occur in plants; thus, they may find their way into the digestive tract and, possibly, internal organs as well. Steroid glucosides probably occur in animals, and glucosidase activity toward a number of synthetic steroid β-glucosides has been demonstrated in rabbit kidney, liver, and small intestine (Mellor and Layne, 1971). During the purification of glucocerebrosidase, Pentchev *et al.* (1973) noted that the ratio of aryl glucosidase to cerebroside glucosidase changed by a factor of 12, from which it would appear that the former assay method (when applied to whole tissue) is derived from a good deal of some other enzyme or enzymes.

No doubt the question of the utility of aryl glucosidase measurements has been confused by the observation that patients with Gaucher's disease exhibit very little of this activity (Patrick, 1965; Brady *et al.*, 1966). Because there is a similar decrease in glucocerebrosidase activity in the tissues of these patients, the two measurements have generally been taken to be derived from the same enzyme. It is very likely that this disease represents a multiple enzyme deficiency, presumably because of a genetic defect in a section of enzyme common to two or more glucosidases. Thus, one must keep in mind the data obtained with both types of assays in thinking of glucocerebrosidase.

4.1. Substrate Preparation and Enzyme Assay

The substrate can be prepared from glucosyl sphingosine (glucopsychosine) and radioactive fatty acid as described in the previous section, which gives our procedure for acylation of sphingosine. See also some details in Erickson and Radin (1973). Glucosyl sphingosine is conveniently prepared in good yield by alkaline hydrolysis of glucocerebroside (Radin, 1974). Glucocerebroside can be obtained from the tissues of patients with Gaucher's disease, particularly from the spleen, which is most readily available. It can be purchased from Supelco, Inc. (Bellefonte, Pa.), and a synthetic preparation (containing DL-dihydrosphingosine as the base) can be purchased from Miles Laboratories (Kankakee, Ill.). Methods for isolating cerebroside from Gaucher spleen have been described by several laboratories, mainly adaptations of the methods used for isolating galactocerebroside from brain. We prefer the following sequence:

> Extraction with chloroform–methanol, filtration, and partition with concentrated saline solution. (Formalin, if present, is removed at this step). Evaporate the lower layer under vacuum, with copious additions of benzene to remove water. When the distillate shows that no water is present (single phase), add methanolic NaOH and let the ester lipids split for 2 hr. Neutralize the NaOH with dilute acetic acid and partition with water and chloroform to remove the glycerol derivatives. Again evaporate the lower layer with benzene until it is water-free and then purify the cerebroside with a Florisil column. The crude cerebroside can probably be used directly for glucopsychosine preparation or be purified further with a silica gel column.

A peculiarity of glucocerebroside is its tendency to form gels when a solution is concentrated. As this gelling can produce serious splashing in the evaporator, it is better to replace the solvent with benzene (by evaporation) and to lyophilize the gel. We have recently found that benzene can be handled very conveniently with a mechanical lyophilizer that is cooled to $-80°C$ (Thermovac FD-ULT-1). Mechanically cooled lyophilizers that cannot cool that well will allow benzene vapors to leak into the pump oil. Of course, Dry Ice traps also work, but they are a nuisance and usually too small for large-scale preparations.

Glucocerebroside has also been prepared synthetically, labeled in the glucose moiety (Brady et al., 1965b). This was made from DL-sphingosine rather than the natural isomer (D), but the natural isomer could be used (Shapiro, 1969).

Incidentally, some publications in the sphingolipid field have obviously been derived from the synthetic (DL) mixture since the authors state that their material came from Miles Laboratories, which sells only the material made by the Shapiro reactions. Other suppliers generally furnish the natural compound. However, one supplier offers DL-sphingosine from beef brain! This unlikely label is certainly confusing. Editors and researchers should pay more attention to this question in the future.

An assay procedure for glucocerebrosidase has been described by Gatt (1969). Nonradioactive cerebroside was used and the liberated glucose was measured with glucose oxidase. Each incubation tube contained 200 nmol of substrate; thus, the procedure seems reasonably sensitive. No details were furnished on the use of the assay procedure with whole tissues or crude enzyme, but the purified enzyme from beef brain exhibited activity proportional to enzyme weight and time for at least 3 hr. Nonradioactive glucose can also be determined by other enzyme methods or with an automatic chromatographic analyzer (Lee, 1972).

A second assay procedure by Weinreb and Brady (1972) was applied to beef spleen. This utilized glucose-labeled substrate, and the unreacted lipid was removed after incubation by precipitation with trichloroacetic acid. In the Gatt assay method, 0.4% taurocholate was the activating bile salt, and in the second method, 0.375% cholate was the activator. Acetate buffer pH 5 was used in the first; phosphate buffer pH 6 was used in the second. There seems to be a disagreement as to the optimum pH, which could arise from the use of different buffers or bile salts.

No statement was made in the second method as to kinetic aspects of the assay system, but in an earlier paper Brady et al. (1965) reported that the time course was linear for about 2 hr and then the enzyme slowed down and assumed a new linear (but slower) time course for about 18 hr. This observation was made with partially purified enzyme from human spleen in a medium lacking bile salt.

A re-examination of the optimal conditions for glucocerebrosidase assay has recently been carried out in my laboratory (Hyun and Radin, 1975). We made a partially purified preparation from human placenta and then assayed it with an emulsion of stearate-labeled glucocerebroside. In this procedure, the unreacted substrate was removed at the end of the incubation by partitioning between hexane, methanol, and boric acid. The optimum bile salt concentration was found to be 1.2% taurocholate, somewhat higher than that used by other researchers. The best buffer proved to be citrate–phosphate–K$^+$, pH 5.4. Both phosphate and K$^+$ proved to be stimulatory, and the pH optimum was lowered by the presence of both phosphate and taurocholate.

Here, too, the rate of hydrolysis was high initially (linear for about 15 min); then it slowed and assumed a new, slower, constant rate for at least 2 hr more. We showed that the triphasic aspect was due to the presence of taurocholate, since preincubation with the bile salt produced the enzyme form with the same, slower rate (i.e., the initial rapid stage was eliminated). When the enzyme was passed through additional purification steps, which involved exposure to taurocholate for prolonged periods, the triphasic time curve was eliminated and normal straight lines were obtained. It therefore appears that bile salt slowly affects the form of the enzyme, and assay procedures with tissue preparations ought to take this into account. One cannot tell from publications derived from tissue homogenates whether the authors checked the kinetic properties of their systems. At present, we are using 10-min incubations to obtain the data from the faster form. However, one can economize on enzyme by preincubating the enzyme with taurocholate and buffer and then adding substrate and incubating for several hours. While the specific activity is lower, the greatly increased incubation time produces higher total hydrolysis.

Incidentally, the sodium taurocholate that is available from virtually every commercial supplier is material of distinctly low purity. Only Calbiochem (as far as I know) furnishes a high-quality product. While the price is high, the cost per assay is low, and assayers ought to use this product. The price is prohibitive for enzyme purification work, however. Observations in my laboratory indicate that the next best product is "taurocholic acid, 70% pure" from Matheson Coleman and Bell. We have made good-quality taurocholate by the procedure of Pope (1967), but the purification is tedious. Sodium cholate is probably quite pure from several commercial sources, but it precipitates at pH 5.4 and this might be a source of difficulty. Unfortunately no one seems to have made a comparison of the efficacy of the various bile salts (types and suppliers). Researchers rarely describe the source or purity of the bile salt that they use.

There is a special problem in assaying glucocerebrosidase when a tissue from a Gaucher patient is used, because the tissue may contain a fairly large amount of endogeneous glucocerebroside which dilutes the radioactive substrate to an indeterminate degree. The problem can be treated by using less tissue and raising the specific activity of the substrate, or by assaying two different weights of tissue and trying to correct for the dilution by a double simultaneous equation analysis. The latter method involves the assumption that endogenous and exogenous cerebroside are treated equally by the enzyme. Perhaps this is a fair assumption if the two cerebrosides are allowed to incubate in detergent for some time before the addition of buffer to speed up the enzymatic reaction. A third approach, which does not seem to have been tried, is the separation of the enzyme from the endogenous cerebroside before assay. Bile salt is a good extractant for the enzyme, and the enzyme is efficiently precipitated from the extract with acetone, probably leaving the cerebroside behind. With any of these methods, one ought certainly to check the enzyme assay at different levels of enzyme to make sure that the problem has been solved.

4.2. Enzyme Purification

This subject has received an appreciable amount of attention. Starting with beef brain, Gatt and Rapport (1966) and Gatt (1969a) achieved a tenfold purification with a 9 % yield. (Since the purification was followed with nitrophenyl glucoside as substrate, the numbers must be pretty rough with respect to glucocerebrosidase activity.) Weinreb and Brady (1972) then reported a purification from beef spleen, with enrichment somewhat over 200-fold and a yield of about 13 % Both procedures called for solubilization with bile salt. In the former, the extraction was rather ineffective, as only 23 % of the activity entered the solution. In the latter, the effectiveness was not reported. An unusual feature of the Weinreb–Brady method is the use of butanol to extract some impurities and to precipitate others.

A more complete study was made by Pentchev *et al.* (1973), who apparently obtained the enzyme in pure form from human placenta. The tissue was washed and ground, washed with water again, and then extracted with phosphate pH 6 and Cutscum (probably Triton X-100) and 1 % taurocholate. The remaining steps involved ammonium sulfate precipitation, gel permeation, and ion exchange. A curious feature of the salt precipitation step is that the enzyme appeared as a film floating on the surface of the solution. Presumably at that stage it is complexed with detergent and some tissue lipid and thus has a low density. Glycerol (20 %) and dithiothreitol were needed in the last steps to maintain the stability of the enzyme. The overall yield from the initial extract was only 5 %, but the enrichment was 4100-fold.

The final product thus obtained showed a single band after electrophoresis in an SDS gel, and the molecular weight was apparently 60,000. When the purified enzyme was permeated through a Sephadex G-200 column, the indicated molecular weight was about 240,000. Thus the form under these conditions appears to be a tetramer.

Dr. Jung Hyun and I have been working on the isolation of the enzyme from the same tissue. We found that a high degree of purification can be achieved with a Concanavalin A–Sepharose column and with a Sepharose affinity column to which has been coupled a moiety closely resembling the substrate. Thus far the column does not seem to have been degraded by contact with the enzyme. Additional purification has also been achieved by use of a related column, in which the glucose is replaced by galactose. Because of the high enzyme yields in the various steps, the method holds much promise for large-scale purification.

Kanfer *et al.* (1974) have obtained glucocerebrosidase purification by use of an affinity column bearing a side chain made from benzidine and gluconolactone. The lactone is presumably bound in amide linkage to one of the amine groups in the benzidine. The principle seems to be useful for other glycosidases, since most or all of them appear to be inhibited by the corresponding lactone.

4.3. Enzyme Characteristics

The most highly purified preparation of glucocerebrosidase (Pentchev *et al.*, 1973) exhibited some activity toward methylumbelliferyl glucoside. The ratio of activities, cerebrosidase/aryl glucosidase, was 2 in the initial tissue extract and 24 in the final product. Thus it would appear that at least one other glucosidase had been considerably removed by the purification process. The enzyme also exhibited slight activity toward glucosyl sphingosine, which has been suggested as an intermediate in glucocerebroside synthesis (Curtino and Caputto, 1974). Since ability to hydrolyze glucosyl sphingosine, as well as glucosyl ceramide, is greatly decreased in spleen and skin fibroblasts from patients with Gaucher's disease (Raghavan *et al.*, 1973), both substrates might be hydrolyzed by the same enzyme. However, more detailed comparisons are needed to determine this question.

K_m values reported are 49 μM for rat intestine (Brady *et al.*, 1965), 25 μM for bovine spleen (Weinreb and Brady, 1972), 65 μM for human placenta (Pentchev *et al.*, 1973), and 180 μM for bovine brain (Gatt, 1966). We found a value of 57 μM when the enzyme from human placenta was incubated only 10 min, and 43 μM after the enzyme had been preincubated with taurocholate.

The enzyme in intestine (Brady *et al.*, 1965) seems to be a hydrolase of low specificity, presumably more suited to digestion than to controlling metabolic processes. It attacks galactocerebroside and is apparently the same enzyme that attacks phlorizin, a plant glucoside (Leese and Semenza, 1973).

A significant discovery arose out of the observation that the specific activity of aryl glucosidase in a Gaucher spleen increased with increasing tissue concentration (Ho and O'Brien, 1971). This result indicated the presence of an endogenous stimulator, which subsequently turned out to be in much higher concentration in the spleen of Gaucher patients, compared with normals. Presumably the increase reflects a control system that normally adjusts the level of the factor (which should probably be called "coglucosidase") to the need for glucosidase activity. The dynamics and mechanism of this interrelationship are yet to be elucidated. A later study (Ho *et al.*, 1973) showed that the factor also acted when glucocerebroside was used as the substrate. The degree of stimulation was not the same for the two substrates, which is further evidence for the existence of two glucosidases.

The mechanism of action of the coglucosidase seems to involve binding to the enzyme, which is largely membrane-bound. When the particulate enzyme is assayed in the absence of bile salt or detergent, its activity is very low. When a solution containing coglucosidase is added, there is considerable stimulation. It could be shown by this assay method that spleen particles absorb the factor from solution, presumably by combination between the factor and glucosidase.

A further development (Ho and Light, 1973) was the finding that the activity toward glucocerebroside was greatly enhanced when an acidic lipid, which could be 0.12 mM phosphatidyl serine, phosphatidic acid, or phosphatidyl inositol, was added to the incubation. Taurocholate interfered with the stimulation. This work was done with glucocerebrosidase which had undergone some degree of purification: Spleen particles were extracted with Triton X-100 and the extract was passed through a column of Sephadex G-150. This preparation of enzyme seemed to be quite stable in the freezer, but a similar preparation (Ho, 1973) was quite unstable. Apparently the main difference in the two preparations was the pH used for the initial solubilization; the use of pH 4 at 37°C produced the unstable enzyme while the use of pH 7 at 4°C for a much briefer time produced a stable enzyme. I wonder if, in the former procedure, there was some degradation of the enzyme by other enzymes in the tissue particles. At pH 4 there is some activity of glycosidases, which could remove carbohydrate residues from the glucosidase. Another possible explanation is that the content of glycoprotein which accompanies the enzyme in the extraction is a factor in stabilization.

The finding of Ho and Light that acidic phospholipids and a glycoprotein were stimulators may explain the puzzle that has intrigued sphingolipid biochemists ever since bile salts were found to be rather general stimulators. Because bile salt concentrations must be very low in the regions where most sphingolipid hydrolases act, it always seemed likely that the true enzyme activators were something different.

If coglucosidase occurs partly in the cytosol and partly in the membranes, bound to glucosidase, it is easy to see how the observed activity of the enzyme will depend greatly on how the tissue is prepared for assay. Ho (1973) states that a low salt concentration and a low pH favor the combination between enzyme and factor, while bile salt favors dissociation.

Some conflicting data on coglucosidase have been published by Pentchev and Brady (1973) and Pentchev *et al.* (1973). The points made are too complex to discuss here, and the assay conditions differed in the different studies. These workers did confirm the existence of a stimulating heat-stable factor in normal and Gaucher tissues, but the stimulation was found only with aryl glucosidase, not glucocerebrosidase. The latter activity did show stimulation at low pH values (5.4 and below), but not at 5.8 or above. The cerebrosidase assays were carried out with added taurocholate, which was found by Ho and Light (1973) to block the action of coglucosidase.

I should like to offer a hypothesis on the mechanism of coglucosidase action which could explain some of the disagreements mentioned above. This was suggested to me by Dr. Jack Distler and subsequently again by Dr. Joel Dain. The glycoprotein might be an acceptor for the glucose released by glucosidase; that is, glucosidase may really be a transferase which can transfer the glucose moiety to water if it has to but which prefers to transfer it to coglucosidase. In general, the assay procedures that have been used to assay glucosidases have not relied on direct measurement of glucose liberation, but rather of ceramide formation or of formation of a TCA-soluble radioactive material, which could be coglucosidase containing glucose. In support of this idea is the observation by Ho and O'Brien (1971) that coglucosidase contains bound glucose. I assume that this glucoprotein is subsequently hydrolyzed to free glucose by a second glucosidase, regenerating the original glycoprotein. The isolation procedure for coglucosidase as described by Ho and O'Brien could not have separated the "aglucosyl" and glucosylated proteins. This hypothesis might also explain why so much coglucosidase was found in Gaucher spleens. The glucosidase that acts on glucosylated glycoprotein may be very deficient in this disorder; thus the heavily glucosylated glycoprotein accumulates, just like glucocerebroside. As I pointed out in the introduction to this section, the disorder appears to involve more than one glucosidase. My laboratory is presently trying to test this hypothesis, which might, moreover, apply to all the glycoprotein coenzymes.

If the hypothesis is correct, the correct assay conditions must eliminate the role of the second glucosidase or of coglucosidase. Probably a high taurocholate concentration does this, and assays carried out with a relatively low bile salt concentration may reflect in part the amount of contaminating coglucosidase.

Carrying the hypothesis to a stage beyond experimental fact, one might propose that a single glycoprotein accounts for the stimulations reported for a series of glycolipid hydrolases. In other words, there might be a protein with a specific polypeptide backbone which has the ability to pick up a series of sugars from a series of transferases. As it picks up one sugar, it becomes an acceptor for a different sugar, and so on. For example, a series of sugars is removed during the degradation of gangliosides and other ceramide polysaccharides. The various glycosidases involved could be lined up in a lysosomal structure, and the accompanying glycoprotein could move down the line together with the glycolipid, picking up each sugar as it is severed from the glycolipid. Moving down another line of glycosidases, the totally glycosylated glycoprotein could then undergo regeneration to its original form.

Some evidence is available on the dynamics of glucocerebrosidase. Radin *et al.* (1969) measured the activity of the enzyme in brain of rats of different ages and found that the specific activity was highest at the earliest time-point studied (4 days) and then declined during the period of most rapid myelination. It remained constant between 90 and 320 days at about 55 % of the maximal activity. Thus there is no great change with age, especially if one were to calculate the specific activity on the basis of protein rather than total brain.

A study by Kampine *et al.* (1967) showed that the level of glucocerebrosidase in spleen could be increased considerably by injecting rats with red cell stroma. This effect was presumably due to the presence of glucocerebroside in the stroma, since injection of methanol-extracted stroma had no effect. It would appear from this that the spleen has a feedback mechanism for controlling the enzyme's concentration as a function of the cerebroside concentration.

Some evidence that glucocerebrosidase also catalyzes hydrolysis of phenolic glucosides comes from Raghavan *et al.* (1974), who showed that a glucosidase preparation could catalyze the transfer of glucose from methyl-umbelliferyl glucoside to ceramide, with formation of glucocerebroside. Since aryl glucosides are compounds of relatively high energy, they can act as glycosyl donors to compounds other than water. An example of this is the galactosylation of glucose by nitrophenyl galactoside and a purified testicular β-galactosidase (Distler and Jourdian, 1973). These reports of trans-glycosidation activity on the part of glycosidases support the hypothesis above (that glycoprotein cofactors act as sugar acceptors from glycolipids).

4.4. Enzyme Inhibitors

Gatt (1966*b*) found that sphingosine and gluconolactone were good inhibitors of the brain enzyme. Pentchev *et al.* (1973) found that *p*-amino-phenyl-β-thioglucoside was a weak inhibitor of the placental enzyme, the

K_i being only 6.25 mM. Erickson and Radin (1973) also found D-erythro-sphingosine to be effective with a preparation of rat brain glucocerebrosidase; the inhibition was 59% at 0.3 mM. Curiously, DL-erythro-*dihydro*sphingosine was a weak inhibitor, but glucosyl D-sphingosine (glucopsychosine) produced 75% inhibition at 0.3 mM. These workers prepared a series of N-alkyl derivatives of glucopsychosine and found that the n-hexyl compound was very effective $(K_i = 0.3 \mu M)$. The compound acted as a competitive inhibitor, a role which is to be expected in view of its very close similarity to glucocerebroside. It appears very likely that the plus-charged secondary amine group combines with an important COOH near the enzyme's active site.

When this inhibitor, N-hexyl-O-glucosyl-sphingosine, was added to cultures containing rat astrocytoma cells (RGC-6) and mouse neuroblastoma cells (NB41A), it produced an accumulation of glucocerebroside (Dawson *et al.*, 1974). The inhibitor, at a concentration of 5 μg/ml in the medium, caused no interference with growth rate and only minor changes in a variety of lysosomal hydrolases, yet the glucocerebroside concentration was raised five- to sixfold. There was also a 63% depression in the level of β-glucuronidase; the inhibitor has not yet been tested with that enzyme *in vitro*. It would appear from these experiments that a model form of Gaucher's disease has been induced in the cultured cells, and further study might be helpful in elucidating the detailed changes that occur.

A number of curious points were observed in the cultured cells. When labeled glucocerebroside was included in the medium, the lipid was taken up fairly rapidly. However, the addition of hexyl glucosyl sphingosine slowed down the uptake considerably. In the case of NB2-A cells, the uptake of labeled cerebroside eventually caught up with the uninhibited cells and the radioactivity in the cells declined in the normal way; that is, the catabolism of the "ingested" cerebroside was not impeded by the inhibitor. This fact could be explained by eventual breakdown of the inhibitor in the cells. In the case of RGC-6 cells, the inhibition of uptake was not as severe, but the blockage of cerebroside degradation was complete in the inhibited cells. These findings raise the possibility that cerebroside uptake by cells is a normal process and that the process requires glucocerebrosidase. It is possible that the enzyme is located (in part) in the plasma membrane, and it can bind the lipid at its active site or some other site, thus bringing the lipid into the plasma membrane. In the normal course of an enzyme's action, there is a moment before attack on the substrate when the substrate can escape (this process is the origin of the K_m). In this example, the escape could be into the plasma membrane milieu.

While lipid uptake from a cell's medium might seem unexpected, there is much evidence to show that this can happen with many lipids. Red cells are known to exchange cholesterol with the cholesterol in plasma, and indirect evidence has shown that red cells do the same with glucocerebroside (Dawson and Sweeley, 1970). *In vitro* studies with isolated brain cells have indicated that neurons can make glucocerebroside but glia cannot (Radin *et al.*, 1972*a*). If these studies are correct, glia must get their glucocerebroside from another source, presumably the neurons, by an uptake phenomenon. The mechanism of the uptake phenomenon is currently under study in my laboratory.

Additional attempts at synthesizing glucocerebrosidase inhibitors in my laboratory (Hyun *et al.*, 1975) have produced several compounds which act as mixed-type inhibitors, that is, they seem to act at the catalytic site and at a second site, presumably an allosteric region. One of the best is a ceramide analog, in which the long side chain of sphingosine is replaced by a benzene ring and in which the acyl group is replaced by an alkyl group. Thus the compound is a secondary amine, like hexyl psychosine, but it lacks the glucosyl moiety. Tested with human placental glucocerebrosidase, 3-(p-decanoyl-amidophenyl)-2-decylamino-1,3-propanediol produced an inhibition of 68% at $6\,\mu M$. It was also very effective with the rat spleen enzyme and with the rat spleen aryl glucosidase. The latter observation is further evidence for the idea proposed early in this section, namely, that aryl and cerebroside glucosidases have an important structural region in common.

Analogs of the above inhibitor, in which an acyl group replaced the alkyl group, were inactive. Deoxycorticosterone β-glucoside was a moderately active noncompetitive inhibitor and thus is unlikely to be a substrate for the enzyme. *p*-Nitrophenyl β-glucoside was a moderately effective inhibitor, acting by mixed modes. *p*-Chloromercuribenzenesulfonate was a good inhibitor, as noted by Kanfer *et al.* (1972). Evidently the enzyme possesses a sensitive mercaptan group.

The finding that glucocerebrosidase seems to possess an allosteric region that recognizes and binds compounds resembling the substrate appears to be a possibly important point. This region may bind glucocerebroside and act as an essential part of the uptake mechanism by which cerebroside enters cells. This region may have originated far back in prehistoric times by an accidental gene duplication, complete or partial, so that the enzyme now had two active sites in the same polypeptide chain. As time went on, mutations took place and eventually the second site lost its catalytic activity, yet still retained its ability to bind substances bearing a resemblance to the original substrate. This hypothesis, which has been offered before in the case of galactocerebrosidase (Arora *et al.*, 1973), might find confirmation when the amino acid sequence of the enzyme is determined.

We have also tested the effect of *N*-hexyl-*O*-glucosyl-sphingosine on human skin fibroblasts in culture (Warren *et al.*, 1974). Glucocerebrosidase was found to be inhibited strongly here, too, while aryl α-glucosidase was not particularly affected. In cells grown for 28 days on inhibitor-augmented medium, the inhibitor could be detected in the cell lipids, together with an amine that was identified as *N*-hexyl sphingosine. Thus it is apparent that glucosidase is able to act slowly on the inhibitor. However, *N*-hexyl sphingosine is itself a rather good inhibitor of glucocerebrosidase. The inhibited cells exhibited a two- to threefold increase in glucocerebroside, a lesser accumulation of trihexosyl ceramide (probably galactosyl galactosyl glucosyl ceramide), and an increased weight of cells per culture plate. Concentrations of cholesterol, protein, and total lipid were unchanged. These changes are much like those seen in Gaucher patients, although the increase in trihexosyl ceramide has not been consistently observed. While the accumulation of cerebroside struck us at first as being disappointingly small, we realized after looking at the limited data on Gaucher spleens that the accumulation *in vivo* is actually quite slow. The *total accumulation* of cerebroside is higher than the increase in concentration because of the considerable enlargement that takes place in the spleen.

A curious feature of these "Gaucher" fibroblasts was the presence of many multilamellar bodies, evidently due to accumulation of something. They could be due to cerebroside accumulation, but the two- to threefold increase does not seem sufficient to produce such bodies and they do not resemble the bodies seen in Gaucher tissues. We are inclined to believe that the lamellae are derived from an accumulation of a complex composed of inhibitor and glucosidase. Similar bodies have been found in animals dosed with excessive amounts of chloroquine (Read and Bay, 1971) and in cultured spinal ganglia that had been exposed to chlorpromazine (Brosnan *et al.*, 1970). Both are lipoidal amines of clinical interest and, while chloroquine does not affect glucocerebrosidase, the other amine is a modest inhibitor (28 % at 0.3 mM).

A similar study carried out by Dr. Kenneth Warren in my laboratory with rats, injected intraperitoneally every 4–5 days, produced no accumulation of glucocerebroside in spleen after 28 days. This disappointing result may have been caused by adaptation of the animals, with induction of some detoxifying enzyme. Shorter periods of inhibitor treatment did produce some cerebroside accumulation. With the aid of radioactive hexyl psychosine it was shown that hydrolysis to hexyl sphingosine occurred, as well as formation of polar products. Hopefully other inhibitors will give more promising results.

Several inhibitors of aryl *β*-glucosidase look interesting and might act on glucocerebrosidase. 5-Amino-5-deoxyglucose exhibited K_i values of 0.6–7 μM with several plant glucosidases (Reese *et al.*, 1971). 1-Aminoglucose (glucosylamine) had a K_i of 2.3 μM with yeast glucosidase (Lai and

Axelrod, 1973). Thus it may be a general characteristic of glucosidases to possess a sensitive cation-binding group near the active site. However, since we found no effect of 2-amino-2-deoxyglucose with glucocerebrosidase, the location of the amino group seems to be quite critical.

Hyun *et al.* (1974) found that one of the compounds tested with placental cerebrosidase produced some stimulation. This was *N*-decanoyl-L-threo-3-phenyl-2-amino-1,3-propanediol, which produced 47% more hydrolysis at a concentration of 1.2 mM. This result suggests the possibility of treating Gaucher patients with an enzyme stimulator, which might bring the defective enzyme up to a useful level of activity. Because heterozygotes with this disorder do not have much more activity than the affected homozygotes, a great deal of stimulation would not be needed.

4.5. Clinical Aspects of Glucocerebrosidase

It is now well-known that Gaucher's disease involves an inherited deficiency in the activity of glucocerebrosidase. The reader might wish to consult the excellent chapter on the disease by Fredrickson and Sloan (1972). The substrate accumulates to a considerable extent, particularly in spleen, liver, and bone marrow. The lipid accumulates in the form of minute twisted bilayers, when visualized by electron micrography, in combination with phospholipid and cholesterol (Glew and Lee, 1973). Also present is some protein and glycoprotein, and a later study showed that the protein includes glucocerebrosidase (Glew *et al.*, 1974). It is possible that the glycoprotein is identical to, or related to the coglucosidase discovered by Ho and O'Brien (1971). Glew *et al.* point out that it is not surprising that an enzyme should be bound to its substrate if the substrate is produced at too high a rate for the inefficient enzyme to handle it.

It is interesting that Glew *et al.* found a good deal of aryl glucosidase activity outside of the deposited particles. Either the unbound enzyme is not the one which acts on cerebroside or much of the glucocerebrosidase is, for some reason, not bound to its substrate. Evidence to support the former possibility comes from a survey of Gaucher tissues for aryl glucosidase activity (Hultberg and Öckerman, 1970). These workers found that the specific activity in white blood cells and urine was reduced only by about half in Gaucher patients, whereas liver and spleen activities were greatly reduced (about 90%). Sephadex chromatography of the liver enzyme from normal individuals produced four peaks of activity, of which two exhibited activity toward glucocerebroside. While improved chromatographic procedures are clearly needed, it seems definite that several types of glucosidase occur in the body, that the ratio varies with the tissue, and that some types are more deficient than others in Gaucher's disease.

Another view of this situation comes from an examination of the relationship between pH and aryl glucosidase activity of white blood cells (Beutler and Kuhl, 1970). When Na citrate buffer was used, the pH optimum lay between 5.0 and 5.5, but a second, smaller peak was observed at 4.0. The enzyme activity at the lower pH was reduced in Gaucher cells to a much greater extent than was the major enzyme activity. It would be valuable to repeat this analysis with glucocerebroside as substrate.

Beutler and Kuhl checked the K_m values with the fluorogenic glucoside and found them to be different at the two pH optima, but the Gaucher enzymes appeared normal in this respect. Presumably the Gaucher enzymes differ in the catalytic efficiencies or are simply made too slowly.

Klibansky et al. (1973) recently examined the stability to heat of glucocerebrosidase from leukocytes. The enzyme was extracted from white cells with Triton X-100 + NaCl + Na cholate, then heated in phosphate–citrate pH 5.3 at 50°C for 20 min, and assayed with labeled substrate. About 77% of the activity remained after this treatment when normal cells were tested. A similar stability was found on testing cells from Gaucher patients in whom the disease had been diagnosed after age 10, but significantly less stability (50%) was found in patients who had been diagnosed earlier in life. This finding introduces a new factor to consider. One might postulate that greater heat lability reflects faster proteolytic attack or faster turnover of an enzyme, and a consequent lower specific activity in the tissue. However, the two groups of patients, both of which come under the category of "adult Gaucher's disease," did not exhibit differing enzyme activities. The range of specific activities was 6 to 20% of normal, with no clear distinction between the two groups. However, the authors did state that they felt there was a correlation between heat lability and severity of the disease, as estimated by age at diagnosis and spleen size.

Heat stability tests can be complicated by the stabilizing or destabilizing effects of substances that accompany the enzyme being stressed. For example, one might expect coglucosidase and cerebroside to stabilize glucocerebrosidase. Thus it is possible that, for some reason, the Gaucher individuals with the lower heat stability had less coglucosidase or glucocerebroside in their leukocytes. In any event, there is a distinct need to assay tissues for both of these factors, as well as the enzyme.

A further study by Klibansky et al. (1974) involved a comparison of cerebroside and aryl glucosidase activities in leukocytes from patients with adult Gaucher's disease. Both activities were found to be equally reduced in the defective cells (also in cells from heterozygotes, but less so). The pH/activity curves were similar for both substrates. These observations seem to indicate that only one glucosidase exists. However, they also found that glucocerebrosidase was more heat-resistant than aryl glucosidase and that mercuric ions (10 μM) inhibited the former enzyme 85% but affected the latter enzyme activity only 30%. The authors conclude that several enzymes may be defective in Gaucher's disease.

This study also included interesting observations on a possible role of cations in glucosidase function. The leukocytes were extracted with Na cholate and Triton X-100; then the soluble enzymes were dialyzed against EDTA and then against saline. About half of the two activities was lost by this procedure, possibly indicating a need for tightly bound cation. Incubation with Ca, Mn, or Cu ions partially restored both glucosidase activities. While few glycosidases have been shown to require a cation, previous tests may have been inadequate. It may also be relevant that Concanavalin A, the protein that binds glucosides and mannosides, requires two different metal ions for activity.

One of the curious features of Gaucher's disease is that the adult form shows no involvement of the central nervous system, while the infantile form shows severe failure of brain development with particular loss of neurons. The peripheral organs in both types accumulate glucocerebroside, yet there is little evidence for lipid accumulation in the affected brain. The most recent study of this subject (Gonzalez-Sastre et al., 1974) offers the finding that total cerebroside concentration is close to normal, possibly a little low, but the glucose content of this cerebroside is abnormally high. In other words, galactocerebroside accumulation is impaired, which would be expected in failure to mature, but glucocerebroside does indeed accumulate to some extent. This study was made with gray matter of brain; previous studies with white matter showed no glucocerebroside accumulation.

Perhaps this difference is related to our previous observation (Radin et al., 1972a) that glial cells—the primary synthesizer of white matter—cannot make glucocerebroside. Glucocerebroside and gangliosides have been found in glial cells and myelin, and we have found good glucocerebrosidase activity in isolated glia (Radin, Erickson, and Sellinger, unpublished results), so there is probably some turnover of glucocerebroside in white matter. Because presumably the synthetic input into the turnover comes from neurons, which could supply glucocerebroside or gangliosides, one ought to expect some glucocerebroside accumulation even in white matter of infants with Gaucher's disease. However, the turnover rate might be relatively slow. Another possibility is that glucocerebrosidase is required for the *transfer* of the lipid from neurons to glia, as proposed in Section 4.4. Such a function could then explain the severity of the brain defect in the infantile form. The noninvolvement of the brain in the adult form might be explained as due to a much slower turnover of gangliosides and glucocerebroside in the mature brain or to the appearance during maturation of a new, second glucosidase which can handle the modest turnover requirements of the adult brain. Unfortunately no one seems to have assayed the brain of an adult victim of Gaucher's disease for glucosidase activities.

Another possible explanation for the brain malfunction in infantile Gaucher's disease is that glucocerebroside normally is metabolized by two routes, primarily through a glucosidase (to form ceramide) and secondarily through some other route which is forcibly augmented in the diseased state, giving rise to accumulation of a toxic product. Against this possibility is the failure, thus far, of any chemist to isolate a seemingly toxic material from the affected tissue. However, the amount accumulated might be too small to detect without a special effort. For example, there might be a weak amidase in brain which removes the fatty acid moiety, leaving glucosyl sphingosine, which might be highly toxic. Lin and Radin (1973) looked for such an enzyme in the brain of young rats but found no clear evidence for it. Stearate-labeled glucocerebroside was incubated with brain homogenate under various conditions. While some free fatty acid was indeed formed, its formation could be blocked by the addition of substances known to inhibit glucocerebrosidase; thus the fatty acid formation could be attributed to ceramidase action during the incubation. Of course, since a negative finding in such a search might be due only to a difference in species or to failure to try the correct conditions, the finding can only be considered tentative.

Some Gaucher spleens have been shown to have an increased amount of some glucocerebroside derivatives. The ganglioside, GM_3, was found augmented by Makita et al. (1966) and Kuske and Rosenberg (1972). The former also found what seemed to be a fatty acid ester of glucocerebroside, previously unknown, and the latter authors also found some accumulation of trihexosyl ceramide, a compound which we found elevated in fibroblasts in which glucocerebrosidase had been blocked chemically. It is difficult to believe that these substances could be toxic at the low levels that were observed, if indeed they accumulate in the infant brain.

We know from the work of Ho and O'Brien (1971) that there is considerable accumulation of coglucosidase in the spleen of people with Gaucher's disease. Perhaps this accumulation is toxic in some way. It would be useful to assay other tissues of Gaucher patients for coglucosidase, particularly the brains of infantile and adult patients.

Glucocerebroside accumulation presumably comes from two sources: membrane-bound cerebroside and ceramide oligosaccharides (gangliosides, globosides, blood group substances, and so forth). The known pathways for degradation of the complex glycosphingolipids involve hydrolysis, ultimately forming glucocerebroside, which presumably is hydrolyzed by the same glucosidase that degrades membrane-bound cerebroside. Because all mammalian cells seem to have both the simple and the complex lipids, both lines of degradation may be assumed to occur everywhere. The spleen has the extra burden of hydrolyzing the cells from other organs, namely red and white cells from blood. Thus it is not surprising to find most cerebroside accumulation in this and related tissues. Kattlove *et al.* (1969) have estimated the amount of glucocerebroside that might be degraded in the course of normal spleen function and concluded, on the basis of analytical data and cell turnover estimates, that most of the glucocerebroside that is handled by the spleen comes from white blood cells. The actual daily amount is appreciable: at least 400 mg "glycolipid" per day. The calculation seems to be derived from the sum of all the glycosphingolipids in the blood cells; thus the amount of glucocerebroside to be expected from this might be 250 mg/day. (This calculation disregards the turnover of membrane-bound glucocerebroside, nongranulocytic white cells, and blood platelets, for which no estimate can be made.) If a Gaucher patient were unable to hydrolyze any of the on-rushing glucocerebroside, the accumulation rate would be $365 \times 0.25 = 91$ g/yr. Because the actual accumulation is far less than this, it is apparent that the residual activity of the defective spleen's glucosidase is sufficient to deal with much of cerebroside turnover needs. In the case of tissues which do not destroy blood cells, such as brain, the accumulation problem may be relatively minor. Because of this I am inclined to attribute the neuropathy of Gaucher infants to a thus far undiscovered function of glucocerebrosidase.

An intriguing question yet to be answered is: How does the accumulation of glucocerebroside in Gaucher spleen stimulate spleen hypertrophy? Hopefully some answers will be obtained from the *in vitro* or *in vivo* use of glucosidase inhibitors.

It would be going too far afield to discuss recent diagnostic and therapeutic approaches in Gaucher's disease, although these may be the most exciting developments on the topic of glucocerebrosidase. For example, one group has recently reported on a preliminary treatment of two Gaucher patients with intravenously administered glucocerebrosidase. The level of cerebroside in liver was drastically reduced by only one or two treatments (Pentchev *et al.*, 1974).

5. GALACTOCEREBROSIDASE

Galactocerebroside → Ceramide + Galactose

Galactocerebrosidase is a β-galactosidase which was found in various rat organs by Hajra *et al.* (1966) and in rat intestine by Brady *et al.* (1965). Some purification of the enzyme was achieved by these workers, and a purification of more than 300-fold was achieved by Bowen and Radin (1968*a*), starting with rat brain. It was noted that aryl galactosidase activity could be considerably separated from the cerebrosidase, and later studies by others have indicated that the assays with aromatic galactosides reflect primarily the activities of the enzymes that hydrolyze the more complex galactolipids, or an enzyme of low specificity. The enzyme is deficient in the genetic human disorder Krabbe's disease or globoid leukodystrophy. It is very likely that the same enzyme hydrolyzes galactosyl diglyceride and galactosyl acyl alkyl glyceride, naturally occurring lipids in brain. There is also a question as to whether it also attacks lactosyl ceramide.

5.1. Substrate Preparation and Enzyme Assay

Galactocerebroside labeled in the fatty acid moiety can be synthesized by the procedure described in the corresponding section on glucocerebrosidase (Section 4.1), in which case the hexane–methanol–water partition system can be used to separate the radioactive enzyme product (ceramide) from unused substrate. Also unlabeled cerebroside can be used and the galactose can be determined enzymatically, using either galactose oxidase (*D. dendroides*) or galactose dehydrogenase (*P. fluorescens*). The former enzyme is obtainable from Worthington Biochemical Corporation or AB Kabi, Stockholm, and the latter enzyme, from Sigma Chemical Co. The use of galactose oxidase for galactocerebrosidase assay was described by Gatt (1969b); under the conditions used the amount measured was about 100 nmol. The hydrolytic reaction was stopped by heating in boiling water, the proteins (and excess substrate?) were removed with a charcoal column, and the eluted sugar was measured enzymatically in a 2-hr incubation.

The galactose dehydrogenase method is described by Meisler (1972) for miscellaneous galactosides. The scale of this assay allows measuring 10–50 nmol with an incubation time of 40 min. Another version of the reaction has been described by Gatt (1970) for use with galactolipids. This version treats the problem of cloudy liquids (due to proteins or lipids). The free galactose is oxidized by the dehydrogenase, forming NADH, and interfering materials are removed by addition of chloroform–methanol, which leaves the NADH in the clear aqueous layer. The unreacted galactolipid need not be removed prior to galactose determination, since the galactosidases show little activity at the preferred pH of the dehydrogenase (8.6). However, when whole tissue is assayed, interfering enzymes must be removed by heat denaturation before adding the galactose dehydrogenase. Assays involving NADH production can often be increased in sensitivity, but no special effort seems to have been made for this application.

It is also possible to measure galactose by adding an aliquot from the reaction with galactosidase to an automatic chromatographic sugar analyzer (Lee, 1972). This convenient procedure can assay 10–80 nmol of sugar in 0.2 ml of the initial hydrolase mixture (from which lipids ought to be removed first, no doubt). While the procedure seems slow, it requires little attention; however, it does not sound too useful for large numbers of samples. Perhaps modern, high-pressure liquid chromatographs will be adapted to this problem. These instruments utilize extremely small ion exchange beads and column pressures in the thousands of pounds; typical simple chromatographic runs take only 15 min each.

Probably the most sensitive and convenient method for galactocerebrosidase assay is the use of galactose-labeled cerebroside, which allows one to isolate the radioactive product by a simple solvent partition between water, methanol, and chloroform. The preparation of labeled substrate is a 2-day procedure, involving oxidation of unlabeled galactocerebroside by galactose oxidase, reduction of the 6-aldehydo carbon with tritium-labeled sodium borohydride, and chromatographic purification (Radin, 1972a; Radin et al., 1969). (This approach has been used for a variety of galactose- and galactosamine-containing lipids and glycoproteins.) Specific activities of a very high order can be obtained (over 50,000 cpm/nmol), allowing one to measure very low enzyme activities. We have settled on a specific activity of about 350 cpm/nmol for most work and aim for about 10 nmol hydrolysis, but assay of fetal amniotic fibroblasts requires about 15 times this specific activity.

Apparently [^{3}H]borohydride is able to insert 1 or 2% of the label into a lipoidal region of the cerebroside molecule; thus for precise work one ought to determine the amount of radioactivity that is not in the galactose moiety and to subtract that in calculating the specific activity.

The details of the assay procedure have been described recently (Radin, 1972b). The cerebroside is emulsified in a mixture of detergents (Tween 20, Myrj 59, Tris oleate, and Na taurocholate), mixed with citrate buffer pH 4.5, and incubated with enzyme for several hours. The emulsion is "broken" with a mixture of castor oil, isopropanol, and chloroform, and the galactose is taken out by the addition of water. The blank, which is normally about 0.15% of the initial substrate activity, can be reduced by a backwash. Occasional repurification of the substrate is necessary to remove breakdown products. The use of castor oil was adopted when we noted a tendency for the usual Folch partition system to develop a slight emulsion, evidently because of the detergents in the assay medium. The emulsion caused a slight amount of cerebroside carryover into the aqueous galactose-containing layer. By "drowning" the detergents with a large amount of lipid, their tendency to form an emulsion was neutralized.

In the case of brain assays, there is a great deal of endogenous cerebroside present except at very early ages. The lipid dilutes the radioactive substrate to an appreciable degree. This problem can be treated by three methods, as described for glucocerebrosidase in Section 4.10. The cerebroside was normally removed from the enzyme by a relatively slow series of steps: extraction with taurocholate and pancreatic enzymes, centrifugation to remove undissolved material, precipitation of the enzyme at pH 3, and solubilization at about pH 6. Perhaps, if many tissue samples are to be assayed, it might pay simply to raise the specific activity of the substrate and to reduce the amount of brain to the point where the endogenous dilution effect becomes negligible. Unused substrate can be recovered from the chloroform layer (Radin and Arora, 1971).

Miyatake and Suzuki (1974b) have introduced a simpler way of removing the enzyme from endogenous cerebroside. The brains are homogenized in water, freeze-thawed, sonicated in a water bath, and then added to ether–methanol 3:1 at −30°. This procedure yields the precipitated protein, which can be dried. Apparently 80–90% of the endogenous cerebroside is removed by the treatment and very little enzyme is denatured.

There seem to be no complications to the kinetic properties of galactocerebrosidase, although they have not been studied in many tissues. Occasionally a slight slowing of the reaction rate with time has been observed (Arora and Radin, 1972a). The choice of bile salt makes a distinct difference in the assayed activity of the enzyme (Bowen and Radin, 1969b). Crude commercial taurocholate was the most stimulatory of those tested, but pure taurocholate yielded a relative activity of only 61%. Taurodeoxycholate was about as active, but the mixture of bile salts produced 82% relative activity. Cholate was moderately stimulating, while deoxycholate and taurochenodeoxycholate were inhibitory. A few other enzymes have been compared in this way and also found to exhibit marked differences in bile salt effects.

5.2. Enzyme Purification

Galactocerebrosidase has been purified somewhat from rat brain (Bowen and Radin, 1968a). One unusual feature in the procedure is the use of a crude preparation of pancreatic lipase, containing proteases, together with Na taurocholate to extract the enzyme. Whether the proteases or other enzymes attack any part of the cerebrosidase during the extraction has not been determined, but the total enzyme activity is increased considerably as the result of the treatment. The other purification steps are conventional, producing over a 300-fold increase in specific activity and 27% yield. The enzyme becomes unstable to storage after DEAE-cellulose chromatography but can then be stabilized by inclusion of 50% glycerol. Much of the aryl galactosidase activity in brain is removed in the course of the various steps. A survey of various animal species and organs was disappointing in terms of finding a better source than rat brain.

Miyatake and Suzuki (1974b) have carried out some cerebrosidase purification starting with their rat brain powder, which had been separated from much of the endogenous lipid. They extracted the powder with water, which solubilizes $\frac{1}{3}$ of the enzyme (with little increase in specific activity), precipitated most of the enzyme with ammonium sulfate, and then applied the enzyme to a DEAE–cellulose column. Two minor peaks of enzyme followed the major one. (A similar multiplicity of enzymes had been reported by Bowen and Radin, 1968a.) An isoelectric focusing treatment with the major peak yielded a nice sharp peak having an isoelectric point of 4.45. Unfortunately the specific activity was not determined, but the method shows promise.

5.3.   Enzyme Characteristics

The rat brain enzyme occurs at a concentration higher in white matter than in gray, and in both isolated neurons and glia (Radin et al., 1972a). The finding of activity in neuronal preparations was a surprise since galacto-cerebroside had been assumed to occur only in myelin and in the manufac-turers of myelin, the glia. However, there have been reports of trace amounts of galactocerebroside in neuronal preparations, and DeVries et al. (1972) have reported finding considerable amounts of the lipid in axonal prepara-tions. Moreover, we have found in neurons fair amounts of the galactosyl-transferase which makes cerebroside. Thus it appears that neurons, as well as glia, carry on synthesis and degradation of galactocerebroside. Perhaps galactocerebroside has a special function besides entering into myelin.

Preliminary subcellular fractionation work has indicated that the enzyme is localized in brain lysosomes (Bowen and Radin, 1968b). However, it has not been sought after in myelin preparations, which might be a fruitful question in view of the histochemical demonstration of a galactosidase in myelin (Mickel and Gilles, 1970). Cerebrosidase occurs in a wide variety of organs, including blood plasma and leukocytes. It has been found in in-vertebrates despite the virtual or complete absence of the substrate (Mraz and Jatzkewitz, 1972).

The molecular weight of the rat brain enzyme appears to be about 50,000, judging by its elution from a Sephadex G-200 column.

The purest cerebrosidase preparation tested still contained some hydrolytic activity toward several other galactosides. Lactosyl ceramide ("lactoside") was about as good a substrate as galactosyl ceramide, *o*-nitrophenyl galactoside was a better substrate, and galactosyl sphingosine was a poor substrate. Lactosyl ceramide was found to be a competitive inhibitor (Arora *et al.*, 1973), which could mean that it is a substrate for the same enzyme. However, Gatt and Rapport (1966) isolated a partially purified galactosidase from rat brain which could hydrolyze lactosyl ceramide without affecting galactocerebroside. Moreover, this enzyme was inhibited by fatty acid, which—by contrast—acts to stimulate galactocerebrosidase. This finding could mean that there are *two* lactosidases, one that is specific for this lipid and one that also acts on galactocerebroside.

Lactoside is an intermediate, synthetic and degradative, in the metabolism of gangliosides and the other complex glycosphingolipids. In the case of the gangliosides, the principal fatty acid is stearic (roughly 88 % in brain) and only traces of palmitic and lignoceric are found. Data on the fatty acids of the other complex glycosphingolipids seem to be unavailable, because of the low concentrations, but a sample of ceramide trihexoside, found in the nervous system of a patient with Fabry's disease by Miyatake and Ariga (1972), can be considered. This material, which is made from lactoside and the higher glycolipids of the globoside series, contained behenic acid (22:0) as the major fatty acid. Lactoside has been isolated from normal brain (Svennerholm, 1966) and found to contain fatty acids closely resembling the nonhydroxy galactocerebrosides (mostly 22–26 carbons). A sample of lactoside isolated from the brain of a patient with GLD (globoid leukodystrophy, or Krabbe's disease) yielded a fatty acid distribution resembling both gangliosides and cerebrosides; that is, it contained 32 % stearate and 56 % 22–26 carbons (Evans and McCluer, 1969). A large amount of lactoside was found in the brain of a patient with Hurler's disease, an iduronidase deficiency (Taketomi and Yamakawa, 1967). In this case, the fatty acid distribution resembled the ganglioside distribution even more closely. Thus it would seem that lactoside can come from two sources, one specializing in stearate production, the other specializing in production of the very long acids. Probably the latter source consists of glial cells, which make galactocerebroside, and the former source consists of neurons, which make glucocerebroside and the polysaccharide lipids. It would then not be surprising to find two different enzymes that hydrolyze lactoside, as suggested above. (Perhaps there is significance in the finding of elevated lactoside levels in a variety of unrelated genetic diseases that involve hydrolysis in the brain. Lactosidase may be rather easily inhibited by the substances that accumulate in the disorders.)

Further evidence that bears on the question of specificity comes from a study of rat brains from animals of different ages (Bowen and Radin, 1969*b*; Radin *et al.*, 1969). The specific activity of galactocerebrosidase at age 4 days was 0.26 nmol/hr/mg of brain, it rose for roughly 90 days to four times that value, and then it dropped slightly over the next 8 mo. By contrast, lactoside galactosidase specific activity was 3.5 of these units at 4 days, rising only 50% to its maximum at about 24 days. This activity too dropped only slightly over the remaining period of time. The assay conditions used were similar to those used by Gatt and Rapport. On the basis of the different developmental patterns one would conclude that lactosidase is a different and somewhat more active enzyme.

Suzuki and Suzuki (1974a) made a comparison of the two enzyme activities in human liver, using the same assay systems described above. An aqueous extract (not entirely free of particles probably) was made from the liver and exposed to electrofocusing, that is, electrophoresis in a vertical density gradient containing ampholytes. Lactosidase appeared in three peaks, two of which also contained galactocerebrosidase. Thus one kind of lactosidase seems totally different from cerebrosidase. Another separation technique, gel filtration with Sephadex G-200, produced two enzyme peaks, one containing both activities, the other containing only lactosidase. Again the same conclusion can be drawn. However, it is not definite from these data that cerebrosidase also shows activity toward lactoside.

Further evidence on the question comes from a study of liver in the human genetic disorder, GLD (Suzuki and Suzuki, 1974b). These workers found a marked lack of cerebrosidase and a slight lack of lactosidase. The latter effect is cloudy because of the few samples available (GLD is a rare disease). Control activities were 4.9, 6.9, 7.9, and 12.8 nmol/hr/g, while the two GLD samples exhibited 3.6 and 5.6 units. This difference is consistent with the hypothesized dual lactosidases, one of the activities being deficient because of the genetic lack of galactocerebrosidase.

A curious point about the normal activities is that cerebrosidase activity was about 49 units and lactosidase activity was about 8 units. In other words, compared with rat brain, the ratio of the two activities was reversed even though it is likely that liver has negligible galactocerebroside content and metabolism.

A similar comparison of liver activities in dogs with a genetic disease resembling GLD (Suzuki et al., 1974) also revealed a serious lack of cerebrosidase, although the degree of deficiency was less than that seen in the human disease. Here too the lactosidase activity seemed low in the affected dogs, but the difference was not statistically significant.

A recent report by Wenger et al. (1974) offers a somewhat different picture of the two enzyme activities. These workers modified the assay for lactosidase, offering different optimum conditions: pH 4.4 instead of 5.0 and oleic acid, which had previously been found to inhibit the rat brain enzyme. Under these conditions, the liver, brain, and cultured fibroblasts of patients with GLD showed very low activities for cerebroside *and* lactoside hydrolysis. On this basis, one might propose that a single enzyme cleaves both galactolipids, or that the two enzymes share a section in common which is defective in the GLD disorder. Alternatively, one might conclude that the use of oleic acid and a lower pH for lactosidase assay prevents action of the normal lactosidase specific enzyme, while still revealing the ability of cerebrosidase to hydrolyze lactoside. Under the assay conditions of Wenger *et al.*, the specific activity of liver was higher for lactoside than for cerebroside, in contrast to the findings of Suzuki and Suzuki, but this is not inconsistent with the two-enzyme theory. A crucial test of the theory could be obtained by assaying with the two substrates in the same GLD tissue but under differing conditions of pH, with and without inhibitors.

The relationship between pH and lactosidase activity was studied in rat brain homogenate with citrate buffer (Miyatake and Suzuki, 1974*a*). The maximum activity was at pH 4.2, but a distinct shoulder was visible in their graph at approximately pH 5. The assay medium in this study included a higher taurocholate concentration than was originally recommended for the purified enzyme (Gatt and Rapport, 1966), as well as some NaCl; it also omitted the Triton. It may be that the specific lactosidase has an optimum at about 5.0 (depending on the concentration of taurocholate, and so forth) and that galactocerebrosidase, when hydrolyzing lactoside, has an optimum at about 4.2. Because the two enzymes may have different requirements for taurocholate, the optimal bile salt concentration will depend on the pH used for the test.

Partial support for lactosidase as a separate enzyme comes from the finding of a genetic disorder in which lactoside accumulation is a dominant feature (Dawson, 1972; Dawson and Stein, 1970). The symptoms were distinctly different from those seen in GLD, and some accumulation also of ganglioside intermediates was seen (including glucocerebroside). Thus the disorder seems to involve a basic neuronal mechanism. This interpretation is consistent with Dawson's observation that lactoside galactosidase was severely deficient in this patient. Unfortunately galactocerebrosidase and hydrolases of ganglioside metabolism were not evaluated with natural substrates.

Two other simple galactolipid hydrolase activities have been found to be abnormally low in GLD patients: hydrolysis of psychosine (galactosyl sphingosine) and galactosyl diglyceride. In the case of the former lipid, which has not been found in nature, Miyatake and Suzuki (1974*b*) concluded that it is hydrolyzed by cerebrosidase. The conclusion was based on a detailed comparison of the properties of the two activities: thermal stability, solubility in ammonium sulfate, DEAE–cellulose chromatography, electrofocusing, developmental changes, and others. Of course the lack of activity in GLD is further evidence for the conclusion. In the case of galactosyl diglyceride galactosidase activity, the only evidence for a single enzyme is the common deficiency in GLD (Wenger *et al.*, 1973), as well as similar subcellular distribution in normal human brain and liver. Unpublished data are mentioned in this study which showed that the ester glycolipid is a competitive inhibitor for cerebroside hydrolysis and vice versa. This result certainly supports the one-enzyme thesis.

Unfortunately for this thesis in the case of the ester lipid and sphingolipid, an earlier study of the former activity (Subba Rao *et al.*, 1970) revealed some differences from reported data on cerebrosidase. In this report there was no direct comparison between the two activities; thus the differences in enzyme properties could be due to interlaboratory technical differences.

Galactocerebrosidase levels have been determined in the brain of mice that carry an important sex-linked mutation, "myelin synthesis deficiency" or *msd* (Brenkert *et al.*, 1972). The specific activity was normal in mice between 8 to 21 days, which covers the period from normal appearance to severe myelin lack. Bowen and Radin (1969*a*) also examined the cerebrosidase level in quaking and jimpy mice, 17 days old. No difference from normal was seen in the *jp* mice but the *qk* mice had a 17% lower activity. A more significant difference was seen in the dispersability of the enzyme; that is, the fraction of the activity that could be rendered soluble by sonicating the tissue homogenate was somewhat higher in the *jp* animals. This fact could mean that the lysosomes in jimpy brain are unusually fragile, but this fragility cannot be true of all the brain lysosomes, since the dispersability of aryl galactosidase and aryl sulfatase was normal. The failure to find a significant lack of hydrolytic activity toward cerebroside is interesting because the ability to *synthesize* the lipid is severely deficient in all three mutants. My tentative hypothesis is that the mice lack some primary ability to make myelin-forming cells, so that a large number of enzymes involved in myelin formation do not form. Since presumably the same cells would make cerebrosidase, this enzyme should be lacking, but the neurons—which also make this enzyme—might react to the situation by making more cerebrosidase that normal. This explanation could be tested by isolating the neurons from normal and defective mice and comparing their contents of cerebrosidase.

A highly purified galactosidase preparation from *E. coli* has been found to have some activity toward galactocerebroside (Brady *et al.*, 1965*a*). However, because it is far more active toward nitrophenyl galactoside, this activity is probably an expression of nonspecificity. A preparation of galactosidase from jack bean meal has also been found to hydrolyze cerebroside (Kanfer *et al.*, 1973).

5.4. Enzyme Inhibitors and Stimulators

Like so many lipid-hydrolyzing enzymes, galactocerebrosidase is greatly stimulated by bile salts. The effect is quite specific for the type of bile salt, as noted in Section 5.1. Under the assay conditions used by Bowen and Radin (1969*b*), oleic acid at a level of 0.2 mg/ml doubled the activity further. It had previously been observed that oleic acid stimulated the enzyme in the absence of bile salt too (Hajra *et al.*, 1966).

A variety of divalent metal cations had no effect nor was EDTA inhibitory. However, because no attempt was made to remove tightly bound cations, as by dialysis against EDTA, the possible role of a metal is still uncertain. *p*-Hydroxymercuribenzoate was reported to inhibit effectively, but it had no effect on the supposedly identical enzyme, the one that hydrolyzes galactosyl diglyceride (Subba Rao *et al.*, 1970). Because of the low solubility of that particular mercury compound at low pH, this question ought to be re-examined with the sulfonate analog. Moreover, one must wonder when crude enzymes are tested whether there are not many sulfhydryl compounds present that could bind the mercurial more strongly than the enzyme under test.

Bowen and Radin (1968*b*) also found that ceramide, the product of hydrolysis, is a weak inhibitor of cerebrosidase. Ceramide trihexoside was inert at the one concentration tested, $65\ \mu M$. Galactonolactone, but not gluconolactone, was a strong inhibitor, as expected. Galactose itself produced only 33% inhibition at a concentration of 60 mM. *o*-Nitrophenyl β-galactoside, at 30 mM, inhibited 62%. This result could mean that the phenolic glycoside is a substrate for the enzyme.

In the course of investigating the effects of a variety of synthetic analogs of ceramide, Arora and Radin (1972*b*) found that a group of branched chain compounds could stimulate cerebrosidase. The most effective one was *N*-decanoyl-2-amino-2-methyl-propanol, which produced 60% stimulation of the rat brain enzyme at about 1.5 mM. Since the amide did not affect the K_m for the enzyme–substrate complex, it may act to improve the efficiency of the enzyme. Removing the branched methyl group destroyed the effect. As was pointed out in Section 4.4, such stimulators offer the promise of therapeutic stimulation of defective enzymes in human genetic disorders. Since cerebrosidase activity is deficient in GLD, one might effect an amelioration of the disorder by regular administration of a cerebrosidase stimulator. One would have to start with the pregnant mother, since the infantile form of the disease produces abnormalities already *in utero*, in all probability. In a test with the stimulator with brain from GLD victims (Radin *et al.*, 1972*b*), the authors were able to show that the amide works on the defective enzyme as well as the normal one (and in human as well as in rat brain). When the chain length of the fatty acid was shortened or lengthened, both the rat and human enzyme showed similar changes in degree of stimulation, suggesting that the two enzymes are rather similar.

Pig brain apparently contains a heat-stable stimulating factor, resembling the glycoprotein factor of Ho and O'Brien (Section 4.3). Dr. Yuh-Nan Lin and I are now characterizing this material, which can be obtained from the cytosol produced from rat brain. Our tentative belief is that this material is also a glycoprotein and could be called a cogalactosidase. It is more active than the highly purified glycoprotein prepared by Li and Li (1974), which stimulates the hydrolysis of the more complex glycosphingolipids. Unlike coglucosidase, it is effective in the presence of bile salt. The assay of brain extracts for the stimulation has been hampered by the presence of what seems to be an inhibitor. Thus the controlling system in tissues may involve both a stimulator and an inhibitor. The fearless reader might wish to examine a hypothesis which explains how such stimulators work, discussed in Section 4.3.

A number of synthetic compounds have been found to inhibit cerebrosidase fairly effectively (Arora and Radin, 1972a; Arora et al., 1973). The most active compound was an analog of hydroxy ceramide in which the long aliphatic side chain of sphingosine was replaced by a benzene ring. Of the various fatty acids tested in this structure, 2-hydroxydodecanoic was most effective; thus the compound has the formula, N-(2-hydroxydodecanoyl)-DL-erythro-3-phenyl-2-amino-1,3-propanediol. It may be recalled that sphingolipids have the chiral structure D-erythro. Changing the structure of the inhibitor by removing the benzene ring; substituting the benzene ring in the para-position; removing one, two, or three of the hydroxyl groups; or inverting the configuration of the 3-hydroxy group resulted in partial or complete loss of inhibitory activity. We were surprised to find that the compound acted as a noncompetitive inhibitor despite the apparent stringent requirements calling for a structure very similar to that of ceramide, the normal product of enzyme action. Maximal inhibition with the rat brain enzyme was 82% attained at a concentration of 0.6 mM. The K_i was 0.1 mM.

A short-chain cerebroside, N-decanoyl galactosyl sphingosine, was found to be a competitive inhibitor, but it turned out to be an excellent substrate for the cerebrosidase. (It might be worth re-examining the optimal assay conditions for cerebrosidase using this as well as the 2-hydroxyacyl homolog.) The acetyl cerebroside homolog was also found to be a good inhibitor (57% at 0.3 mM), but here the inhibition was of the mixed type. Thus it is possible that acetyl psychosine binds to the active site of the enzyme and is also a substrate, but apparently the second, allosteric site also binds the compound. Perhaps this is the same site that binds the ceramide analogs mentioned above.

Galactocerebroside in which the amide group had been reduced to a secondary amine was an active inhibitor. N-(n-hexyl)-O-galactosyl sphingosine produced 68% inhibition at 0.3 mM while the glucosyl analog, which had proved to be an excellent inhibitor for glucocerebrosidase, yielded 36% inhibition at this level. The glucosyl compound acted as a noncompetitive inhibitor, while the galactosyl compound acted as a mixed-type inhibitor. Again there is evidence for two sensitive sites. Galactosyl sphingosine, the primary amine, was rather inert at 0.3 mM, showing the importance of a residue attached to the nitrogen atom.

To summarize the known properties of cerebrosidase, galactonolactone, lactosyl ceramide, and modified cerebrosides can bind to the catalytic site, while some modified cerebrosides and modified ceramides can bind to a secondary, rate-modifying site. The situation is thus rather similar to that seen with glucocerebrosidase (see Section 4.4) and the same hypothesis can safely be proposed that was given in that section. This is the gene duplication hypothesis, which proposes that there was formed at some time during evolution a partially duplicated enzyme molecule bearing two catalytic sites. Both sites recognized cerebroside, but one site mutated in time to the point where its recognition properties had become warped and catalytic activity was no longer possible. This then constitutes the allosteric site for this enzyme.

Some biological tests have been conducted with cerebrosidase inhibitors (Benjamins et al., 1974). Explants of newborn rat brain were cultured under conditions which normally led to myelination of the axons. In the case of the experimental explants, small amounts of inhibitor or synthetic stimulator were added to the culture medium at the time at which myelination actively began (8–9 days). Using compounds of varying effectiveness in vitro (with purified cerebrosidase), we found a rather distinct correlation with ability to prevent myelination. Thus, in the case of the enzyme inhibitors, it would appear that a lesion similar to that seen in the human cerebrosidase disorder, GLD, had been produced in explanted brain. Similar results were obtained with cerebrosidase stimulators, such as decanoyl aminomethylpropanol; thus it would appear that cerebrosidase had been stimulated in these exposed tissues to the point where excessive destruction of cerebroside had occurred.

In some experiments, explants were allowed to myelinate and then were exposed to cerebrosidase inhibitors. Demyelination occurred, again related in intensity to in vitro efficacy of the enzyme inhibitors. The microscopic appearance of the demyelinating cells resembled that seen when explants are exposed to anticerebroside containing antisera (Bornstein and Appel, 1961; Fry *et al.*, 1974).

The tentative interpretation for these findings is that interference with cerebrosidase, whether through inhibition or overstimulation, produces a severe interference in the formation and maintenance of myelin. Antibodies against cerebroside may be harmful because they keep the substrate from being attacked by cerebrosidase. Indeed one might speculate that some of the compounds which accumulate in various genetic diseases are inhibitory to cerebrosidase and thereby inhibit myelin development.

If this galactosidase is so important in myelin metabolism, and if its modification produces so rapid a change in myelin integrity, one would expect galactocerebroside to have a high turnover rate. In a detailed study in young rats with [^{3}H]acetate, Hajra and Radin (1963) showed that there were two cerebroside components. One component exhibited a rapid turnover (less than 0.5 day) while the other exhibited a very slow turnover (too slow to measure). Actually a precise figure for turnover cannot readily be obtained for this substance because its total weight per brain and its concentration in brain continue to rise for a very long time.

A recent study by Berthold (1973) may offer a clue to the significance of the rapidly hydrolyzed cerebrosides. He examined the myelin of peripheral nerve fibers microscopically and came to the conclusion that local regions may normally undergo what seemed like demyelination. This "demyelination" may involve hydrolysis of cerebroside at nodes of Ranvier or regions in which "remodeling" of myelin is occurring. Perhaps cerebroside is a stiffening agent in the myelin complex of proteins and lipids, and it must be periodically hydrolyzed and resynthesized to enable myelin to envelop axon fibers.

The long-term persistence of galactocerebrosidase with age (Section 5.3) makes sense in the light of this hypothesis, since cerebroside accumulation (also myelin formation and winding) persists for a long time too.

5.5.   Clinical Aspects of Galactocerebrosidase

A fine summary of this topic has been prepared by Suzuki and Suzuki (1972). As noted in the previous sections on this enzyme, a deficiency in cerebrosidase seems to underlie GLD (globoid cell leukodystrophy or Krabbe's disease). In most cases of the disorder the afflicted child soon develops a degeneration of the central nervous system, with death ensuing within 2 yr of age. Several longer living cases are known; thus there appears to be a milder form of the disorder. The brain is characterized by lack of myelin and oligodendroglia, astrocytic gliosis, and the appearance of globoid cells containing several nuclei. The globoid cells seem to contain some galactocerebroside, which is present in the form of helical tubules similar to those seen in Gaucher cell deposits, which contain glucocerebroside (Yunis and Lee, 1970). Peripheral nerves show degeneration of the axons, as well as the myelin. Since cerebrosidase is present in neurons, it is not surprising to see some of the disease symptoms in axons.

The globoid cells, which give the disorder its name, are apparently elicited by the presence of free cerebroside, which may form when the lipid fails to undergo hydrolysis. This idea comes from the observations that animals given an injection of cerebroside directly into the brain produce globoid cells (Austin and Lehfeldt, 1965; Anzil *et al.*, 1972) and that cultured cells of the nervous system also generate globoid cells when exposed to cerebroside (Sourander *et al.*, 1966). Whether the globoid cells produce toxic materials which cause demyelination is not clear yet, but no demyelination was observed in the above studies.

Despite the apparent presence of small amounts of cerebroside in the globoid cells of GLD patients, there is no accumulation of the lipid in the brain as a whole. The situation is thus very similar to that seen in the infantile form of Gaucher's disease, and the same question arises: If cerebroside does not hydrolyze at an adequate speed, why does it not accumulate? Presumably synthesis must be slowed down, possibly as the result of degeneration of the cells that are the prime source of the glycolipid. When the brains of dogs bearing the GLD trait were assayed for ceramide:galactosyltransferase (the enzyme which makes cerebroside), the synthetic capability appeared to be close to normal (Radin *et al.*, 1972*b*). The step prior to that (sphingosine:acyltransferases) was also assayed, but in human GLD brain; here the enzyme activities of the different transferases were found to be somewhat higher than normal. Perhaps the GLD brain contains increased amounts of hydrolases which reduce UDP–galactose or acyl–CoA concentrations and thus slow down ceramide or cerebroside synthesis. It would clearly be of interest to assay also the other enzymes involved in cerebroside synthesis, such as the hydroxylase which makes the hydroxy fatty acids that are so characteristic of galactocerebroside.

A test was made of the hypothesis that cerebroside can be diverted, as the result of cerebrosidase lack, to a minor degradative pathway that produces a myelination toxin. Under normal circumstances this metabolic route might produce too little of the toxin to be harmful. Stearate-labeled galactocerebroside was incubated with brain homogenates from 12-day-old rats under various conditions and novel metabolic products were sought (Lin and Radin, 1973). No evidence for deacylation (with formation of psychosine) could be obtained, but over 1 % of the cerebroside was converted to two polar products which were alkali-labile. The compounds were not identified and further work is needed to determine whether such compounds actually occur in GLD brain tissue. A search for a dehydrogenase acting on the six-position of the galactose moiety and a search for a transacylase that might transfer the fatty acid to sphingomyelin both gave negative results.

As mentioned in the previous sections, cerebrosidase seems to occur in more than one form. Whether the forms differ only with respect to the presence or absence of a binding material or with respect to a distinct structural difference cannot yet be stated. Suzuki and Suzuki (1974b) have studied the cerebrosidase in human liver of normals and GLD patients. Electrofocusing, followed by assay for enzyme activity, showed two cerebrosidase fractions in normal liver but only a single fraction, as a broad peak, in GLD liver. The broad peak corresponded to a band of precipitated material not seen in normal liver; thus one cannot say that it corresponded to either one of the two normal peaks. (This is a weakness of electrofocusing, because the supporting liquid is too fluid to support precipitated proteins.)

When a similar study was carried out with dog liver, using the canine GLD mutant (Suzuki et al., 1974a), two overlapping peaks were seen in normals and affected dogs, but the ratios of the two peaks were reversed. Another feature which distinguishes the canine and human forms of the disease is distribution of the affected enzyme: In the human forms the enzyme was found to be quite deficient in every tissue tested, but in the canine form the activity in serum was normal (Suzuki et al., 1972). Again we see evidence for multiple forms of the enzyme and the possibility that a mutation may affect one or two forms.

The assay of cerebrosidase in cultured fibroblasts from human amniotic fluid is now proving useful in determining the presence or absence of GLD in a fetus known to be at risk. At present there seems to be little hope of enzyme therapy for children who have already been born with the disorder, especially since the seriousness of the disorder seems to be concentrated in the brain and a method would have to be devised for bringing the enzyme to the brain cells. However, it is possible that chemotherapy with a stimulator for cerebrosidase and an inhibitor of cerebroside synthesis might bring the disorder under control.

6. REFERENCES

Agranoff, B. W., Radin, N. S., and Suomi, W., 1962, Enzymatic oxidation of cerebrosides: studies on Gaucher's disease, *Biochim. Biophys. Acta* **57**:194–196.

Anzil, A. P., Blinzinger, K., Mehraein, P., Dorn, G., and Neuhäuser, G., 1972, Cytoplasmic inclusions in a child afflicted with Krabbe's disease (globoid leucodystrophy) and in the rabbit injected with galactocerebrosides, *J. Neuropath. Exp. Neurol.* **31**:370–388.

Arora, R. C., and Radin, N. S., 1972a, Ceramide-like synthetic amides that inhibit cerebroside galactosidase, *J. Lipid Res.* **13**:86–91.

Arora, R. C., and Radin, N. S., 1972b, Stimulation *in vitro* of galactocerebroside galactosidase by N-decanoyl 2-amino-2-methylpropanol, *Lipids* **7**:56–59.

Arora, R. C., Lin, Y.-N., and Radin, N. S., 1973, The inhibitor-sensitive sites of galactosyl ceramide galactosidase, *Arch. Biochem. Biophys.* **156**:77–83.

Austin, J. H., and Lehfeldt, D., 1965, Studies in globoid (Krabbe) leukodystrophy. 3. Significance of experimentally produced globoidlike elements in rat white matter and spleen, *J. Neuropathol. Exptl. Neurol.* **24**:265–289.

Benjamins, J. A., Fitch, J., and Radin, N. S., Effects of ceramide analogs on myelinating organ cultures. Submitted for publication.

Bergsma, D., 1973, *Enzyme Therapy in Genetic Diseases*, The Williams and Wilkins Co., Baltimore.

Bernsohn, J., and Grossman, H. J., eds., 1971, *Lipid Storage Diseases: Enzymatic Defects and Clinical Implications*, Academic Press, New York.

Berthold, C.-H., 1973, Local "demyelination" in developing feline nerve fibres, *Neurobiol.* **3**:339–352.

Beutler, E., and Kuhl, W., 1970, The diagnosis of the adult type of Gaucher's disease and its carrier state by demonstra·ion of deficiency of β-glucosidase activity in peripheral blood leukocytes, *J. Lab. Clin. Med.* **76**:747–755.

Bornstein, M. B., and Appel, S. H., 1961, The application of tissue culture to the study of experimental "allergic" encephalomyelitis. I. Patterns of demyelination, *J. Neuropathol. Exptl. Neurol.* **20**:141–157.

Bowen, D. M., and Radin, N. S., 1968a, Purification of cerebroside galactosidase from rat brain, *Biochim. Biophys. Acta* **152**:587–598.

Bowen, D. M., and Radin, N. S., 1968b, Properties of cerebroside galactosidase, *Biochim. Biophys. Acta* **152**:599–610.

Bowen, D. M., and Radin, N. S., 1969a, Hydrolase activities in brain of neurological mutants: Cerebroside galactosidase, nitrophenyl glucoside hydrolase, and sulfatase, *J. Neurochem.* **16**:457–460.

Bowen D. M., and Radin, N. S., 1969b, Cerebroside galactosidase: A method for determination and a comparison with other lysosomal enzymes in developing rat brain, *J. Neurochem.* **16**:501–511.

Brady, R. O., Kanfer, J. N., Bradley, R. M., and Shapiro, D., 1966, Demonstration of a deficiency of glucocerebroside-cleaving enzyme in Gaucher's disease, *J. Clin. Invest.* **45**:1112–1115.

Brady, R. O., Gal, A. E., Kanfer, J. N., and Bradley, R. M., 1965a, Purification and properties of a glucosyl- and galactosylceramide-cleaving enzyme from rat intestinal tissue, *J. Biol. Chem.* **240**:3766–3770.

Brady, R. O., Kanfer, J., and Shapiro, D., 1965b, Purification and properties of a glucocerebroside-cleaving enzyme from spleen tissue, *J. Biol. Chem.* **240**:39–43.

Brenkert, A., Arora, R. C., Radin, N. S., Meier, H., and MacPike, A. D., 1972, Cerebroside synthesis and hydrolysis in a neurological mutant mouse (msd), *Brain Res.* **36**:195–202.

Brosnan, C. F., Bunge, M. B., and Murray, M. R., 1970, The response of lysosomes in cultured neurons to chlorpromazine, *J. Neuropath. Exp. Neurol.* **29**:337–353.

Burton, R. M., and Guerra, F. C., eds., 1974, *Fundamentals of Lipid Chemistry*, BI-Science Publ. Div., Webster Groves, Mo.

Curtino, J. A., and Caputto, R., 1974, Enzymic synthesis of cerebroside from glycosylsphingosine and stearoyl–CoA by an embryonic chicken brain preparation, *Biochem. Biophys. Res. Commun.* **56**:142–147.

Dawson, G., 1974, Glycolipid biosynthesis and catabolism, *in Mammalian Glycoproteins and Glycolipids* (W. Pigman and M. I. Horowitz, eds.), Academic Press, New York.

Dawson, G., 1972, Glycosphingolipid levels in an unusual neurovisceral storage disease characterized by lactosylceramide galactosyl hydrolase deficiency: Lactosylceramidosis, *J. Lipid Res.* **13**:207–219.

Dawson, G., and Stein, A. O., 1970, Lactosyl ceramidosis: Catabolic enzyme defect of glycosphingolipid metabolism, *Science* **170**:556–558.

Dawson, G., and Sweeley, C. C., 1970, *In vivo* studies on glycosphingolipid metabolism in porcine blood, *J. Biol. Chem.* **245**:410–416.

Dawson, G., Stoolmiller, A. C., and Radin, N. S., 1974, Inhibition of β-glucosidase by *N*-(*n*-hexyl)-*O*-glucosylsphingosine in cell strains of neurological origin, *J. Biol. Chem.* **249**:4634–4646.

DeVries, G. H., Norton, W. T., and Raine, C. S., 1972, Axons: Isolation from mammalian central nervous system, *Science* **175**:1370–1372.

Distler, J. J., and Jourdian, G. W., 1973, The purification and properties of β-galactosidase from bovine testes, *J. Biol. Chem.* **248**:6772–6780.

Erickson, J. S., and Radin, N. S., 1973, *N*-Hexyl-*O*-glucosyl sphingosine, an inhibitor of glucosyl ceramide β-glucosidase, *J. Lipid Res.* **14**:133–137.

Evans, J. E., and McCluer, R. H., 1969, The structure of brain dihexosylceramide in globoid cell leukodystrophy, *J. Neurochem.* **16**:1393–1399.

Fredrickson, D. S., and Sloan, H. R., 1972, Glucosyl ceramide lipidoses: Gaucher's disease, *in The Metabolic Basis of Inherited Disease* (J. B. Stanbury, J. B. Wyngaarden, and D. S. Fredrickson, eds.), pp. 730–759, McGraw-Hill Book Co., New York.

Fry, J. M., Weissbarth, S., Lehrer, G. H., and Bornstein, M. B., 1974, Cerebroside antibody inhibits sulfatide synthesis and myelination and demyelinates in cord tissue cultures, *Science* **183**:540–542.

Gatt, S., 1966*a*, Hydrolysis and synthesis of ceramides by an enzyme from rat brain, *J. Biol. Chem.* **241**:3724–3730.

Gatt, S., 1966*b*, Enzymic hydrolysis of sphingolipids: Hydrolysis of ceramide glucoside by an enzyme from ox brain, *Biochem. J.* **101**:687–691.

Gatt, S., 1969*a*, β-Glucosidase from bovine brain, *in Methods in Enzymology* (J. M. Lowenstein, ed.), Vol. 14, pp. 152–155, Academic Press, New York.

Gatt, S., 1969*b*, β-Galactosidase from rat brain, *in Methods in Enzymology* (J. M. Lowenstein, Vol. 14, pp. 157–158, Academic Press, New York.

Gatt, S., 1970, Enzymatic estimation of galactose in the presence of galactolipids, *Biochim. Biophys. Acta* **218**:173–175.

Gatt, S., 1973, *in Glycolipids, Glycoproteins, and Mucopolysaccharides of the Nervous System* (V. Zambotti, G. Tettamanti, and M. Arrigoni, eds.), Plenum Press, New York.

Gatt, S., and Barenholz, Y., 1973, Enzymes of complex lipid metabolism, *Ann. Rev. Biochem.* **42**:61–90.

Gatt, S., and Rapport, M. M., 1966, Hydrolysis of ceramide lactoside by an enzyme from rat brain, *Biochem. J.* **101**:680–686.

Gatt, S., and Yavin, E., 1969, Ceramidase from rat brain, *in Methods in Enzymology* (J. M. Lowenstein, ed.), Vol. 14, pp. 139–144, Academic Press, New York.

Glew, R. H., and Lee, R. E., 1973, Composition of the membranous deposits occurring in Gaucher's disease, *Arch. Biochem. Biophys.* **156**:626–639.

Glew, R. H., Christopher, A. R., Schnure, F. W., and Lee, R. E., 1974, The occurrence of beta-glucocerebrosidase activity in the glucocerebroside-rich deposits of Gaucher's disease, *Arch. Biochem. Biophys.* **160**:162–167.

Gonzalez-Sastre, F., Pampols, T., and Sabater, J., 1974, Infantile Gaucher's disease: A biochemical study, *Neurology* **24**:162–167.

Hajra, A. K., and Radin, N. S., 1963, Isotopic studies of the biosynthesis of the cerebroside fatty acids in rats, *J. Lipid Res.* **4**:270–278.

Hajra, A. K., Bowen, D. M., Kishimoto, Y., and Radin, N. S., 1966, Cerebroside galactosidase of brain, *J. Lipid Res.* **7**:379–386.

Hammarström, S., 1971, A convenient procedure for the synthesis of ceramides, *J. Lipid Res.* **12**:760–765.

Hickman, S., Shapiro, L. J., and Neufeld, E. F., 1974, A recognition marker required for uptake of a lysosomal enzyme by cultured fibroblasts, *Biochem. Biophys. Res. Commun.* **57**:55–61.

Ho, M. W., 1973, Identity of "acid" β-glucosidase and glucocerebrosidase in human spleen, *Biochem. J.* **136**:721–729.

Ho, M. W., and Light, N. D., 1973, Glucocerebrosidase: Reconstitution from macromolecular components depends on acidic phospholipids, *Biochem. J.* **136**:821–823.

Ho, M. W., and O'Brien, J. S., 1971, Gaucher's disease: Deficiency of "acid" β-glucosidase and reconstitution of enzyme activity *in vitro, Proc. Nat. Acad. Sci. (U.S.)* **68**:2810–2813.

Ho, M. W., O'Brien, J. S., Radin, N. S., and Erickson, J. S., 1973, Glucocerebrosidase: Reconstitution of activity from macromolecular components, *Biochem. J.* **131**:173–176.

Hultberg, B., and Öckerman, P. A., 1970, β-Glucosidase activities in human tissues; findings in Gaucher's disease, *Clin. Chim. Acta* **28**:169–174.

Hyun, J. C., and Radin, N. S., 1975, The assay of glucocerebroside β-glucosidase. Submitted for publication.

Hyun, J. C., Misra, R. S., Greenblatt, D., and Radin, N. S., 1975, Synthetic inhibitors of glucocerebroside β-glucosidase. *Arch. Biochem. Biophys.* **166** (in press).

Kampine, J. P., Kanfer, J. N., Gal, A. E., Bradley, R. M., and Brady, R. O., 1967, Response of sphingolipid hydrolases in spleen and liver to increased erythrocytorhexis, *Biochim. Biophys. Acta* **137**:135–139.

Kanfer, J. N., Stein, M., and Spielvogel, C., 1972, Recent observations on Gaucher's disease, in *Sphingolipids, Sphingolipidoses and Allied Disorders* (B. W. Volk and S. M. Aronson, eds.), pp. 225–236, Plenum Press, New York.

Kanfer, J. N., Petrovich, G., and Mumford, R. A., 1973, Purification of α- and β-galactosidases by affinity chromatography, *Anal. Biochem.* **55**:301–305.

Kanfer, J. N., Mumford, R. A., Raghavan, S. S., Friedman, R., and Byrd, J., 1974, Purification of β-glucosidase activities from bovine spleen by affinity chromatography, *Federation Proc.* **33**:1299.

Kattlove, H. E., Williams, J. C., Gaynor, E., Spivack, M., Bradley, R. M., and Brady, R. O., 1969, Gaucher cells in chronic myelocytic leukemia: An acquired abnormality, *Blood* **33**:379–390.

Klibansky, Ch., Hoffman, J., Zaizov, R., and Matoth, Y., 1974, Gaucher's disease, chronic adult type: A comparative study of glucocerebroside and methylumbelliferyl–glucopyranoside cleaving potency in leukocytes, *Biomed.* **20**:24–30.

Klibansky, Ch., Hoffman, J., Zaizov, R., Matoth, Y., Pinkhas, J., and de Vries, A., 1973, Chronic Gaucher's disease: Heat-resistance of leukocyte glucocerebrosidase in relation to some clinical parameters, *Biomed.* **19**:345–348.

Kopaczyk, K. C., and Radin, N. S., 1965, *In vivo* conversions of cerebroside and ceramide in rat brain, *J. Lipid Res.* **6**:140–145.

Kuske, T. T., and Rosenberg, A., 1972, Quantity and fatty acyl composition of the glycosphingolipids of Gaucher spleen, *J. Lab. Clin. Med.* **80**:523–529.

Lai, H.-Y. L., Axelrod, B., 1973, 1-Aminoglycosides, a new class of specific inhibitors of glycosidases, *Biochem. Biophys. Res. Comm.* **54**:463–468.

Lee, Y. C., 1972, Analysis of sugars by automated liquid chromatography, in *Methods in Enzymology* (V. Ginsburg, ed.), Vol. 28, pp. 63–73, Academic Press, New York.

Leese, H. J., and Semenza, G., 1973, On the identity between the small intestinal enzymes phlorizin hydrolase and glycosylceramidase, *J. Biol. Chem.* **248**:8170–8173.

Li, S.-C., and Li, Y.-T., 1974, Isolation and characterization of a heat-stable glycoprotein activating the hydrolysis of sphingoglycolipids, *Federation Proc.* **33**:1299.

Lin, Y.-N., and Radin, N. S., 1973, Alternate pathways of cerebroside catabolism, *Lipids* **8**:732–736.

Makita, A., Suzuki, C., Yosizawa, Z., and Konno, T., 1966, Glycolipids isolated from the spleen of Gaucher's disease, *J. Exptl. Med.* **88**:277–288.

Meisler, M., 1972, β-Galactosidase from human liver, *in Methods in Enzymology* (V. Ginsburg, ed.), Vol. 28, pp. 820–824, Academic Press, New York.

Mellor, J. D., and Layne, D. S., 1971, Steroid β-D-glucosidase activity in rabbit tissues, *J. Biol. Chem.* **246**:4377–4380.

Mickel, H. S., and Gilles, F. H., 1970, Changes in glial cells during human telencephalic myelogenesis, *Brain* **93**:337–346.

Miyatake, T., and Ariga, T., 1972, Sphingoglycolipids in the nervous system in Fabry's disease, *J. Neurochem.* **19**:1911–1916.

Miyatake, T., and Suzuki, K., 1974a, Glycosphingolipid β-galactosidases in rat brain: Properties and the standard assay procedures of the enzymes in whole homogenate, *Biochim. Biophys. Acta* **337**:333–342.

Miyatake, T., and Suzuki, K., 1974b, Galactosylsphingosine galactosyl hydrolase in rat brain: Probable identity with galactosylceramide galactosyl hydrolase, *J. Neurochem.* **22**:231–237.

Morell, P., and Braun, P., 1972, Biosynthesis and metabolic degradation of sphingolipids not containing sialic acid, *J. Lipid Res.* **13**:293–310.

Morell, P., and Radin, N. S., 1969, Synthesis of cerebroside by brain from uridine diphosphate galactose and ceramide-containing hydroxy fatty acid, *Biochem.* **8**:506–512.

Morell, P., and Radin, N. S., 1970, Specificity in ceramide biosynthesis from long chain bases and various fatty acyl Coenzyme A's by brain microsomes, *J. Biol. Chem.* **245**:342–350.

Morell, P., Costantino-Ceccarini, E., and Radin, N. S., 1970, The biosynthesis by brain microsomes of cerebrosides containing nonhydroxy fatty acids, *Arch. Biochem. Biophys.* **141**:738–748.

Moser, H. W., Prensky, A. L., Wolfe, H. J., and Rosman, N. P., 1969, Farber's lipogranulomatosis: Report of a case and demonstration of an excess of free ceramide and ganglioside, *Amer. J. Med.* **47**:869–890.

Mraz, W., and Jatzkewitz, H., 1974, Cerebroside sulphatase activity of arylsulphatases from various invertebrates, *Z. Physiol. Chem.* **355**:33–44.

Nilsson, Å., 1969, The presence of sphingomyelin- and ceramide-cleaving enzymes in the small intestinal tract, *Biochim. Biophys. Acta* **176**:339–347.

Ong, D. E., and Brady, R. N., 1972, Synthesis of ceramides using N-hydroxysuccinimide esters, *J. Lipid Res.* **13**:819–822.

Patrick, A. D., 1965, A deficiency of glucocerebrosidase in Gaucher's disease, *Biochem. J.* **97**:17c–18c.

Pentchev, P. G., and Brady, R. O., 1973, The effect of a heat-stable factor in human spleen on glucocerebrosidase and acid β-glucosidase activities, *Biochim. Biophys. Acta* **297**:491–496.

Pentchev, P. G., Brady, R. O., Hibbert, S. R., Gal, A. E., and Shapiro, D., 1973, Isolation and characterization of glucocerebrosidase from human placental tissue, *J. Biol. Chem.* **248**:5256–5261.

Pentchev, P. G., Brady, R. O., Gal, A. E., Hibbert, S. R., and Dekaban, A. S., 1974, Infusion of purified glucocerebrosidase into patients with Gaucher's disease, *Federation Proc.* **33**:1300.

Pope, J. L., 1967, Crystallization of sodium taurocholate, *J. Lipid Res.* **8**:146–147.

Radin, N. S., 1970, Cerebrosides and sulfatides, *in Handbook of Neurochemistry* (A. Lajtha, ed.), Vol. 3, pp. 415–424, Plenum Press, New York.

Radin, N. S., 1972a, Labeled galactosyl ceramide and lactosyl ceramide, *in Methods in Enzymology* (V. Ginsburg, ed.), Vol. 28, pp. 300–306, Academic Press, New York.

Radin, N. S., 1972*b*, Galactosyl ceramide (galactocerebroside) β-galactosidase from brain, *in Methods in Enzymology* (V. Ginsburg, ed.), Vol. 28, pp. 834–839, Academic Press, New York.

Radin, N. S., 1974, Preparation of psychosines (1-*O*-hexosylsphingosine) from cerebrosides, *Lipids* 9:358–360.

Radin, N. S., and Arora, R. C., 1971, A simplified assay method for galactosyl ceramide β-galactosidase, *J. Lipid Res.* 12:256–257.

Radin, N. S., Hof, L., Bradley, R. M., and Brady, R. O., 1969, Lactosylceramide galactosidase: Comparison with other sphingolipid hydrolases in developing rat brain, *Brain Res.* 14:497–505.

Radin, N. S., Brenkert, A., Arora, R. C., Sellinger, O. Z., and Flangas, A. L., 1972*a*, Glial and neuronal localization of cerebroside-metabolizing enzymes, *Brain Res.* 39:163–169.

Radin, N. S., Arora, R. C., Ullman, M. D., Brenkert, A. L., and Austin, J., 1972*b*, A possible therapeutic approach to Krabbe's globoid leukodystrophy and the status of cerebroside synthesis in the disorder, *Res. Comm. Chem. Pathol. Pharmacol.* 3:637–644.

Raghavan, S. S., Mumford, R. A., and Kanfer, J. N., 1973, Deficiency of glucosylsphingosine β-glucosidase in Gaucher's disease, *Biochem. Biophys. Res. Commun.* 54:256–263.

Raghavan, S. S., Mumford, R. A., and Kanfer, J. N., 1974, Synthesis of glucosylceramide by purified calf spleen β-glucosidase, *Biochem. Biophys. Res. Commun.* 58:99–106.

Read, W. K., and Bay, W. W., 1971, Basic cellular lesion in chloroquine toxicity, *Lab. Invest.* 24:246–259.

Reese, E. T., Parrish, F. W., and Ettlinger, M., 1971, Nojirimycin and D-glucono-1,5-lactone as inhibitors of carbohydrases, *Carbohyd. Res.* 18:381–388.

Rosenberg, A., 1970, Sphingomyelin: enzymatic reactions, *in Handbook of Neurochemistry* (A. Lajtha, ed.), Vol. 3, pp. 453–466, Plenum Press, New York.

Shapiro, D., 1969, *Chemistry of Sphingolipids*, Hermann Publ., Paris.

Sourander, P., Hansson, H.-A., Olsson, Y., and Svennerholm, L., 1966, Experimental studies on the pathogenesis of leukodystrophies. II. The effect of sphingolipids on various cell types in cultures from the nervous system, *Acta Neuropath.* 6:231–242.

Subba Rao, K., Wenger, D. A., and Pierenger, R. A., 1970, The metabolism of glyceride glycolipids. IV. Enzymatic hydrolysis of monogalactosyl and digalactosyl diglycerides in rat brain, *J. Biol. Chem.* 245:2520–2524.

Sugita, M., Dulaney, J. T., and Moser, H. W., 1972, Ceramidase deficiency in Farber's disease (lipogranulomatosis), *Science* 178:1100–1102.

Sugita, M., Connolly, P., Dulaney, J. T., and Moser, H. W., 1973, Fatty acid composition of free ceramides of kidney and cerebellum from a patient with Farber's disease, *Lipids* 8:401–406.

Suzuki, K., and Suzuki, Y., 1972, Galactosyl ceramide lipidosis: globoid cell leukodystrophy (Krabbe's disease), *in The Metabolic Basis of Inherited Disease* (J. B. Stanbury, J. B. Wyngaarden, and D. S. Fredrickson, eds.), pp. 760–782, McGraw-Hill Book Co., New York.

Suzuki, K., Suzuki, Y., and Fletcher, T. F., 1972, *in Sphingolipids, Sphingolipidoses and Allied Disorders* (B. W. Volk and S. M. Aronson, eds.), pp. 478–498, Plenum Press, New York.

Suzuki, Y., and Suzuki, K., 1974*a*, Glycosphingolipid β-galactosidases. I. Standard assay procedures and characterization by electrofocusing and gel filtration of the enzymes in normal human liver, *J. Biol. Chem.* 249:2098–2104.

Suzuki, Y., and Suzuki, K., 1974*b*, Glycosphingolipid β-galactosidases. II. Electrofocusing characterization of the enzymes in human globoid cell leukodystrophy (Krabbe's disease), *J. Biol. Chem.* 249:2105–2108.

Suzuki, Y., Miyatake, T., Fletcher, T. F., and Suzuki, K., 1974, Glycosphingolipid β-galactosidases. III. Canine form of globoid cell leukodystrophy; comparison with the human disease, *J. Biol. Chem.* **249**:2109–2112.

Svennerholm, L., 1966, The metabolism of gangliosides in cerebral lipidoses, *in Inborn Disorders of Sphingolipid Metabolism* (S. M. Aronson and B. W. Volk, eds.), p. 173, Pergamon Press, New York.

Taketomi, T., and Yamakawa, T., 1967, Glycolipids of the brain in gargoylism, *Jap. J. Exptl. Med.* **37**:11–21.

Ullman, M. D., and Radin, N. S., 1972, Enzymatic formation of hydroxy ceramides and comparison with enzymes forming nonhydroxy ceramides, *Arch. Biochem. Biophys.* **152**:767–777.

Volk, B. W., and Aronson, S. M., eds., 1972, *Sphingolipids, Sphingolipidoses and Allied Disorders*, Plenum Press, New York.

Warren, K. R., Schafer, I. A., Sullivan, J. C., Petrelli, M., and Radin, N. S., 1974, Induction of a chemical model of Gaucher's disease in normal cultured human fibroblasts. Submitted for publication.

Weinreb, N. J., and Brady, R. O., 1972, Glucocerebrosidase from bovine spleen, *in Methods in Enzymology* (V. Ginsburg, ed.), Vol. 28, pp. 830–834, Academic Press, New York.

Weiss, B., and Raizman, P., 1958, Synthesis of long chain fatty acid amides of sphingosine and dihydrosphingosine, *J. Am. Chem. Soc.* **80**:4657–4658.

Wenger, D. A., Sattler, M., and Markey, S. P., 1973, Deficiency of monogalactosyl diglyceride β-galactosidase activity in Krabbe's disease, *Biochem. Biophys. Res. Commun.* **53**:680–685.

Wenger, D. A., Sattler, M., and Hiatt, W., 1974, Globoid cell leukodystrophy: deficiency of lactosyl ceramide beta-galactosidase, *Proc. Nat. Acad. Sci. (U.S.)* **71**:854–857.

Yavin, E., and Gatt, S., 1969, Enzymatic hydrolysis of sphingolipids. VIII. Further purification and properties of rat brain ceramidase, *Biochemistry* **8**:1692–1698.

Yunis, E. J., and Lee, R. E., 1970, Tubules of globoid leukodystrophy: A right-handed helix, *Science* **169**:64–66.

CHAPTER 3

BASIC PROTEINS OF CENTRAL AND PERIPHERAL NERVOUS SYSTEM MYELIN

PATRICK R. CARNEGIE AND PETER R. DUNKLEY

The Russell Grimwade School of Biochemistry
University of Melbourne
Parkville, Australia

Studies on the ultrastructure and physiological function of myelin have generally been with peripheral nervous system (PNS) tissue, while chemical studies on the composition of myelin have more often used central nervous system (CNS) tissue. In addition, because of immunological studies on multiple sclerosis, there has been a rapid growth in knowledge of some of the proteins of CNS myelin.

This chapter reviews one of the major proteins of CNS myelin—the basic protein—with regard to its history, isolation, properties, synthesis, and possible role. In contrast to the extensive literature on CNS basic proteins there is little information on the PNS basic proteins, but very recently their composition has been clarified.

1. BASIC PROTEINS OF CENTRAL NERVOUS SYSTEM MYELIN

1.1. Historical Introduction

1.1.1. *Encephalitogens*

An experimentally induced disease with clinical and histological signs similar to acute disseminated encephalomyelitis was first induced in monkeys by repeated injections of an aqueous emulsion of rabbit central nervous system (CNS) tissue (Rivers and Schwentker, 1935). This disease, later referred to as experimental autoimmune (or autoallergic) encephalomyelitis (EAE), was shown to be a truly autoimmune disease when monkeys, injected with autologous brain tissue together with appropriate adjuvants, became paralyzed (Kabat *et al.*, 1947). EAE has been extensively studied during the last 30 years, as it was thought that it might be a model for human demyelinating diseases such as multiple sclerosis (Alvord, 1970). More recently, although the disease has become important as a model for organ specific autoimmune diseases, EAE has been shown to be inadequate in many respects as a model for multiple sclerosis (Mackay *et al.*, 1973).

An important step in understanding the nature of EAE was the elucidation of the CNS antigen responsible for disease induction. In early studies a number of protein and lipid fractions were claimed to possess EAE-inducing (encephalitogenic) activity. However, a "salt-" or acid-extracted protein (Roboz and Henderson, 1959; Kies and Alvord, 1959) and a diffusible polypeptide fraction (Robertson *et al.*, 1962; Kibler *et al.*, 1964; Nakao and Einstein, 1965; Nakao and Einstein 1966*a,b*; Carnegie *et al.*, 1967) were later shown to be the most potent encephalitogens. The comparatively low activity of the other CNS tissue fractions was due to contamination with the acid-extracted protein and/or the polypeptide fraction (Kies, 1965; Kies *et al.*, 1965; Lumsden *et al.*, 1966).

The polypeptide encephalitogens were produced by the action of a brain acid proteinase (Marks and Lajtha, 1965) which digested the acid-extractable protein at pH 3 (Nakao *et al.*, 1966*a*; Einstein *et al.*, 1968), the pH normally used for preparation of encephalitogens. This degradation of the acid-extractable protein during preparation could be overcome by defatting the CNS tissue with chloroform–methanol (2:1, by vol.) which inhibits the acid proteinase activity, rather than with acetone which does not (Carnegie *et al.*, 1967). Thus the polypeptide encephalitogens resulted from the use of acetone for defatting, and the encephalitogenic activity of the CNS tissue was shown to reside in a single basic protein of high isoelectric point.

Although it has been known for a decade that fragments of the basic protein were capable of inducing EAE, it was only recently that these fragments were first characterized. A number of peptides are now known to be capable of inducing EAE, but the potency of each peptide depends on the species used to test the antigen. The major peptide determinants responsible for induction of EAE in guinea pigs (Hashim and Eylar, 1969a; Lennon et al., 1970; Westall et al., 1971; Burnett and Eylar, 1971), rabbits (Shapira et al., 1971a; Bergstrand, 1972), monkeys (Eylar et al., 1972; Kibler et al., 1972; Brostoff et al., 1974), and rats (Dunkley et al., 1973; McFarlin et al., 1973) have been determined. Peptides from basic protein were used in studies on cellular (Bergstrand and Kallen, 1973a,b; Hashim et al., 1973) and humoral (Driscoll et al., 1974) immune responses in guinea pigs and rabbits. It is likely that the encephalitogenic activity of basic protein is a composite effect caused by a number of immunological responses to different peptide determinants. It is not our intention to review this complex field in this chapter.

1.1.2. Location of Encephalitogen

An important step in understanding the immunological reactions to the encephalitogenic protein which occur in EAE was the elucidation of the protein's location in the CNS. Morgan (1947) and Kabat et al. (1947) indicated that CNS white matter was more encephalitogenic than CNS gray matter, non-CNS tissue, and fetal tissue which contained no myelin. Scheinberg and Korey (1958) and Olson et al. (1962) indicated that myelin contained encephalitogenic activity. The first definitive studies using purified myelin and quantitation of EAE induction indicated that, among the various CNS fractions, myelin contained the greatest encephalitogenic activity (Kies et al., 1961; Laatsch et al., 1962). This localization of encephalitogenic activity in myelin was also supported by the subsequent isolation studies of Hulcher et al. (1963) and Soto (1964).

Immunochemical studies using fluorescent- or peroxidase-labeled antibody against basic protein have in general substantiated the myelin localization of basic protein (Rauch and Raffels, 1964; McFarland, 1970; Whittingham et al., 1972; Herndon et al., 1973). Developmental studies indicated that little basic protein was detected in CNS tissue before myelination began (Einstein et al., 1970; Matthieu et al., 1973a; Adams and Osborne, 1973) and that the increase in content of the basic protein followed the increase in myelin content (Gaitonde and Martenson, 1970). In strains of mutant mice such as the Jimpy mouse, which contains only immature myelin, the content of basic protein was negligible (Matthieu et al., 1973b). In the Quaking mouse, which contains small amounts of myelin, basic protein was present but only in small quantities (Greenfield et al., 1971). The level of basic protein and myelin in these mutant mice was consistent with the basic proteins being a myelin component (see review by Mandel *et al.*, 1972). Thus it was established that the encephalitogenic activity of the CNS tissue resided in the basic protein and that the protein was a myelin component.

1.1.3. *Reviews*

Throughout this section the encephalitogenic protein will be referred to as the "myelin basic protein" or simply the "basic protein." Other terms used in the literature for this protein include encephalitogenic basic protein, encephalitogenic protein, encephalitogenic factor, the A1 protein of myelin, and CNS basic protein. Aspects of the chemistry of myelin basic protein have previously been reviewed by Shooter and Einstein (1971), Einstein (1972), Eylar (1972, 1973), and Kies (1973).

1.2. Isolation

1.2.1. *Procedures*

Methods for the routine isolation and purification of basic protein from whole CNS tissue are well established (Eylar *et al.*, 1969; Deibler *et al.*, 1972; Dunkley and Carnegie, 1974*a*). Dunkley and Carnegie (1974*a*) reviewed each of the isolation procedures that have been used to prepare basic protein, and details of a procedure which can be followed without reference to other reports was provided. Brief reviews of methods used to isolate basic protein from purified myelin, and the criteria for estimating basic protein purity, were also included.

Myelin basic protein has been isolated from a number of species including man (Caspary and Field, 1965; Einstein *et al.*, 1965); ox (Eylar *et al.*, 1969); rabbit (Deibler *et al.*, 1972); guinea pig (Kies, 1965); sheep (Quelin and Brahic, 1973); and chicken, turtle, and frog (Martenson *et al.*, 1972*a*). In addition, CNS tissue of monkey, horse, dog (Eylar, 1973), and chinchilla (Martenson *et al.*, 1971*a*) origins are reported to contain basic protein. Tomasi and Kornguth (1967) isolated a protein from pig brain which they believed to be a histone but which has since been shown to be the basic protein of pig myelin (Kornguth *et al.*, 1972; Martenson *et al.*, 1971*b*). Myelin from each of the above-mentioned species contains a single basic protein with similar electrophoretic and/or chromatographic properties to the human basic protein.

Not all species contain a single myelin basic protein. Rodents of the suborders *Myomorpha* (rat, mouse, and hamster) and *Scuiromorpha* (prairie dog, woodchuck, and squirrel) all have a basic protein with the same electrophoretic mobility as the human basic protein, but in addition they have a smaller myelin basic protein (approx. 14,000 daltons) (Martenson *et al.*, 1971*a*). Both the large and small forms of basic protein have been isolated from the rat (Martenson *et al.*, 1970; Dunkley and Carnegie, 1974*b*). Examination of CNS tissue isolated from carp (Mehl and Halaris, 1970), shark (Martenson *et al.*, 1972*a*), and dogfish (Agrawal *et al.*, 1971) indicated that these species also have more than one basic protein, but no protein with the same electrophoretic properties as the human basic protein was found. It is known that myelin isolated from fish is morphologically unusual, but myelin from rodents (especially rats) appears to be similar to myelin from other vertebrates (Bunge, 1968; Bear, 1971).

1.2.2. Content of Basic Protein

1.2.2a. Myelin Composition. The chemical composition of myelin has been the subject of a large number of qualitative and quantitative studies, the results of which have recently been reviewed (Davison, 1970; Norton, 1972; Bear, 1971). There is considerable variation between myelin from different species, from different regions of CNS, from animals of different ages, and myelin from the same source prepared by different techniques (see also Adams and Osborne, 1973; Morell *et al.*, 1973; Matthieu *et al.*, 1973*c*). However, in contrast to other membrane fractions, myelin is characterized by a low content of water and protein, and a high content of lipid. Other nervous system fractions have approximately 80% water content, while for myelin the water content is thought, from X-ray diffraction studies, to be approximately 40% (Bear, 1971; Norton, 1972). The solids of myelin comprise 25–30% myelin protein (Banik and Davison, 1973) and 70–75% myelin lipids. Myelin contains very little nucleic acid, and polysaccharides are not found (Norton, 1972) although some glycoproteins may be present (Quarles *et al.*, 1973). Discussion of the lipid composition of myelin is beyond the scope of this chapter, but a brief account of the other myelin proteins is presented here before the relative proportions of these proteins are discussed.

The protein content of myelin varies depending on the procedure used for its preparation. Myelin of varying densities can be separated by gradient centrifugation, and the protein composition of each fraction is extremely variable (Mehl, 1972). Osmotically shocked myelin contains fewer proteins of high molecular weight than does isotonically prepared myelin (Agrawal *et al.*, 1972); also, solubilization of myelin in chloroform–methanol (2:1, by vol.) is known to select for proteins of lower molecular weight and to exclude some basic protein, depending on the concentration of salts in the solution (Adams and Osborne, 1973; Gonzalez-Sastre, 1970).

The proteins that are subject to the greatest variation with the different isolation procedures are the myelin proteins of high molecular weight. However, even the most highly purified myelin samples still contain some of these proteins (Morell *et al.*, 1972) and they therefore cannot be considered as contaminants, as has been the case in the past. Of the myelin proteins of high molecular weight which have been partially characterized, perhaps the best known is Wolfgram's protein. Finch and Moscarello (1972) have suggested that the Wolfgram protein was not homogeneous and this view is supported by Morell *et al.* (1973). Myelin is also known to contain a number of enzymic activities. A highly active 2',3'-cyclic nucleotide 3'-phosphohydrolase was localized in myelin, and it has since been shown to correspond to a protein band of high molecular weight after gel electrophoresis of whole myelin (Braun and Barchi, 1972). In addition, cholesterol ester hydrolase, amino peptidase, and other enzymic activities are present in myelin, and some of these activities may correspond to the protein bands of high molecular weight seen on gel electrophoresis (Davison, 1970; Carnegie and Sims, 1975).

A major myelin protein which is soluble in chloroform–methanol at neutral and acidic pH values has been partially characterized. This protein, called the Folch-Lees proteolipid protein, has been isolated from myelin by a number of procedures each of which provides material with a different lipid content. These lipids have been characterized and methods for preparation of the apo-protein in a water-soluble form are available (reviewed by Folch-Pi, 1972). This protein is very resistant to enzymic digestion, has a low content (20%) of acidic and basic amino acids, and has a high content (60%) of nonpolar amino acids, especially leucine, alanine, and valine (see Figure 3). A second, but quantitatively less important, myelin-specific proteolipid has also been described (Agrawal *et al.*, 1972; Morell *et al.*, 1973; Banik and Davison, 1973).

1.2.2b. Proportions of the Myelin Proteins. The relative proportions of the three major protein fractions of myelin (basic protein; proteolipid proteins; high molecular weight proteins) have been determined for a number of species and the results obtained depend on the methods used (Table 1). One procedure was to separate the myelin proteins and to estimate the content of each fraction by the Folin method; this could result in some high molecular weight proteins being included in the proteolipid fraction (Banik and Davison, 1973), thus falsely elevating the content of the proteolipid protein; it is also probable that the recovery of each protein fraction was not the same. A second procedure was to calculate the proportions of each myelin protein from their relative dye-binding capacities after gel electrophoresis of whole myelin; this avoids the criticisms leveled at the fractionation procedure, but it depends on the accurate determination of the relative

TABLE 1.   Relative Proportions of the Proteins Present in CNS Myelin[a]

Source of adult myelin		Basic protein	Proteolipid protein(s)	Other proteins (high molecular weight)	References
Human	Brain	1.0	2.2, 1.9, 1.4, 0.8	0.6, 0.7, ND, 1.3	1[b], 2[b], 3[c], 4[c]
	Spinal cord	1.0	0.7	1.1	4[d]
Bovine	Brain	1.0	2.4, 1.4, 0.8	0.4, ND, 1.2	5[b], 3[a], 4[a]
	Spinal cord	1.0	0.4	0.7	4[c]
Rat[d]	Brain	1.0	1.5, 1.2, 1.1, 1.0	0.5, 2.0, ND, ND	6[c], 4[c], 7[c], 3[c]
	Spinal cord	1.0	1.1	1.1	4[c]
Mouse[d]	Brain	1.0	0.7, 0.7	ND, ND	8[e], 9[c]
Rabbit	Brain	1.0	1.4, 1.0	ND, 1.8	3[c], 4[c]
	Spinal cord	1.0	0.9	1.1	4[c]
Guinea pig	Brain	1.0	1.4, 0.7	ND, 1.3	3[c], 4[c]
	Spinal cord	1.0	0.6	0.8	4[c]

[a] Most results presented in the literature have been quoted as a percentage of the total myelin protein and have been recalculated for this table.
[b] Values calculated from protein contents after fractionation of myelin proteins.
[c] Values calculated from dye binding of myelin proteins after gel electrophoresis of whole myelin.
[d] Values for both basic proteins included together.
[e] Values calculated from protein content of bands after gel electrophoresis of whole myelin.

References: 1, Banik and Davison (1973); 2, Eng et al. (1968); 3, Mehl and Halaris (1970); 4, Morell et al. (1973); 5, Gonzales-Sastre (1970); 6, Einstein (1974); 7, Adams and Osborne (1973); 8, Greenfield et al. (1971); 9, Nussbaum and Mandel (1973).

dye-binding capacity of each protein. When differences in dye-binding capacities of the myelin proteins were taken into account (refs. 3 and 9, Table 1) the amount of proteolipid protein was estimated to be lower than that of basic protein, while in other studies (refs. 3, 6 and 7, Table 1) where these differences were not accounted for the amount of proteolipid protein was higher. Greenfield et al. (1971) used a combination of both procedures and found a greater proportion of basic protein than that of proteolipid protein in mouse brain myelin (ref. 8, Table 1). Thus the relative contents of the proteolipid protein and basic protein are not precisely known, but a consensus of the data in Table 1 would suggest approximately equal proportions. In all species the relative content of basic protein in spinal cord tissue was greater than in brain tissue.

The proportion of "other proteins" to basic protein and proteolipid protein depends on the method used for preparing myelin. Thus, as discussed in Section 1.2.2a certain procedures yield data with a greater content of proteins with high molecular weight than do others.

1.2.2c. Yield of Basic Protein. A number of studies have shown that in myelin from adult rat, the larger basic protein is quantitatively less important than the smaller protein. The exact ratio varied depending on whether the proteins were extracted from whole brain (Martenson *et al.*, 1970) or from isolated myelin (Sammeck *et al.*, 1971; Adams and Osborne, 1973; Einstein, 1974), but it was always between 1:1.7 and 1:3. The ratio did not vary in preparations from different regions of the adult CNS (Sammeck *et al.*, 1971), but in developing brain there was a greater content of the larger basic protein and the proportions varied with age (see Section 1.6.2). As there are between 50 and 60 mg myelin per gram adult rat (calculated from Norton and Poduslo, 1973*a*,*b*), and as myelin is approximately 40% water and 25–30% protein in the dry matter, there are 8–11 mg myelin protein per gram adult rat brain. From the results presented in Table 1 for myelin from adult rat brain, the basic proteins account for 30–40% of the total myelin protein. Thus the theoretical content of basic protein is 2–4 mg per gram adult rat brain. Of the values used for the above calculation, the water content of myelin from adult rat is most open to question (Bear, 1971; Norton, 1972). The content of basic proteins in the CNS of other species will vary depending on the myelin content of the tissue (Deibler *et al.*, 1972), and bovine spinal cord was estimated to contain 10 mg per gram tissue (Eylar, 1972).

1.3. Physical and Chemical Properties

Unless otherwise indicated, the results described below were obtained with either human or bovine basic proteins.

1.3.1. *Molecular Weight*

1.3.1a. Gel Filtration. The basic protein has a high net positive charge and is slightly retarded on Sephadex columns, which were generally used for gel filtration studies, because of the slight net negative charge on the Sephadex. This retardation tends to increase the apparent molecular weight of the basic protein when compared to other proteins which are less positively charged. To overcome this effect, proteins were generally eluted with solutions of low pH or high ionic strength (Deibler *et al.*, 1970). The unusual conformation of the basic protein also contributed to overestimation of its molecular weight, as globular proteins were satisfactory standards of molecular weight only when the basic protein and the standards were run under denaturing conditions, such as those used by Chao and Einstein (1969). These authors obtained a molecular weight of 19,000 daltons.

1.3.1b. Sedimentation Velocity and Equilibrium. Sedimentation velocity experiments, in conjunction with measurement of the diffusion coefficient of basic proteins ($D^{\circ}_{20,w}$ 7.80 $\times$ 10^{-7} cm^2/sec) and the estimation of the specific volume from amino acid analysis (0.72 g/ml), indicated that its $S^{\circ}_{20,w}$ value was between 1.33 S (Palmer and Dawson, 1969*a*) and 1.72 S (Eylar and

Thompson, 1969). Sedimentation equilibrium studies (Chao and Einstein, 1970) indicated a molecular weight of 18,000 daltons.

1.3.1c. Gel Electrophoresis. The molecular weight of the basic protein estimated by gel electrophoresis also depends on the conditions and the standards used for electrophoresis (Mehl, 1972).

1.3.1d. Chemical Methods. Estimates of the molecular weight of the basic protein obtained from amino acid analysis and tryptic peptide maps were in reasonable agreement with values obtained by other methods. More precise molecular weights were obtained from the complete amino acid sequence of the human (18,500), bovine (18,300), and rat (14,100) basic proteins (Figure 1). However, because of enzymic modification (Section 1.5), these values are still only approximate.

1.3.2. Spectral Properties

The ultraviolet absorption maximum for the bovine basic protein in 0.2 M KCl at 276 nm was 5.89 for a 1% solution. The absorbance at 276 nm did not vary with ionic strength, and no time-dependent conformational changes were observed. The absorption of the basic protein in the ultraviolet was accounted for entirely by the tryptophan and tyrosine content of the protein (Eylar and Thompson, 1969). The u.v. absorption pattern for the basic protein of pig (Kornguth and Perrin, 1971) was essentially identical in water, 0.1 M NaCl and 90% (by vol.) trifluoroethanol, while the pattern differed slightly in 50% (by vol.) aqueous *n*-propanol.

1.3.3. Isoelectric Point

The basic protein was so named because of its unusually high content of basic amino acids, and the isoelectric point was found to be greater than pH 10.6. From the amino acid composition of the basic protein from bovine, the iso-ionic point was calculated to be pH 12–13 (Eylar and Thompson, 1969). Thus the basic protein exists as a polyvalent cation over virtually the entire pH range.

1.3.4. Conformation

No evidence for the existence of polymer forms of the basic protein have been found during the gel filtration, sedimentation, or sequence studies. The basic protein does, however, aggregate and precipitate from aqueous solutions at pH values of 7–10, especially in the presence of polyvalent anions such as phosphate.

The conformation of myelin-basic protein has been deduced mainly from viscometric studies (Eylar and Thompson, 1969; Chao and Einstein,

1970; Kornguth and Perrin, 1971). Axial ratios for the basic protein of 10:1 and 15:1 have been calculated assuming either a prolate ellipsoid or an oblate ellipsoid, respectively. This rodlike shape was maintained in all aqueous solutions tested, and the ellipticity was increased in organic solvents. Calculation of the frictional ratio for the basic protein from its sedimentation and diffusion coefficients confirmed the asymmetric nature of the protein (Palmer and Dawson, 1969a). Recently Epand et al. (1974), using a number of techniques, obtained results consistent with a prolate ellipsoid structure with approximate dimensions of 15 × 150 Å.

Aqueous solutions of basic protein contain almost no secondary structure in the pH range 1.4–12 as determined by optical rotatory dispersion studies (Anthony and Moscarello, 1971; Palmer and Dawson, 1969a; Oshira and Eylar, 1970; Chao and Einstein, 1970). The basic protein was shown by circular dichroism to have very little helical structure in aqueous solutions of varying ionic strengths and in the presence of different electrolytes (Anthony and Moscarello, 1971; Kornguth and Perrin, 1971; Block et al., 1973). From these earlier studies, the basic protein was assumed to be essentially random coil; however, subsequent work has shown it to have a nonrandom structure which has some as yet unspecified folding (Epand et al., 1974), which could be of the type visualized by Eylar (1973). The open conformation was supported by thermal perturbation studies which showed that the tryptophan residue behaved like free tryptophan (Leach and Smith, 1972). Helical structure could be induced in the basic protein by dissolution in 50% (by vol.) n-propanol (20% α-helix) or in 2-chloroethanol (40% helical structure) (Kornguth and Perrin, 1971; Block et al., 1973).

Almost all the studies relating to the quaternary, tertiary, and secondary structure of the basic protein have been performed in aqueous solutions, while in vivo the basic protein is associated with a hydrophobic proteolipid protein, and lipids. The fact that the conformation of the basic protein can be altered in the presence of negatively charged lipids such as sodium dodecylsulfate, sodium oleate, and triphosphoinositide (Anthony and Moscarello, 1971; Palmer and Dawson, 1969b), and in organic solvents, indicates that the protein's conformation in vivo is unknown. A novel approach to this problem is that of the late Dr. London and his colleagues, who studied the interactions of proteins and lipids of myelin in a model system (London et al., 1973; see also Section 1.7.2).

1.3.5. Amino Acid Composition

The amino acid composition of human basic protein (Table 2) is characteristic of all myelin basic proteins, and the marked difference with the proteolipid protein composition is depicted in Figure 3. The amino acid

TABLE 2. Amino Acid Composition
(Moles %) of Basic Protein Isolated from
Human Myelin[a]

Asp	6.5	Ile	2.4
Thr	4.7	Leu	4.7
Ser	11.2	Tyr	2.4
Glu	5.3	Phe	5.3
Pro	7.1	Lys	7.1
Gly	14.7	His	5.9
Ala	7.6	Arg	11.2
Val	2.4	Trp	0.6
Met	1.2		

[a] Calculated from the primary sequence of the human
basic protein (Figure 1).

analysis is consistent with the properties of the basic protein discussed in
Section 1.3.4. As glycine and proline are known to be helix breakers, the low
helical content of the protein is not unexpected. The lack of disulfide bridges,
the low content of hydrophobic residues, and the charge repulsion of the
basic amino acids are all consistent with the formation of a disordered
elongated protein. From its amino acid analysis, Krigbaum and Knutton
(1973) calculated that the bovine basic protein would have 14% helix and
29% β-sheet. These predictions are not borne out by the experimental data
discussed above; however, the amino acid analysis of the protein is obviously
not consistent with a high content of α-helix and β-sheet.

1.4.   Amino Acid Sequence

1.4.1.   Complete

The complete amino acid sequences of the basic protein from human
(Carnegie, 1971a), bovine (Eylar et al., 1971), and rat (small) (Dunkley and
Carnegie, 1974b) have been determined (Figure 1). In subsequent reference
to an amino acid, the number given will indicate the position of that residue
in the human basic protein sequence as shown in Figure 1. The significance
of the amino acid sequence of the basic protein is discussed elsewhere in this
review in connection with evolution of basic proteins (Section 1.4.4.);
enzymic modification (Section 1.5); encephalitogenic determinants (Section
1.1.1); and interaction with other myelin components (Section 1.6). Eylar et
al. (1971) have commented on the distribution of polar and nonpolar regions
in the protein and how these might form templates for the attachment of
phospholipids.

Bovine
          Ala
Human
Ac-Ala-Ser-Gln-Lys-Arg-Pro-Ser-Gln-Arg-His-Gly-Ser-Lys-Tyr-Leu-Ala-Ser-Thr-Met-Asp-His-Ala-
                  5   10   15   20
Rat (small)

Bovine
  25   30   35   40   Ser 45
Human
Arg-His-Gly-Phe-Leu-Pro-Arg-His-Arg-Asp-Thr-Gly-Ile-Leu-Asp-Ser-Ile-Gly-Arg-Phe-Phe-Gly-Gly-Asp-Arg-
Rat (small)
                                                Ser

Bovine
                    Gly   Ala   Thr
Human
Gly-Ala-Pro-Lys-Arg-Gly-Ser-Gly-Lys-Asp-Ser-His-His-Pro-Ala-Arg-Thr-Ala-His-Tyr-Gly-Ser-Leu-Pro-Gln-
    50   55   60   65   70
Rat (small)
                                      —   Thr   Thr

Bovine
          Ala Gln   His Pro   Glu Asn
                    ↑
Human
Lys-Ser-His-Gly-Arg-Thr-Gln-Asp-Gln-Asp-Pro-Val-Val-His-Phe-Phe-Lys-Asn-Ile-Val-Thr-Pro-Arg-Thr-Pro-
    75   80   85   90   95
Rat (small)
          Gln —   Glu Asn

Bovine
                                                Lys
Human
Pro-Pro-Ser-Gln-Gly-Lys-Gly-Arg-Gly-Leu-Ser-Leu-Ser-Arg-Phe-Ser-Trp-Gly-Ala-Glu-Gly-Gln-Arg-Pro-Gly-
   100   105 (MeArg)   110   115   120
Rat (small)
                (Me₂Arg)   —

Bovine
                              Leu   His
Human
Phe-Gly-Tyr-Gly-Gly-Arg-Ala-Ser-Asp-Tyr-Lys-Ser-Ala-His-Lys-Gly-Phe-Lys-Gly-Val-Asp-Ala-Gln-Gly-Thr-
  125   130   135   140   145
Rat (small)
            —   —   —

Bovine
Human
Leu-Ser-Lys-Ile-Phe-Lys-Leu-Gly-Gly-Arg-Asp-Ser-Arg-Ser-Gly-Ser-Pro-Met-Ala-Arg-Arg
  150   155   160   165   170
Rat (small)
            —   —   —   —

FIGURE 1. Amino acid sequence of myelin basic proteins. The full sequence of the human protein is shown in the center with changes in the bovine above and the rat below. The bovine sequence differs from that frequently published in that an error at residue 2 has been corrected (see Brostoff et al., 1974). The sequences of the bovine and rat proteins are the same as that of the human protein except where substitutions, insertions (↑), or deletions (—) are shown. The residue numbers used in the text refer to the human protein.

1.4.2. *Incomplete*

1.4.2a. Larger Basic Protein from Rats. Martenson *et al.* (1972*b*) isolated and obtained amino acid compositions for the tryptic peptides present in the larger basic protein from rats, that were not present in the smaller basic protein. These peptides had amino acid compositions and mobilities comparable to the peptides from the human basic protein and were equivalent to residues 114–159, except for an arginine-to-lysine replacement at position 122 and a valine-to-alanine replacement at position 144. Amino acid analysis of the remaining tryptic peptides from the larger rat protein, and a comparison of the mobilities and cadmium ninhydrin colors with tryptic peptides from the smaller rat protein, indicated that the larger protein contains all of these peptides and that their compositions are identical (P. R. Dunkley, unpublished data). Thus the larger rat protein differs from basic proteins isolated from human and bovine myelin only by a few minor amino acid replacements and deletions.

1.4.2b. Other Species. Incomplete amino acid sequence data are available on peptides and basic proteins from a number of other species including guinea pigs (Shapira *et al.*, 1971*b*; Martenson *et al.*, 1975), rabbits (Shapira *et al.*, 1971*b*; Brostoff and Eylar, 1972), monkeys (Shapira *et al.*, 1971*b*), pigs (Kornguth *et al.*, 1972; Martenson *et al.*, 1971*b*), and chickens (Eylar, 1973). Dunkley and Carnegie (1974*b*) have tabulated these data.

1.4.3. *Errors and Disputed Sequences*

Historical developments leading to the amino acid sequences of the bovine and human proteins were summarized by Kies (1973), who also discussed some of the earlier errors which have since been corrected.

1.4.3a. Human. Eylar (1970) published a summary of the sequence of the human protein which differed at five residues from the sequence shown in Figure 1; these differences have been discussed by Carnegie (1971*a*). Subsequently, in another summary of the human protein sequence (Brostoff and Eylar, 1972), three of these differences were altered to that shown in Figure 1. Full details of Eylar's characterization of the sequence of the human basic protein have yet to be published. The remaining points of disagreement are the order of the histidine and glycine residues at positions 76 and 77, and the assignment of amides at residues 83 and 84.

1.4.3b. Bovine. An error occurred in sequencing the bovine protein at residue 2 in the original sequence (Eylar, 1970; Eylar *et al.*, 1971). More accurate analysis of this region of the protein showed that there was no serine in the *N*-terminal tryptic peptide (Brostoff *et al.*, 1974) and that the sequence should read acetyl-Ala-Ala-Gln-Lys. Kornguth *et al.*, 1972, suggested that there may be a histidine-to-leucine substitution at residue 23 in a small proportion of the protein.

1.4.3c. Rat. Part of the amino acid sequence of the smaller protein from rats has been reported in connection with studies on localization of the determinant which induces EAE in rats (McFarlin *et al.*, 1973). There is disagreement at four residues between the McFarlin *et al.* sequence and that presented in Figure 1 for the smaller basic protein from rats. The glycine at position 83 and alanine at position 50 reported by McFarlin *et al.* (1973) are printing errors and should read, as in Figure 1, glutamic acid and glycine, respectively (**R. F. Kibler**, personal communication). The assignment of serine and glycine at positions 46 and 47, respectively, rather than glycine and serine, was clearly demonstrated in our study (Dunkley and Carnegie, 1974*b*).

1.4.4. *Evolution of Basic Protein*

1.4.4a. Smaller Protein from Rat. The smaller basic protein from rat CNS myelin differs from all other myelin basic proteins in having a major internal deletion of 40 amino acid residues equivalent to residues 118–157 in the larger proteins. Whether it is glycine-117 or glycine-157 which is deleted cannot be resolved. However, the central position of the deletion ensures that the smaller protein is not derived from the larger protein by proteolysis. As both basic proteins are normally expressed in inbred and outbred rat strains, each must be products of nonallelic genes (Martenson *et al.*, 1972*b*).

How could the smaller basic protein gene have been formed in the ancestor of the *Myomorpha* and *Sciuromorpha*? It was probably derived by a gene duplication similar to that which occurred to produce the hemoglobin variants which have been characterized, but the shorter length of the basic protein necessitates that there must have been excision of a portion of the gene at the time of duplication, or at some later stage. At least two possible mechanisms could explain the formation of the smaller basic protein gene. The first involves unequal crossover at partially homologous DNA regions during synapsis, and the second involves misrepair of a strand of DNA coding for the larger basic protein after breakage by either enzymic or mechanical action. These possibilities are discussed in more detail by Dunkley and Carnegie (1974*b*).

1.4.4b. Minor Sequence Variations. The close homology in sequence between basic proteins from human and bovine shown in Figure 1 also extends to basic proteins from other species (Dunkley and Carnegie, 1974*b*), and a large proportion of the basic protein sequence appears to be invariant. Dayhoff (1972) calculated the mutation acceptance rate and showed that the rate was low for myelin basic proteins when compared to hemoglobins and growth hormones, but was higher than that for cytochrome c's. Recent more extensive data from other species are consistent with her conclusion.

In the few regions of sequence variability, the amino acid replacements are generally typical of those found in other proteins and require only single-base changes to be expressed. With other proteins, deletions are frequently found at the N- and C-terminal ends (Dayhoff, 1972), but the relatively conservative sequence at the N- and C-terminal ends of the myelin basic proteins suggests that these regions may be of functional importance and mutants would be lethal. The forty residues which are deleted in the smaller protein from rats may not be required for whatever structural or functional role the basic protein plays in myelin. However, if this region were unimportant it might be expected to be variable in sequence and this is not the case (Dunkley and Carnegie, 1974b). Perhaps there is an advantage in retaining two basic proteins with common sequence as mutational errors leading to loss of function would be minimized.

A conservative region of the basic protein (residues 90–120) contains a number of interesting residues: a triproline sequence (amino acid residues 99–101, Figure 1), a single tryptophan residue (116) which interacts with serotonin *in vitro* (Carnegie *et al.*, 1972), and a number of residues (98, 103, 107, 110) which have been found to exist in more than one form on isolation of the basic protein. These latter residues are discussed in Section 1.5.

1.5. Enzymic Modification of Amino Acid Residues

The basic protein contains a number of amino acid residues which have been shown to be modified by acetylation, methylation, phosphorylation, glycosylation, and deamidation.

1.5.1. *Acetylation*

The basic proteins for human and bovine have blocked N-terminal amino acid residues, and analysis of the blocking group indicated that it was acetyl–alanine for both proteins (Carnegie, 1969; Hashim and Eylar, 1969b). No unblocked form of the human protein was found and basic proteins from other species also appear to have blocked N-terminal residues (Dunkley and Carnegie, 1974b).

1.5.2. *Methylation*

Human basic protein is actually a mixture of three inseparable proteins (Figure 1); at position 107 the first contains arginine; the second, ω-N-monomethylarginine; and the third ω-N,N'-dimethylarginine (Baldwin and

Carnegie, 1971*a,b*). Partial methylation of a single arginine residue was subsequently found in basic proteins from a number of other species (Brostoff and Eylar, 1971; Deibler and Martenson, 1973*a,b*). The ratio of monomethyl to dimethylarginine in the basic protein varies with the species studied, but it appears to be constant for a given species. However, published values for the ratio of methylated-to-unmethylated forms of the basic protein from a single species varied considerably (Baldwin and Carnegie, 1971*b*; Deibler *et al.*, 1973*b*), and this difference in results may be a reflection only of the methods used to estimate unmethylated arginine. Baldwin and Carnegie (1971*b*) isolated small peptides containing arginine 107 which allowed accurate analysis of unmethylated arginine at this position, while Deibler *et al.* (1973*b*) used the whole protein and had difficulty resolving monomethylarginine from the large amount of arginine present in the hydrolysate.

Arginine residue 107 in the basic protein can act as an acceptor for methyl groups, donated from S-adenosylmethionine, in the presence of an S-adenosylmethionine:protein arginine methyl transferase (Baldwin and Carnegie, 1971*a*; Sundarraj and Pfeiffer, 1973). This enzyme has been localized mainly in the cytosol fraction of rat brain (Paik and Kim, 1971; Paik and Kim, 1973; Miyake and Kakimoto, 1973; Jones and Carnegie, 1974). Strong product inhibition was caused by S-adenosylhomocysteine (Jones and Carnegie, 1974). The physiological role of basic protein methylation is not known. It is possible that the dysmyelination which is observed in vitamin B12 deficiency is a result of defective methylation (Baldwin and Carnegie, 1971*a*).

1.5.3. *Phosphorylation*

1.5.3a. Substrate for Cyclic AMP-Dependent Protein Kinases. The basic protein of myelin has been shown to act as a good substrate for the transfer of radioactivity from $[\gamma\text{-}^{32}P]$-ATP, by protein kinases isolated from rabbit muscle (Carnegie *et al.*, 1973), bovine brain (Miyamoto *et al.*, 1974; Miyamoto and Kakiuchi, 1974), and rat skeletal muscle (Steck and Appel, 1974). Carnegie *et al.* (1973) identified the major sites on the human and smaller rat basic proteins which were phosphorylated by the rabbit muscle enzyme; these were serine residue 13, threonine residue 35, and serine residue 110. Daile and Carnegie (1975) found a wide variety of soluble kinases produced a similar labeling pattern with human basic protein as substrate.

As a substrate, basic protein was similar to histones in that it activated soluble protein kinases in the absence of cyclic AMP (Carnegie *et al.*, 1973; Miyamoto and Kakiuchi, 1974). Preliminary evidence indicated that the presence of dimethylarginine at residue 107 inhibited phosphorylation of residue 110 (Carnegie *et al.*, 1973, 1974).

1.5.3b.   Substrate for Endogenous Myelin Kinase. Studies using myelin from bovine (Carnegie *et al.*, 1974) and rat (Miyamoto and Kakiuchi, 1974; Steck and Appel, 1974) showed that the basic protein was also phosphorylated by an endogenous myelin kinase which was not activated by cyclic AMP. Both of the basic proteins from rat were phosphorylated and young rats appeared to have less active endogenous kinase than did adults (Steck and Appel, 1974). With myelin from bovine, label was incorporated mainly into one site, which was tentatively identified as serine residue 56 (Carnegie *et al.*, 1974).

A rapid dephosphorylation of myelin basic protein was observed and it was shown that myelin also contains a phosphoprotein phosphatase (Miyamoto and Kakiuchi, 1974; Steck and Appel, 1974).

1.5.3c.   In Vivo Phosphorylation. In order to establish that phosphorylation of myelin basic protein occurs *in vivo*, Miyamoto and Kakiuchi (1974) isolated basic protein from bovine spinal cord and demonstrated the presence of small amounts of phosphoserine and phosphothreonine. The incorporation of low levels of ^{32}P into rat basic protein *in vivo* has also been demonstrated (Miyamoto and Kakiuchi, 1974; Steck and Appel, 1974), but the site(s) on basic protein that is phosphorylated *in vivo* has not yet been established. One difficulty in this work is the high activity of phosphoprotein phosphatase which could rapidly remove label from the protein.

If phosphorylation of basic protein were controlled, for example, in response to fluctuations in cyclic AMP levels or phosphoprotein phosphatase activity, rapid changes in basic protein conformation could occur. Such changes could alter myelin structure in a controlled manner and thus may be important for whatever role the basic protein does play in myelin (see Section 1.7.3).

1.5.4.   *Glycosylation*

Basic protein from bovine has been shown to be a good substrate for acetylgalactosaminyl transferases from bovine submaxillary glands (Hagopian and Eylar, 1968) and rat brain (Ko and Raghupathy, 1972), and these enzymes formed an acetylgalactosaminyl-*O*-threonine linkage at threonine 98 (Hagopian *et al.*, 1971). However, the basic protein, as normally isolated, contains no detectable carbohydrate (Eylar and Thompson, 1969). There may be a glycosylated form of the basic protein *in vivo* which is not isolated under the conditions normally used for extraction of basic protein. For example, a glycoprotein with an amino acid analysis comparable to a peripheral nervous system basic protein was not extracted by acid from rat sciatic nerves (Wood and Dawson, 1973*a*; Section 2.2.3). It remains to be determined if the glycoprotein from CNS myelin (Quarles *et al.*, 1973) is related to the basic protein.

1.5.5. *Deamidation*

Modification of amino acids by deamidation is not necessarily an enzymically catalyzed reaction and may be entirely a result of the acidic conditons used to prepare the basic protein.

Partial deamidation of glutamine residue 103 has been detected after washing basic protein with 5% TCA (Hagopian *et al.*, 1971), and after preparing basic proteins from human, rat, and bovine by the usual isolation procedures (Dunkley and Carnegie, 1974*b*), which involve extraction at pH 3. A deamidated form of the tryptic peptide containing glutamine residue 74 was found for the larger basic protein from rats (P. R. Dunkley, unpublished data). Deamidation of glutamine and asparagine has been shown to occur spontaneously with peptides of similar sequence to regions of the basic protein (Westall, 1972), and Westall (1974) has suggested a link between deamidation of basic protein with its turnover and role in autoimmune disease.

1.5.6. *Heterogeneity of Myelin Basic Protein*

Myelin basic proteins that appear homgeneous on polyacrylamide gel electrophoresis at acid pH's show heterogeneity at alkaline pH values. Five bands of protein are usually seen and these have been isolated (Deibler and Martenson, 1973*a*). The basis of this heteroegeneity is unknown although a number of suggestions have been made; these include methylation of arginine residue 107 (Carnegie, 1971*b*), deamidation of glutamine or asparagine residue(s) (Deibler and Martenson, 1973*a*), and limited proteolysis at the C-terminal end of the protein (Bergstrand, 1971).

Amino acid analysis of the separated protein fractions suggests that partial methylation of arginine residue 107 does not account for the basic proteins heterogeneity at alkaline pH values (Deibler and Martenson, 1973*a*). However, phosphorylation of basic protein may be important in this regard (Dunkley and Carnegie, 1974*b*). Perhaps the heterogeneity of basic protein is not due to a single type of modification but rather to a combination of the modifications that have been discussed above. During sequencing of the rat basic proteins no evidence for single amino acid changes within each protein, such as that suggested by Kornguth *et al.* (1972) (Section 1.4.3*b*), or proteolysis of the C-terminal end of the proteins, was found (Dunkley and Carnegie, 1974*b*).

1.6. Synthesis and Turnover

1.6.1. *Myelinogenesis*

In the PNS bundles of nerve axons are initially surrounded by a single Schwann cell. A process of multiplication of Schwann cells and invasion of the axon bundles follows so that each axon becomes surrounded by an individual Schwann cell (Peters and Vaughn, 1970). Only then can ensheathment of the axon occur by a wrapping of the Schwann cell around the axon to form a lamellar structure in which the cytoplasm has been "lost" from the Schwann cell, this procedure causes internal membrane surfaces to be apposed and thus to form major dense lines, and external surfaces to be apposed and thus to form intraperiod lines. The number of lamellae formed varies from 5 to 90 depending on the axon diameter (Bunge, 1968; Peters and Vaughn, 1970); as the axon expands, the lamellae also expand and lengthen by insertion of new material and slippage over each other. When it was eventually shown that in the CNS the interfascicular oligodendroglial cell membrane was continuous with the myelin lamellae, it was generally accepted that a similar process of myelin formation occurred in the CNS. However, a number of important differences between CNS and PNS myelin preclude this simplistic assumption. Most importantly, one glial cell is responsible for myelination of a number of CNS internodes (Bunge, 1968) and is therefore not free to rotate about each individual axon as the Schwann cell does. In the CNS, loss of cytoplasm and formation of major dense lines (see Figure 2) often precede compaction to form intraperiod lines, and these are not observed in the PNS (Peters and Vaughn, 1970). Also, myelination in the CNS appears to be an irregular process compared to PNS myelination as two lots of lamellae may surround the same segment of axon. Thus more myelin than is required is often synthesized to surround a single axon (Peters and Vaughn, 1970). How this transition from glial cell plasma membrane to myelin membrane occurs, has not yet been accounted for by the wrapping mechanisms proposed for CNS myelin formation. Processes other than wrapping of the glial cell around the axon have been envisioned for myelin formation (Bunge, 1968). Adams and Osborne (1973) recently suggested that a "crystalization process," using preformed components, might occur within an annulus of glial cytoplasm which was formed by "pincers" of glial membrane. This proposal would circumvent the need to invoke a mechanism for transition from glial cell membrane to myelin membrane.

When myelin was isolated from developing rats and subjected to osmotic shock, followed by density gradient centrifugation, two membrane fractions were found. The lighter fraction was chemically and morphologically similar to adult myelin, while the heavier fraction, referred to as the myelin-like fraction, was composed of single-membrane vesicles similar to microsomal subfractions (Agrawal *et al.*, 1970). The content of the myelin-like fraction was maximal at 16 days of age, a time which suggested that it may be implicated in myelin formation. Characterization of the myelin-like fraction (Banik and Davison, 1969; Davison, 1971) indicated a different lipid composition to adult myelin, a lack of basic protein, but the presence of myelin marker enzymes such as the 2'3'-cyclic nucleotide 3'-phosphohydrolase. In contrast, Adams and Osborne (1973) and Agrawal *et al.* (1973) found basic protein in the myelin-like fraction. It has been suggested that the myelin-like fraction may represent the transition form from an oligodendroglial cell plasma membrane to myelin, or perhaps even the first few layers that the glial cell produces during myelination (Davison, 1971; Norton, 1972). However, no precursor–product relationship was established for the myelin-like and myelin fractions (Agrawal *et al.*, 1970).

1.6.2. Basic Protein During Development

To study the formation of myelin components, species such as rats, mice, cats, and rabbits are particularly useful as in these species myelin formation occurs postnatally (Bunge, 1968; Davison, 1970). Also, in considering the process of myelinogenesis, one must remember that myelin is not laid down in all regions of the CNS at the same time. Initially, deposition of myelin occurs in phylogenetically older areas of the CNS, such as the spinal cord, and progresses to the hind brain; finally, the forebrain is myelinated (Norton, 1972; Peters and Vaughn, 1970). Investigations using whole brain have shown that rat myelin was first isolated at day 10 after birth. The rate of myelin synthesis then rapidly increased to a maximum (3.5 mg per brain per day) at day 20, decreased rapidly to half the maximal rate at day 25, and continued slowly to decrease (Norton and Poduslo, 1973*b*). An almost identical pattern was found in mice (Morell *et al.*, 1972), and both species appeared to continue myelination throughout their lifetime, with the increase in brain weight after 100 days being due almost solely to myelin deposition (Norton and Poduslo, 1973*b*). In other species, myelinogenesis starts before birth and does not appear to continue throughout life (Davison, 1970).

Because of difficulty in obtaining fetal and neonatal material from larger mammals, there have been only limited studies on the appearance of basic protein in the human (Eng *et al.*, 1968; Savolainen *et al.*, 1972), bovine (Hergstrand and Kornguth, 1973), and rabbit (Einstein *et al.*, 1970). Thorough electrophoretic studies using rats and mice clearly show the relationship of the two myelin basic proteins to myelinogenesis. Rat basic proteins were first detected at approximately 7 days after birth (Gaitonde and Martenson, 1970;

Adams and Osborne, 1973). At day 7, the larger basic protein from rats was present, whereas the smaller protein appeared after day 12; only after 25 days was the smaller protein found at higher contents than the large protein (Adams and Osborne, 1973). Einstein (1974) independently obtained almost identical ratios to those of Adams and Osborne (1973) for the levels of the two basic proteins during development of the rat CNS myelin. In contrast, the smaller basic protein was always found in higher content than the larger protein in mouse myelin from day 8 onward (Morell et al., 1972). The maximum rate of appearance of the basic proteins was between days 10 and 17 in the mouse (Morell et al., 1972; Matthieu et al., 1973a), and days 10 and 40 in the rat (Gaitonde and Martenson, 1970), after which the level of basic protein continued slowly to increase throughout life. The transition from rapid to slow rate of synthesis of basic protein in the rat depended upon the CNS region studied (Sammeck, 1973).

There is disagreement about whether the proteolipid appears before (Einstein et al., 1970; Savolainen et al., 1972) or after (Morell et al., 1972; Adams and Osborne, 1973) the appearance of the basic protein. It is possible, however, that the early proteolipid detected by the former workers was a nonmyelin contaminant (Nussbaum and Mandel, 1973).

1.6.3.   Mode and Site of Basic Protein Synthesis

From electrophoretic studies, Adams and Osborne (1973) suggested that basic protein was synthesized in the endoplasmic reticulum, transferred to large granule structures, and subsequently deposited in myelin. Sammeck et al. (1971), however, provided evidence which indicated that in myelin from adult rats a precursor may have been formed prior to basic protein deposition in myelin. One way of determining whether a precursor of basic protein exists is to isolate the mRNA responsible for basic protein synthesis. Such a study was undertaken by Lim et al. (1974); after injection of the isolated mRNA into Xenopus laevis oocytes, a nonoocyte basic protein was produced. This preliminary report indicated that the protein product had the characteristics of myelin basic protein.

The above-mentioned studies are important in understanding how basic protein is synthesized, but they give no indication of the cellular origin of the basic protein, which is as yet unknown. As the glial cell plasma membrane is continuous with the myelin sheath and the basic protein is thought to be localized in the major dense line of myelin, it is probable that basic protein is synthesized in the oligodendroglia. However, attempts to detect basic protein on glial plasma membranes were unsuccessful (Savolainen and Palo, 1972; Herndon et al., 1973). In studies on axonal flow of proteins in the optic nerve it appears that certain myelin proteins came from the axon, but basic protein did not appear to be neuronally derived (Giorgi *et al.*, 1973). Pfeiffer and Wechsler (1972) have isolated a neoplastic clone of Schwann cells which, although of peripheral origin (see Section 2), produced a single basic protein closely similar in amino acid composition and electrophoretic properties to the larger protein from rat brain. These results would further indicate that the myelin basic proteins are not neuronally derived and suggest that there exist separate controls over synthesis of the two basic proteins of rat.

1.6.4. *Turnover of Basic Protein*

That basic protein is turned over *in vivo* is shown by a large number of incorporation studies. However, the exact rate of turnover is still uncertain, although it is clearly much slower than, for example, that of synaptosomal membrane proteins. A variety of half-lives have been quoted for basic proteins from both mouse and rat (Table 3). In these studies various radio-active precursors, routes of injection, ages of animals, and purities of labeled basic protein products were used. These differences, together with the fact that some studies did not account for dilution of labeled basic protein with newly synthesized protein, make comparison difficult (Lajtha and Marks, 1971; Smith, 1973*a*). In addition, it is known that different regions of CNS tissue from rat metabolize basic protein at different rates (Sammeck *et al.*, 1971; Sammeck, 1973), and it is possible that there are differences in basic protein metabolism in different myelin "compartments" within the CNS. Another difficulty with these studies is that re-utilization of precursors or labeled basic protein cannot be accounted for in the type of studies performed. Fischer and Morell (1974*a*) discussed these problems in detail and found quite different results depending on the radioactive precursor used in the experiments. They suggested that there may be two pools of myelin, one turning over rapidly and the other turning over slowly (Fischer and Morell, 1974*a,b*).

An important consideration is the control over normal degradation of basic protein (Smith, 1973*b*). Basic protein is readily hydrolyzed *in vitro* by acid proteinase (Marks and Lajtha, 1971; Sammeck and Brady, 1972; Einstein, 1972), yet the normal function of this enzyme *in vivo* is unknown. However, in demyelinating disease such as multiple sclerosis, Einstein *et al.* (1972) have shown an increase in acid proteinase associated with plaques and selective disappearance of basic protein. Westall (1973, 1974) has made the interesting suggestion that turnover of myelin basic protein could be related to deamidation of selected amide residues in basic protein.

TABLE 3. Turnover of Myelin Basic Protein

Author and comments	Half-life	Species (Age[a])	Route injection	Precursor
Davison (1961)[b]	Stable	Rats (11 and 150 days)	Intraperitoneal	[1-^{14}C]-glycine
Rodriguez de Lores Arnaiz et al. (1971)[b]	95 days	Rats (35–40 days)	Intraventricular	[1-^{14}C]-leucine
Fischer and Morell (1974a)[c]	Stable	Mice (14 days)	Intraperitoneal	[4,5-^{3}H]-leucine
	95 days	Mice (60 days)	Intraperitoneal	[4,5-^{3}H]-leucine
Fischer and Morell (1974b)[d]	45 days	Mice (15 days)	Intraperitoneal	[^{14}C]-glucose
	95 days	Mice (60 days)	Intraperitoneal	[4,5-^{3}H]-leucine
Smith (1972)[e]	42–44 days	Rats (38 days)	Intracisternal	[^{14}C]-leucine
Smith (1968)	35 days	Rats (85 days)	Intraperitoneal	[^{14}C]-glucose
Wood and King (1971)[f]	21 days	Rats (10 and 70 days)	Subcutaneous (dorsum–neck)	[4,5-^{3}H]-leucine
D'Monte et al. (1971)[g]	11–21 days	Rats (40–50 days)	Intracisternal	[^{14}C]-lysine
Gaitonde and Martenson (1970)[h]	Not done	Rats (0–90 days)	Intraperitoneal	[^{14}C]-lysine
Sammeck et al. (1971)[i]	Not done	Rats (20–25 days)	Intracisternal	[2-^{14}C]-tryptophan
Smith (1973b)[j]	Not done	Rats (60 days)	Intracisternal	[1-^{14}C]-leucine

[a] Age in days after birth.
[b] Observed total myelin protein turnover.
[c] Observed half lives for basic proteins of 15 and 19 days with myelin-like fraction.
[d] Mice injected at day 60 after birth had previously been injected with [^{14}C]-glucose at day 15 after birth.
[e] Found greater uptake [1-^{14}C]-glycine compared with [1-^{14}C]-leucine into basic protein.
[f] See Smith (1972) and Fischer and Morell (1974a) for comments.
[g] Studied uptake of label rather than loss over a long time period.
[h] Studied incorporation of [^{14}C]-lysine into basic proteins at various ages.
[i] Incorporation studies which suggest a possible precursor for basic protein.
[j] Marked increase in incorporation after triethyl tin administration.

1.7.   Basic Protein as a Myelin Component

1.7.1.   *Localization Within Myelin*

Electron microscopy of myelin showed a lamellar structure of alternating dark and light lines separated by unstained zones (see Figure 2). The stained lines are the protein layers and the unstained zones the lipid hydrocarbon chains. The less dark or intraperiod lines are thought to represent two

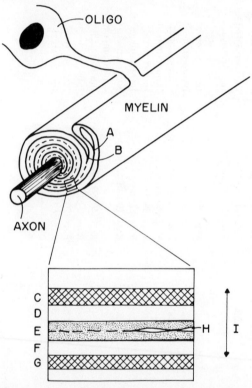

FIGURE 2. The ultrastructure of CNS myelin. The exact mechanism by which mature CNS myelin is formed is unknown, but it is generally accepted that the lamellar structure of myelin is a result of the apposition of inner and outer membrane surfaces of the oligodendroglial cell. Top: In mature myelin the inner or cytoplasmic membrane surfaces come together (A) to form the major dense lines (often called the period lines) of myelin, while the outer membrane surfaces (B) form the intraperiod (or interperiod) lines. Bottom: Electron microscope photos of myelin show the major dense lines (C, G) separated by a repeat distance (I) of approximately 120 Å. Between are areas of light and dark staining. Regions D and F are thought to be the lipid bilayers, which are not electron dense, and apposed outer membrane surfaces (E), which together make up the intraperiod line of myelin. Under high magnification (× 350,000) the two outer membranes are seen to be separated by a gap (H) (see Norton, 1972).

fused outer protein coats of the original membrane, while the dark major dense line is the fused inner protein coats of the cell membrane (Norton, 1972). Under certain conditions the intraperiod line is seen to be a double structure presumably because the outer protein coats of the original membrane have become separated. Freeze fracture studies have indicated the presence of protein within the lipid layers of a number of membranes, but with myelin no such penetration of lipids by protein has been observed (Bear, 1971). Thus the basic protein can reside in only two possible locations within the myelin lamellae—the major dense line or the intraperiod line.

After using histochemical staining procedures on intact myelin and extraction of the tissue with anionic and cationic salts, Wolman (1971) suggested that the intraperiod line of myelin was anionically charged and the major dense line was cationically charged, and that basic protein was in the latter. Herndon et al. (1973) used an immunoelectron microscopic technique in which antibody to basic protein was coupled to peroxidase. The tissue sections used in this method were not frozen. Basic protein was not labeled by antibody except where the myelin sheath was disrupted during processing and if labeling was observed it was found on the major dense line. With PNS myelin again the basic proteins appear to be in the major dense line (Section 2.3).

Dickinson et al. (1970) found that incubation of isolated myelin caused release of basic protein into the incubation medium and the intraperiod line was replaced by a dense line. From this they concluded the basic protein was in the intraperiod line. Basic protein in isolated myelin is readily accessible to tryptic digestion, and almost all of the protein is liberated from myelin within 30 min (Kies et al., 1965). No other myelin protein appears to be altered, and in contrast to the results of Dickinson et al. (1970) the gross morphology of the myelin is unaffected by this loss of basic protein (Wood and Dawson, 1973b). Lipids, in particular the highly acidic phospholipids, are also released on tryptic digestion (Raghavan et al., 1973).

Mehl (1972) used a water-soluble carbodiimide to cross-link lysine residues in isolated myelin and found that all the basic protein molecules present in myelin were cross-linked, while no other protein was affected. This result indicated that in isolated myelin all the basic protein molecules are accessible to carbodiimide and are in close association with each other.

The results discussed above indicate that with isolated myelin the basic protein is readily accessible to carbodiimide, trypsin, and even such bulky molecules as fluorescent-labeled antibodies. With intact myelin (i.e., unhomogenized myelin observed histochemically) basic protein was also accessible to trypsin and fluorescent-labeled antibody, but only when processing procedures caused disruption of myelin's native conformation, particularly methods such as freezing the intact tissue (Herndon et al., 1973).

If the basic protein were in the major dense line of myelin, as evidence now suggests, then accessibility of the basic protein requires that "aqueous channels" be present in myelin to allow the water-soluble carbodiimide, trypsin, or antibody to penetrate without having to cross lipid barriers. The exact location and the accessibility of basic protein within myelin are important in understanding the demyelinating diseases.

1.7.2. *Interaction with Myelin Lipids*

The high content of lipid and the accepted distribution of components within the myelin lamellae ensure that basic protein will be in direct contact with lipid *in vivo*, and a number of *in vitro* studies have shown that the protein can interact with myelin lipids. Complexes between basic protein and acidic phospholipids such as phosphatidyl serine, phosphatidyl inositol, and triphosphoinositide can be formed; these complexes are largely stabilized by electrostatic bonds (Palmer and Dawson, 1969b). However, stable complexes are not formed between basic protein and phosphatidyl choline or phosphatidyl ethanolamine, a fact suggesting that factors other than charge must also be involved. Some of the aqueous insoluble complexes dissolve in chloroform–methanol, a behavior which is characteristic of proteolipids. In aqueous solutions the basic protein takes up a disordered rodlike conformation under various conditions of pH and ionic strength, while with negatively charged lipids a more ordered structure prevails (Section 1.3.4).

Demel *et al.* (1973) found that at an air–water interface the most avid interaction was between basic protein and cerebroside sulfatide, or phosphatidyl serine, while phosphatidyl ethanolamine and neutral lipids showed markedly less affinity for basic protein. Although ionic interactions again appeared to predominate, hydrophobic interactions were important. In contrast to the specificity of basic protein, the proteolipid protein interacted with a large number of myelin lipids including cholesterol (London *et al.*, 1974). The relative affinity of the two myelin proteins for cholesterol and cerebroside sulfatide was demonstrated by competition experiments. The proteolipid protein was able to interact with a cholesterol monolayer even in the presence of basic protein by expelling the latter from the interface, while with cerebroside sulfatide monolayers both proteins showed similar affinities and basic protein was not expelled by proteolipid. Using proteolytic enzymes, London and Vossenberg (1973) and London *et al.* (1973) indicated that certain segments within the N-terminal 100 amino acid residues of basic protein interacted with lipids, while the C-terminal end of the protein remained exposed to the aqueous environment.

Using glucose-loaded liposomes prepared from both PNS and CNS myelin lipids, Gould and London (1972) showed that specific interaction with basic protein caused release of the glucose and the phenomenon could not be duplicated with other similar proteins (e.g., P2 from the PNS, see Section 2). Also, the addition of basic protein to liposomes caused an increase in spacing and electron density of the lamellar structure.

1.7.3. *Speculation on Role of Basic Protein*

1.7.3a. Is Basic Protein a "Structural Cement?" The most obvious function for basic protein is that of a structural component. No matter what other role the protein plays, it must be involved in maintaining the normal conformation of myelin. In this respect basic protein is peculiarly suited. The amino acid sequence of the protein (Figure 1) indicates that charged amino acids are distributed throughout its length and that certain regions between these residues are hydrophobic. This distribution of charged residues causes the protein to become disordered and expanded in aqueous solution and precludes the formation of polymer structures. In myelin, because of the high ratio of lipid to protein, the latter are sparsely distributed between lipid bilayers with little penetration occurring (Bear, 1971). Thus basic protein could "spread" over the surface of the lipid bilayer and interact ionically with the negative regions of certain lipids, as well as form some hydrophobic bonds with neutral lipids. Charge repulsion between basic protein molecules and the limited amount of protein compared to the area required to be covered would suggest that only a single layer of basic protein exists between lipid bilayers. Thus the protein would act as a "cement" and bind the two cytoplasmic surfaces of the oligodendroglia. The ability of carbodiimide to cross-link basic protein molecules within myelin *in vitro* (Mehl, 1972) further suggests that each molecule is in close proximity and possibly a "sheet" of basic protein exists between the lipid bilayers. Unfortunately the residues cross-linked by carbodiimide were not identified, and no conclusion can yet be reached as to the existence of "sheets" of basic protein within myelin.

The three facts, (a) that basic protein causes an increase in the lamellar size of lipid liposomes with a concomitant release of glucose (Gould and London, 1972), (b) that it is localized in the major dense line of myelin, and (c) that when it interacts with lipids certain regions remain exposed to enzymes, suggest a further structural role for basic protein. It may in fact be required in order to maintain an "aqueous channel" by which the inner lamellae of myelin can maintain contact with the glial cytoplasm and thus allow exchange of metabolites. The observed early loss of basic protein in conditions such as Wallerian degeneration, EAE, and multiple sclerosis (Adams, 1972) could results in a subsequent degeneration of myelin.

1.7.3b. Does Basic Protein Have a Receptor Function? Although the basic protein is present throughout the CNS, the paralysis and incontinence associated with EAE suggest localization of the autoimmune attack to certain regions of the CNS. The similarity of the main antigenic determinant for guinea pigs, and the requirements (Smythies *et al.*, 1970) for a binding site for serotonin, led Carnegie (1971*b*) to speculate that an immune response to the tryptophan region of the basic protein might induce an immunopharmacological block of serotonin receptors. Although some additional evidence has been obtained for the involvement of serotonin receptors in EAE (White *et al.*, 1973; Lennon, 1972; Lycke and Roos, 1973), and for the interaction of the basic protein with serotonin and hallucinogenic indoles (Carnegie *et al.*, 1972; Carnegie, 1974), there is no definitive evidence that myelin basic protein *in vivo* interacts with serotonin. If such interaction did occur, it would be most likely at the nodal regions. However, any hypothesis on the role of basic protein in myelin will have to explain the marked clinical symptoms which follow immunization with this protein, but not with other brain or even myelin proteins. Moreover, the proximity of the tryptophan residue to the site phosphorylated by cyclic AMP-dependent protein kinase (Section 1.5.3) raises intriguing questions regarding the possible dynamic role of the basic protein in the brain.

2. BASIC PROTEINS OF PERIPHERAL NERVOUS SYSTEM MYELIN

Until recently there was considerable confusion over the nature and composition of the PNS proteins which have been less extensively studied than the myelin proteins from the CNS. More work is required on the characterization of these proteins. This summary represents our interpretation of data from a number of papers, and our nomenclature and conclusions may well be different from those of the original authors.

2.1. Isolation

Because of the high content of connective tissue, myelin is more difficult to prepare from PNS material. However, proteins have been isolated from PNS tissue obtained from bovine (Bencina *et al.*, 1969; London, 1971; London, 1972; Uyemura *et al.*, 1972), pig (Uyemura *et al.*, 1970), rabbit (Brostoff *et al.*, 1972; Brostoff and Eylar, 1972), and human (Paty, 1971; Palo *et al.*, 1972). PNS myelin has been studied by polyacrylamide gel electrophoresis in either phenolic solvents (Mehl and Wolfgram, 1969; Csejtey *et al.*, 1972) or detergents (Morris *et al.*, 1971; Greenfield *et al.*, 1973). In both systems, a number of proteins were observed. The proteins which have been

TABLE 4. Properties of Partially Characterized PNS Proteins

	Total myelin protein, %[a]		Electrophoretic mobility		Approximate molecular weight	Comment
	Rabbit	Bovine	Phenol[b]	Detergent[a]		
P0	55	54	0.86	0.69	20,000[c]	Probably a glycoprotein derivative of P2
P1	13	7	1.00	1.00	18,000	Same as CNS basic protein
P2	7	15	1.15	1.14	12,000	Does *not* induce auto-immune disease of PNS

[a] Results from Greenfield et al. (1973); proportion of P0 molecules includes "Y" component.
[b] Calculated from data on 7.5 % acrylamide gel (Mehl and Wolfgram, 1969); all mobilities are relative to CNS basic protein.
[c] Our estimate from mobility of phenolic gels.

isolated and partially characterized are referred to as P0, P1, and P2 (Table 4) following the coding used by Greenfield et al. (1973). In all species so far examined, P0 is the major component accounting for 50–60% of the total protein of PNS myelin. However, the content of the other proteins varies markedly between species and even between different areas of the PNS from one animal (Greenfield et al., 1973).

2.2. Properties

The amino acid composition of the PNS proteins is illustrated in Figure 3. Their properties are given in Table 4. There is reasonable agreement between estimates of the molecular weight (Table 4) of the P1 and P2 proteins from both phenolic and detergent gels, and these values are supported by data from amino acid composition and ultracentrifugation. The molecular weight of the P0 protein is less certain, and the estimate given is based on its mobility relative to P1 protein in phenolic gels.

2.2.1. P2 Protein

The P2 protein has been obtained by acid extraction of defatted PNS myelin, whole sciatic nerve, or intradural spinal roots (Bencina et al., 1969; London, 1971; Uyemura et al., 1970, 1972, 1975; Brostoff et al., 1972). It has a molecular weight of approximately 12,000 daltons and an amino acid composition quite different from that of the CNS basic protein (Figure 3), especially in the lysine-to-arginine ratio and the glycine-to-alanine ratio. No

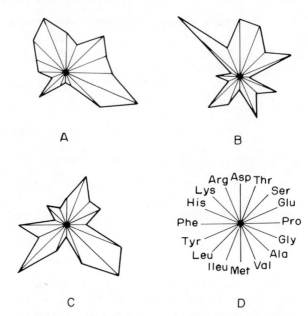

FIGURE 3. Amino acid composition of myelin proteins. Molar percentage of each amino acid is shown as a distance from the center; equimolar proportions are shown in the key to the lines (**D**). (Adapted from Uyemura *et al.*, 1975.)

A is typical of CNS myelin basic protein and PNS P1 protein. B is typical of PNS P2 and P0 proteins. C is typical of the proteolipid of CNS myelin.

methylarginine was detected in the protein in our study (Bencina *et al.*, 1969, and unpublished data). PNS tissue from bovine contains a protein of approximately 14,000 daltons which is closely similar in amino acid composition to the P2 protein (Bencina *et al.*, 1969; London, 1971). Peptide maps of the P2 protein and CNS basic protein were markedly different in appearance although both are highly basic proteins (Uyemura *et al.*, 1975). An earlier report (Brostoff *et al.*, 1972) which claimed that the P2 protein shared a large section of sequence in common with the CNS basic protein has been completely withdrawn (a fragment of P1 protein contaminated their preparation of P2 protein: S. W. Brostoff, personal communication; E. H. Eylar, discussion at 4th Meeting International Society for Neurochemistry, 1973).

2.2.2. *P1 Protein*

The P1 protein from rabbit sciatic nerve was isolated and partially sequenced (Brostoff and Eylar, 1972). At least in this species, the P1 protein appeared to be closely similar to the CNS basic protein in amino acid composition and sequence. Methylarginine was also found to be present. Other species have a protein with the same electrophoretic properties as the P1 protein, but it has not been characterized. In addition, some species have a higher proportion of a minor component, labeled "X" by Greenfield et al. (1973), which moves slightly slower than the P1 protein on gel electrophoresis. It is of great interest that a tumor derived from Schwann cells of the rat produced P1 protein (i.e., CNS-type basic protein), but neither the smaller form of the CNS protein nor the P2 protein appeared to be synthesized (Pfeiffer and Wechsler, 1972).

The presence of the CNS-type protein in the PNS gives a logical explanation for the well-known ability of PNS tissue to induce autoimmune disease of the CNS (Brostoff et al., 1973). PNS myelin can induce an autoimmune attack on the PNS, but the antigen is neither the P1 nor the P2 proteins. It is possibly a minor component of the basic protein fraction (Uyemura et al., 1975).

2.2.3. P0 Protein

The P0 protein is the major protein in PNS myelin. Although it has an electrophoretic mobility similar to CNS proteolipid protein under the same conditions, it has quite different solubility properties and is not extracted by dilute acid nor chloroform–methanol (Csejtey et al., 1972). Recently it was shown that the P0 proteins in PNS myelin from human (Savolainen, 1972) and rat (Everly et al., 1973; Wood and Dawson, 1973a) were glycoproteins. The amino acid composition of the P0 protein (Wood and Dawson, 1973a; Greenfield et al., 1973) is similar to the P2 protein, but it remains to be proved that the P0 protein is simply a glycosylated derivative of the P2 protein. In some species there is a substantial proportion of a protein (Y) which migrates slightly faster than P0 (Greenfield et al., 1973).

2.3. Conclusion

There is obviously a need for more information on the amino acid sequence of the PNS proteins and especially the characterization of the site of glycosylation in the P0 protein. Little information on the biosynthesis and development of the individual PNS proteins exists. Embryonic chicken nerves can be used to study their biosynthesis in vitro and its inhibition by diphtheria toxin (Pleasure et al., 1973). With regard to localization within PNS myelin, there is little information apart from the histochemical studies of

Adams *et al.* (1971) which suggest basic proteins are present in the major dense line.

ACKNOWLEDGMENTS

Our studies on myelin basic protein have been supported by grants from the National Multiple Sclerosis Society, New York, and the Australian Research Grants Committee.

3. REFERENCES

Adams, C. W. M., Bayliss, O. B., Hallpike, J. F., and Turner, D. R., 1971, Histochemistry of myelin, XII, anionic staining of myelin basic proteins for histology, electrophoresis and electron microscopy, *J. Neurochem.* **18**:389–394.

Adams, C. W. M., 1972, *in Research on Multiple Sclerosis* (C. W. M. Adams and U. Leibowitz, eds.), pp. 19–60, Charles C. Thomas, Illinois.

Adams, D. H., and Osborne, J., 1973, A developmental study of the relationship between the protein components of rat CNS myelin, *Neurobiology* **3**:91–112.

Agrawal, H. C., Banik, N. L., Bone, A. H., Davison, A. N., Mitchell, R. F., and Spohn, M., 1970, The identity of a myelin-like fraction isolated from developing brain, *Biochem. J.* **120**:635–642.

Agrawal, H. C., Banik, N. L., Bone, A. H., Cuzner, M. L., Davison, A. N., and Mitchell, R. F., 1971, The chemical composition of dogfish myelin, *Biochem. J.* **124**:70P.

Agrawal, H. C., Burton, R. M., Fishman, M. A., Mitchell, R. F., and Prensky, A. L., 1972, Partial characterization of a new myelin protein component, *J. Neurochem.* **19**:2083–2089.

Agrawal, H. C., Trotter, J. L., Mitchell, R. F., and Burton, R. M., 1973, Criteria for identifying a myelin-like fraction from developing brain, *Biochem. J.* **136**:1117–1119.

Alvord, E. C., Jr., 1970, Acute disseminating encepholomyelitis and "allergic" neuro-encephalopathies, *in Handbook of Clinical Neurology* (P. J. Viken and G. W. Bruyn, eds.), Vol. 9, pp. 500–571, North-Holland Publ. Co., Amsterdam.

Anthony, J. S., and Moscarello, M. A., 1971, A conformation change induced in the basic encephalitogen by lipids, *Biochim. Biophys. Acta* **243**:429–433.

Baldwin, G. S., and Carnegie, P. R., 1971*a*, Specific enzymic methylation of an arginine in the experimental allergic encephalomyelitis protein from human myelin, *Science* **171**:579–581.

Baldwin, G. S., and Carnegie, P. R., 1971*b*, Isolation and partial characterization of methylated arginines from the encephalitogenic basic protein of myelin, *Biochem. J.* **123**:69–74.

Banik, N. L., and Davison, A. N., 1969, Enzyme activity and composition of myelin and subcellular fractions in the developing rat brain, *Biochem. J.* **115**:1051–1062.

Banik, N. L., and Davison, A. N., 1973, Isolation of purified basic protein from human brain, *J. Neurochem.* **21**:489–494.

Bear, R. S., 1971, The structure of the myelin sheath, *Neurosciences Res. Prog. Bull.* **9**:507–598.

Bencina, B., Carnegie, P. R., McPherson, T. A., and Robson, G., 1969, Encephalitogenic basic protein from sciatic nerve, *FEBS Letters* **4**:9–12.

Bergstrand, H., 1971, Isolation and partial characterization of some proteolytically and chemically derived fragments of bovine encephalitogenic protein, *Eur. J. Biochem.* **21**:116–124.

Bergstrand, H., 1972, Encephalitogenic activity in rabbits of the C-terminal region of bovine basic myelin protein: Localization to two different regions, *FEBS Letters* **23**:195–198.

Bergstrand, H., and Kallen, B., 1973*a*, Is there a cross-reactivity between different parts of the bovine encephalitogenic protein in the macrophage migration inhibition assay? *Immunochemistry* **10**:471–476.

Bergstrand, H., and Kallen, B., 1973*b*, Antigenic determinants on bovine encephalitogenic protein: Studies in rabbits with derivatives of fragment 1–43 and the lymph node cell transformation test, *Neurobiology* **3**:246–255.

Block, R. E., Brady, A. H., and Joffe, S., 1973, Conformation and aggregation of bovine myelin proteins, *Biochem. Biophys. Res. Commun.* **54**:1595–1602.

Braun, P. E., and Barchi, R. L., 1972, 2′, 3′-Cyclic nucleotide 3′-phosphodiesterase in the nervous system: Electrophoretic properties and developmental studies, *Brain Res.* **40**:437–444.

Brostoff, S., and Eylar, E. H., 1971, Localization of methylated arginine in the A_1 protein from myelin, *Proc. Nat. Acad. Sci. (U.S.A.)* **68**:765–769.

Brostoff, S. W., and Eylar, E. H., 1972, The proposed amino acid sequence of the P1 protein of rabbit sciatic nerve myelin, *Arch. Biochem. Biophys.* **153**:590–598.

Brostoff, S., Burnett, P., Lampert, P., and Eylar, E. H., 1972, Isolation and characterization of a protein from sciatic nerve myelin responsible for experimental allergic neuritis, *Nature (New Biol.)* **235**:210–212.

Brostoff, S. W., Wisneiwski, H. M., Greenfield, S., Morell, P., and Eylar, E. H., 1973, Immunopathologic response in guinea pigs sensitized with peripheral nervous system myelin, *Brain. Res.* **58**:500–505.

Brostoff, S. W., Reuter, W., Hichens, M., and Eylar, E. H., 1974, Specific cleavage of the A_1 protein from myelin with cathepsin D, *J. Biol. Chem.* **249**:559–567.

Bunge, R. P., 1968, Glial cells and the central myelin sheath, *Physiological Reviews* **48**:197–251.

Burnett, P. R., and Eylar, E. H., 1971, Allergic encephalomyelitis. Oxidation and cleavage of the single tryptophan residue of the A_1 protein from bovine and human myelin, *J. Biol..Chem.* **246**:3425–3430.

Carnegie, P. R., 1969, N-terminal sequence of an encephalitogenic protein from human myelin, *Biochem. J.* **111**:240–242.

Carnegie, P. R., 1971*a*, Amino acid sequence of the encephalitogenic basic protein of human myelin, *Biochem. J.* **123**:57–67.

Carnegie, P. R., 1971*b*, Properties, structure and possible neuroreceptor role of the encephalitogenic protein of human brain, *Nature (London)* **229**:25–28.

Carnegie, P. R., 1974, Interaction of 5-hydroxytryptamine with the encephalitogenic protein of myelin, *in Neurosciences Third Study Program* (F. O. Schmitt and G. Wordin, eds.), pp. 925–928, MIT Press, Cambridge.

Carnegie, P. R., and Sims, N. R., 1975, Properties of myelin proteins and enzymes and their possible role in multiple sclerosis, *in Current Studies in Multiple Sclerosis* (E. J. Field, ed.), Medical and Technical Publishing Co., Oxford, England, in preparation.

Carnegie, P. R., Bencina, B., and Lamoureux, G., 1967, Experimental allergic encephalomyelitis, *Biochem. J.* **105**:559–568.

Carnegie, P. R., Symthies, J. R., Caspary, E. A., and Field, E. J., 1972, Interaction of hallucinogenic drugs with encephalitogenic protein of myelin, *Nature (London)* **240**:561–563.

Carnegie, P. R., Kemp, B. E., Dunkley, P. R., and Murray, A. W., 1973, Phosphorylation of myelin basic protein by a cyclic AMP-dependent protein kinase, *Biochem. J.* **135**:589–591.

Carnegie, P. R., Dunkley, P. R., Kemp, B. E., and Murray, A. W., 1974, Phosphorylation of selected serine and threonine residues in myelin basic protein by endogenous and exogenous protein kinases, *Nature (London)* **249**:147–150.

Caspary, E. A., and Field, E. J., 1965, An encephalitogenic protein of human origin: some chemical and biological properties, *Ann. N.Y. Acad. Sci.* **122**:182–198.

Chao, L. P., and Einstein, E. R., 1969, Estimation of molecular weight of flexible disordered proteins by exclusion chromatography, *J. Chromatography* **42**:485–492.

Chao, L. P., and Einstein, E. R., 1970, Physical properties of the encephalitogenic protein: Molecular weight and conformation, *J. Neurochem.* **17**:1121–1132.

Csejtey, J., Hallpike, J. F., Adams, C. W. M., and Bayliss, O. B., 1972, Histochemistry of myelin. XIV. Peripheral nerve myelin proteins: Electrophoretic and histochemical correlations, *J. Neurochem.* **19**:1931–1935.

Daile, P., and Carnegie, P. R., 1975, Sites of phosphorylation by cyclic AMP-dependent protein kinases, in preparation.

Davison, A. N., 1961, Metabolically inert proteins of the central and peripheral nervous system, muscle, and tendon, *Biochem. J.* **78**:272–282.

Davison, A. N., 1970, The biochemistry of the myelin sheath, *in Myelination* (A. N. Davison and A. Peters, eds.), pp. 80–161, Charles C. Thomas, Illinois.

Davison, A. N., 1971, The biochemistry of myelinogenesis in the central nervous system, *in Chemistry and Brain Development* (R. Paoletti and A. N. Davison, eds.), pp. 375–380, Plenum Press, New York.

Dayhoff, M. D., 1972, *in Atlas of Protein Sequence and Structure*, Vol. 5, National Biochemical Research Foundation, Silver Spring, Md.

Deibler, G. E., and Martenson, R. E., 1973a, Chromatographic fractionation of myelin basic protein: Partial characterization and methylarginine contents of the multiple forms, *J. Biol. Chem.* **248**:2392–2396.

Deibler, G. E., and Martenson, R. E., 1973b, Determination of methylated basic amino acids with the amino acid analyser: Application to total acid hydrolysates of myelin basic proteins, *J. Biol. Chem.* **248**:2387–2391.

Deibler, G. E., Martenson, R. E., and Kies, M. W., 1970, Gel filtration of proteins at acid pH application to molecular weight estimation of myelin basic proteins, *Biochim. Biophys. Acta* **200**:342–352.

Deibler, G. E., Martenson, R. E., and Kies, M. W., 1972, Large scale preparation of myelin basic protein from central nervous tissue of several mammalian species, *Prep. Biochem.* **2**:139–165.

Demel, R. A., London, Y., Geurts Van Kessel, W. S., Vossenberg, F. G., and Deenen, L. L. Van, 1973, The specific interaction of myelin basic protein with lipids at the air–water interface, *Biochim. Biophys. Acta* **311**:507–519.

Dickinson, J. P., Jones, K. M., Aparicio, S. R., and Lumsden, C. E., 1970, Localization of encephalitogenic basic protein in the intraperiod line of lamellar myelin, *Nature (London)* **227**:1133–1134.

D'Monte, B., Mela, P., and Marks, N., 1971, Metabolic instability of myelin protein and proteolipid fractions, *Eur. J. Biochem.* **23**:355–365.

Driscoll, B. F., Kramer, A. J., and Kies, M. W., 1974, Myelin basic protein: location of multiple independent antigenic regions, *Science* **184**:73–75.

Dunkley, P. R., and Carnegie, P. R., 1974a, Isolation of myelin basic proteins, *in Research Methods in Neurochemistry* (N. Marks and R. Rodnight, eds.), Vol. 2, pp. 219–245, Plenum Press, New York.

Dunkley, P. R., and Carnegie, P. R., 1974b, Sequence of a rat myelin basic protein, *Biochem. J.* **141**:243–255.

Dunkley, P. R., Coates, A. S., and Carnegie, P. R., 1973, Encephalitogenic activity of peptides from the smaller basic protein of rat brain myelin, *J. Immunol.* **110**:1699–1701.

Einstein, E. R., 1972, Basic protein of myelin and its role in experimental allergic encephalomyelitis and multiple sclerosis, *Handbook of Neurochemistry* 7:107–129.

Einstein, E. R., 1974, Protein and enzyme changes with brain development, *in Drugs and the Developing Brain* (A. Vernadakis and N. Weiner, eds.), pp. 375–393, Plenum Press, New York.

Einstein, E. R., Csejtey, J., Davis, W., and Rauch, M., 1965, Studies on encephalitogenic protein of human brain origin, *Proc. 8th Int. Cong. Neurol.* 4:137–153.

Einstein, E. R., Csejtey, J., and Marks, N., 1968, Degradation of encephalitogen by purified brain acid proteinase, *FEBS Letters* 1:191–195.

Einstein, E. R., Dalal, K. B., and Csejtey, J., 1970, Biochemical maturation of the central nervous system. II. Protein and proteolytic enzyme changes, *Brain Res.* 18:35–49.

Einstein, E. R., Csejtey, J., Dalal, K. B., Adams, C. W. M., Bayliss, O. B., and Hallpike, J. F., 1972, Proteolytic activity and basic protein loss in and around multiple sclerosis plaques: Combined biochemical and histochemical observations, *J. Neurochem.* 19:653–662.

Eng, L. F., Chao, F. C., Gerstl, B., Pratt, D., and Tavaststjerna, M. G., 1968, The Maturation of human white matter myelin: Fractionation of the myelin membrane proteins, *Biochemistry* 7:4455–4465.

Epand, R. M., Moscarello, M. A., Zierenberg, B., and Vail, W. J., 1974, The folded conformation of the encephalitogenic protein of human brain, *Biochemistry* 13:1264–1267.

Everly, J. L., Brady, R. O., and Quarles, R. H., 1973, Evidence that the major protein in rat sciatic nerve myelin is a glycoprotein, *J. Neurochem.* 21:329–334.

Eylar, E. H., 1970, Amino acid sequence of the basic protein of myelin membrane, *Proc. Nat. Acad. Sci. (U.S.A.)* 67:1425–1431.

Eylar, E. H., 1972, The structure and immunologic properties of basic proteins of myelin, *Ann. N.Y. Acad. Sci.* 195:481–491.

Eylar, E. H., 1973, Myelin-specific proteins, *in Proteins of the Nervous System* (D. J. Schneider, R. H. Angeletti, R. A. Bradshaw, A. Grasso, and B. W. Moore, eds.), pp. 27–44, Raven Press, New York.

Eylar, E. H., and Thompson, M., 1969, Allergic encephalomyelitis: The physicochemical properties of the basic protein encephalitogen from bovine spinal cord, *Arch. Biochem. Biophys.* 129:468–479.

Eylar, E. H., Salk, J., Beveridge, G. C., and Brown, L. V., 1969, Experimental allergic encephalomyelitis: An encephalitogenic basic protein from bovine myelin, *Arch. Biochem. Biophys.* 132:34–48.

Eylar, E. H., Brostoff, S., Hashim, G., Caccam, J., and Burnett, P., 1971, Basic A_1 protein of the myelin membrane: The complete amino acid sequence, *J. Biol. Chem.* 246:5770–5784.

Eylar, E. H., Brostoff, S., Jackson, J., and Carter, H., 1972, Allergic encephalomyelitis in monkeys induced by a peptide from the A_1 protein. *Proc. Nat. Acad. Sci. (U.S.A.)* 69:617–619.

Finch, P. R., and Moscarello, M. A., 1972, A myelin protein fraction extracted with thioethanol, *Brain Res.* 42:177–187.

Fischer, C. A., and Morell, P., 1974a, Turnover of proteins in myelin and myelin-like material of mouse brain, *Brain Res.* 74:51–65.

Fischer, C. A., and Morell, P., 1974b, Precursor dependent turnover measures of proteins in myelin and myelin-like material during development, *Society for Neuroscience* (Abstract).

Folch-Pi, J., 1972, Proteolipids, *in Functional and Structural Proteins of the Nervous System* (A. N. Davison, P. Mandel, and I. G. Morgan, eds.), pp. 171–199, Plenum Press, New York.

Gaitonde, M. K., and Martenson, R. E., 1970, Metabolism of highly basic proteins of rat brain during postnatal development, *J. Neurochem.* **17**:551–563.

Giorgi, P. P., Karlsson, J. O., Sjostrand, J., and Field, E. J., 1973, Axonal flow and myelin protein in the optic pathway, *Nature (London)* **244**:121–124.

Gonzalez-Sastre, F., 1970, The protein composition of isolated myelin, *J. Neurochem.* **17**:1049–1056.

Gould, R. M., and London, Y., 1972, Specific interaction of central nervous system myelin basic protein with lipids: Effects of basic protein on glucose leakage from liposomes, *Biochim. Biophys. Acta* **290**:200–218.

Greenfield, S., Norton, W. T., and Morell, P., 1971, Quaking mouse: Isolation and characterization of myelin protein, *J. Neurochem.* **18**:2119–2128.

Greenfield, S., Brostoff, S., Eylar, E. H., and Morell, P., 1973, Protein composition of myelin of the peripheral nervous system, *J. Neurochem.* **20**:1207–1216.

Hagopian, A., and Eylar, E. H., 1968, Glycoprotein biosynthesis: Studies on the receptor specificity of the polypeptidyl *N*-acetylgalactosaminyl transferase from bovine submaxillary glands, *Arch. Biochem. Biophys.* **128**:422–433.

Hagopian, A., Westall, F. C., Whitehead, J. S., and Eylar, E. H., 1971, Glycosylation of the A$_1$ protein from myelin by a polypeptide *N*-acetylgalactosaminyl transferase: Identification of the receptor sequence, *J. Biol. Chem.* **246**:2519–2523.

Hashim, G. A., and Eylar, E. H., 1969a, Allergic encephalomyelitis: Isolation and characterization of encephalitogenic peptides from the basic protein of bovine spinal cord, *Arch. Biochem. Biophys.* **129**:645–654.

Hashim, G. A., and Eylar, E. H., 1969b, The structure of the terminal regions of the encephalitogenic A$_1$ protein, *Biochem. Biophys. Res. Comm.* **34**:770–776.

Hashim, G. A., Hwang, F., and Schilling, F. J., 1973, Experimental allergic encephalomyelitis: Basic protein regions responsible for delayed hypersensitivity, *Arch. Biochem. Biophys.* **156**:298–309.

Hergstrand, L. R., and Kornguth, S. E., 1973, Isolation and partial characterization of the myelin basic protein from foetal calf brains, *Biochim. Biophys. Acta* **317**:380–393.

Herndon, R. M., Rauch, H. C., and Einstein, E. R., 1973, Immuno-electron microscopic localization of the encephalitogenic basic protein in myelin, *Immunol. Commun.* **2**:163–172.

Hulcher, F., Spudis, E., and Netsky, M. G., 1963, Encephalomyelitis induced by the white matter fraction, *Arch. Neurol. (Chic.)* **8**:1–7.

Jones, G., and Carnegie, P. R., 1974, Methylation of myelin basic protein by enzymes from rat brain, *J. Neurochem.* **23**:1231–1237.

Kabat, E. A., Wolf, A., and Bozer, A. E., 1947, The rapid production of acute disseminated encephalomyelitis in rhesus monkeys by injection of heterogeneous and homologous brain tissue with adjuvants, *J. Exptl. Med.* **85**:117–131.

Kibler, R. F., Fox, R. H., and Shapira, R., 1964, Isolation of a highly purified encephalitogenic protein from bovine cord, *Nature (London)* **204**:1273–1275.

Kibler, R. F., Re, P. K., McKneally, S., and Shapira, R., 1972, Biological activity of an encephalitogenic fragment in the monkey, *J. Biol. Chem.* **247**:969–972.

Kies, M. W., 1965, Chemical studies on an encephalitogenic protein from guinea pig brain, *Ann. N.Y. Acad. Sci.* **122**:161–170.

Kies, M. W., 1973, Experimental allergic encephalomyelitis, *in Biology of Brain Dysfunction* (G. E. Gaul, ed.), Vol. II, pp. 185–224, Plenum Press, New York.

Kies, M. W., and Alvord, E. C., Jr., 1959, Encephalitogenic activity in guinea pigs of water soluble protein fractions of nervous tissue, *in Allergic Encephalomyelitis* (M. W. Kies, and E. C. Alvord, Jr., eds.), pp. 293–299, Charles C. Thomas, Illinois.

Kies, M. W., Gordon, S., Laatsch, R. H., and Alvord, E. C., Jr., 1961, Cellular localization of allergic encephalomyelitic activity in guinea pig brain, *in Proceedings International Congress of Neuropathology* (H. Jacob, ed.), pp. 20–29, Georg Thieme Verlag, Stuttgart.

Kies, M. W., Thompson, E. B., and Alvord, E. C., Jr., 1965, The relationship of myelin proteins to experimental allergic encephalomyelitis, *Ann. N.Y. Acad. Sci.* **122**:148–160.

Ko, G. K. W., and Raghupathy, E., 1972, Glycoprotein biosynthesis in the developing rat brain. II. Microsomal galactosaminyl transferase utilizing endogenous and exogenous protein acceptors, *Biochim. Biophys. Acta* **264**:129–143.

Kornguth, S. E., and Perrin, J. H., 1971, Circular dichroism and viscometric studies on a basic protein from pig brain, *J. Neurochem.* **18**:983–988.

Kornguth, S. E., Kozel, L. R., and Smithies, O., 1972, Tissue specific histone, probable identity with encephalitogenic protein, *Nature (New Biol.)* **237**:49–50.

Krigbaum, W. R., and Knutton, S. P., 1973, Prediction of the amount of secondary structure in a globular protein from its amino acid composition, *Proc. Nat. Acad. Sci. (U.S.A.)* **70**:2809–2813.

Laatsch, R. H., Kies, M. W., Gordon, S., and Alvord, E. C., Jr., 1962, The encephalitogenic activity of myelin isolates by ultracentrifugation, *J. Exptl. Med.* **115**:777–788.

Lajtha, A., and Marks, N., 1971, Protein turnover, *Handbook of Neurochemistry* **5B**:551–630.

Leach, S. J., and Smith, J. A., 1972, Thermal perturbation difference spectroscopy of proteins, *Int. J. Protein Research*, **4**:11–19.

Lennon, V. A., 1972, Cellular and humoral immune responses in experimental autoimmune encephalomyelitis, Ph.D. Thesis, Melbourne University.

Lennon, V. A., Wilks, A. V., and Carnegie, P. R., 1970, Immunologic properties of the main encephalitogenic peptide from the basic protein of human myelin, *J. Immunol.* **10**:1223–1230.

Lim, L., White, J. O., Hall, C., Berthold, W., and Davison, A. N., 1974, Isolation of microsomal poly(A)-RNA from rat brain directing the synthesis of the myelin encephalitogenic protein in *Xenopus* oocytes, *Biochim. Biophys. Acta* **361**:241–247.

London, Y., 1971, Ox peripheral nerve myelin membrane: Purification and partial characterization of two basic proteins, *Biochim. Biophys. Acta* **249**:188–196.

London, Y., 1972, Preparation of purified myelin from ox intradural spinal roots by rate-isopycnic zonal centrifugation, *Biochim. Biophys. Acta* **282**:195–204.

London, Y., and Vossenberg, F. G. A., 1973, Specific interaction of central nervous system myelin basic protein with lipids: Specific regions of the protein sequence protected from proteolytic action of trypsin, *Biochim. Biophys. Acta* **307**:478–490.

London, Y., Demel, R. A., Geurts Van Kessel, W. S., Vossenberg, F. G., and Deenen, L. L. Van, 1973, The protection of A_1 myelin basic protein against the action of proteolytic enzymes after interaction of the protein with lipids at the air–water interface, *Biochim. Biophys. Acta* **311**:520–530.

London, Y., Demel, R. A., Geurts Van Kessel, W. S., Zahler, P., and Deenen, L. L. Van, 1974, The interaction of the "Folch–Lees" protein with lipids at the air–water interface, *Biochim. Biophys. Acta* **332**:69–84.

Lumsden, C. E., Robertson, D. M., and Blight, R., 1966, Chemical studies on experimental allergic encephalitogenic "antigens," *J. Neurochem.* **13**:127–162.

Lycke, E., and Roos, B.-E., 1973, Brain monoamines in guinea pigs with experimental allergic encephalomyelitis, *Int. Arch. Allergy* **45**:341–351.

McFarland, H. F., 1970, Immunofluorescent study of circulating antibody in experimental allergic encephalomyelitis, *Proc. Soc. Exptl. Biol. Med.* **133**:1195–1200.

McFarlin, D. E., Blank, S. E., Kibler, R. F., McKneally, S., and Shapira, R., 1973, Experimental allergic encephalomyelitis in the rat: Response to encephalitogenic proteins and peptides, *Science* **179**:478–480.

Mackay, I. R., Carnegie, P. R., and Coates, A. S., 1973, Immunopathological comparisons between experimental autoimmune encephalomyelitis and multiple sclerosis: A review, *Clin. Exp. Immunol.* **15**:471–482.

Mandel, P., Nussbaum, J. L., Neskovic, N. M., Sarlieve, L. L., and Kurihara, T., 1972, Regulation of myelinogenesis, *Advances in Enzyme Regulation* **10**:101–117.

Marks, N., and Lajtha, A., 1965, Separation of acid and neutral proteinases in brain, *Biochem. J.* **97**:74–83.

Marks, N., and Lajtha, A., 1971, Protein and polypeptide breakdown, *Handbook of Neurochemistry* **5A**:49–140.

Martenson, R. E., Deibler, G. E., and Kies, M. W., 1970, Myelin basic proteins of the rat central nervous system, *Biochim. Biophys. Acta* **200**:353–362.

Martenson, R. E., Deibler, G. E., and Kies, M. W., 1971*a*, The occurrence of two myelin basic proteins in the central nervous system of rodents in the suborders *Myomorpha* and *Sciuromorpha*, *J. Neurochem.* **18**:2427–2433.

Martenson, R. E., Deibler, G. E., and Kies, M. W., 1971*b*, Comparison of amino acid sequences of hypothalamic peptide, brain-specific histone and myelin basic protein, *Nature (New Biol.)* **234**:87–89.

Martenson, R. E., Deibler, G. E., Kies, M. W., Levine, S., and Alvord, E. C., Jr., 1972*a*, Myelin basic proteins of mammalian and submammalian vertebrates: Encephalitogenic activities in guinea pigs and rats, *J. Immunol.* **109**:262–270.

Martenson, R. E., Deibler, G. E., Kies, M. W., McKneally, S. S., Shapira, R., and Kibler, R. F., 1972*b*, Differences between the two myelin basic proteins of the rat central nervous system, *Biochim. Biophys. Acta* **263**:193–203.

Martenson, R. E., Kramer, A. J., Deibler, G. E., and Levine, S., 1975, Comparative studies of guinea pig and bovine myelin basic proteins: Partial characterization of chemically derived fragments and their encephalitogenic activities in Lewis rats, *J. Neurochem.* **24**:173–182.

Matthieu, J. M., Widmer, S., and Herschkowitz, N., 1973*a*, Biochemical changes in mouse brain composition during myelination, *Brain. Res.* **55**:391–402.

Matthieu, J. M., Widmer, S., and Herschkowitz, N., 1973*b*, Jimpy, an anomaly of myelin maturation: biochemical study of myelination phases, *Brain Res.* **55**:403–412.

Matthieu, J. M., Quarles, R. H., Brady, R. O., and Webster, H., 1973*c*, Variation of proteins, enzyme markers and gangliosides in myelin subfractions, *Biochim. Biophys. Acta* **329**:305–317.

Mehl, E., 1972, Separation and characterization of myelin proteins, *in Functional and Structural Proteins of the Nervous System* (A. N. Davison, P. Mandel, and I. G. Morgan, eds.), pp. 157–170, Plenum Press, New York.

Mehl, E., and Halaris, A., 1970, Stoichiometric relation of protein components in cerebral myelin from different species, *J. Neurochem.* **17**:659–668.

Mehl, E., and Wolfgram, E., 1969, Myelin types with different protein components in the same species, *J. Neurochem.* **16**:1091–1097.

Miyake, M., and Kakimoto, Y., 1973, Protein methylation by cerebral tissue, *J. Neurochem.* **20**:859–871.

Miyamoto, E., and Kakiuchi, S., 1974, In vitro and in vivo phosphorylation of myelin basic protein by exogenous and endogenous adenosine 3',5'-monophosphate-dependent protein kinases from brain, *J. Biol. Chem.* **249**:2769–2777.

Miyamoto, E., Kakiuchi, S., and Kakimoto, Y., 1974, *In vitro* and *in vivo* phosphorylation of myelin basic protein by cerebral protein kinase, *Nature (London)* **249**:150.

Morell, P., Greenfield, S., Costantino-Ceccarini, E., and Wisniewski, H., 1972, Changes in the protein composition of mouse brain myelin during development, *J. Neurochem.* **19**:2545–2554.

Morell, P., Lipkind, R., and Greenfield, S., 1973, Protein composition of myelin from brain and spinal cord of several species, *Brain Res.* **58**:510–514.

Morgan, I. M., 1947, Allergic encephalomyelitis in monkeys in response to injection of normal monkey nervous tissue, *J. Exptl. Med.* **85**:131–140.

Morris, S. J., Louis, C. F., and Shooter, E. M., 1971, Separation of myelin proteins on two different polyacrylamide gel systems, *Neurobiology* **1**:64–67.

Nakao, A., and Einstein, E. R., 1965, Chemical and immunochemical studies with the dialyzable encepholitogenic compound from bovine spinal cord, *Ann. N.Y. Acad. Sci.* **122**:171–181.

Nakao, A., Davis, W. J., and Einstein, E. R., 1966a, Basic proteins from the acidic extract of bovine spinal cord, *Biochim. Biophys. Acta* **130**:171–179.

Nakao, A., Davis, W. J., and Einstein, E. R., 1966b, Basic proteins from the acidic extract of bovine spinal cord, *Biochim. Biophys. Acta* **130**:163–170.

Norton, W. T., 1972, Myelin, *in Basic Neurochemistry* (R. W. Albers, G. J. Siegel, R. Katzman, and B. W. Agranoff, eds.), pp. 365–386, Little, Brown & Co., Boston.

Norton, W. T., and Poduslo, S. E., 1973a, Myelination in rat brain: Method of myelin isolation, *J. Neurochem.* **21**:749–757.

Norton, W. T., and Poduslo, S. E., 1973b, Myelination in rat brain: Changes in myelin composition during brain maturation, *J. Neurochem.* **21**:759–773.

Nussbaum, J. L., and Mandel, P., 1973, Brain proteolipids in neurological mutant mice, *Brain Res.* **61**:295–310.

Olson, R. E., Klay, M., Good, R. A., and Condie, R. M., 1962, The encephalitogenic properties of bovine central nervous tissue fractions, *J. Neuropath. Exptl. Neurol.* **21**:461–470.

Oshiro, Y., and Eylar, E. H., 1970, Allergic encephalomyelitis: Preparation of the encephalitogenic basic protein from bovine brain, *Arch. Biochem.* **138**:392–396.

Paik, W. K., and Kim, S., 1971, Protein methylation: Enzymatic methylation of proteins after translation may take part in control of biological activities of proteins, *Science* **174**:114–119.

Paik, W. K., and Kim, S., 1973, Protein methylases during development of rat brain, *Biochim. Biophys. Acta* **313**:181–189.

Palmer, F. B., and Dawson, R. M. C., 1969a, The isolation and properties of experimental allergic encephalitogenic protein, *Biochem. J.* **111**:629–636.

Palmer, F. B., and Dawson, R. M. C., 1969b, Complex formation between triphosphoinositide and experimental allergic encephalitogenic proteins, *Biochem. J.* **111**:637–646.

Palo, J., Savolainen, H., and Haltia, M., 1972, Proteins of peripheral nerve myelin in diabetic neuropathy, *J. Neurol. Sci.* **16**:193–199.

Paty, D. W., 1971, An encephalitogenic basic protein from human peripheral nerve, *Europ. Neurol.* **5**:281–287.

Peters, A., and Vaughn, J. E., 1970, Morphology and development of the myelin sheath, *in Myelination* (A. N. Davison, and A. Peters, eds.), pp. 3–79, Charles C. Thomas, Illinois.

Pfeiffer, S. E., and Wechsler, W., 1972, Biochemically differentiated neoplastic clone of Schwann cells, *Proc. Natl. Acad. Sci. (U.S.A.)* **69**:2885–2889.

Pleasure, D. E., Feldmann, B., and Prockop, D. J., 1973, Diphtheria toxin inhibits the synthesis of myelin proteolipid and basic proteins by peripheral nerve *in vitro*, *J. Neurochem.* **20**:81–90.

Quarles, R. H., Everly, J. L., and Brady, R. O., 1973, Evidence for the close association of a glycoprotein with myelin in rat brain, *J. Neurochem.* **21**:1177–1191.

Quelin, S., and Brahic, M., 1973, Purification of basic encephalitogenic protein from brain of sheep, *C. R. Acad. Sci. (Paris)* **277**:2565–2568.

Raghavan, S. S., Rhoads, D. B., and Kanfer, J. N., 1973, The effects of trypsin on purified myelin, *Biochim. Biophys. Acta* **328**:205–212.

Rauch, H. C., and Raffels, S., 1964, Immunofluorescent localization of encephalitogenic protein in myelin, *J. Immunol.* **92**:452–455.

Rivers, T. M., and Schwentker, F. F., 1935, Encephalomyelitis accompanied by myelin destruction experimentally produced in monkeys, *J. Exptl. Med.* **61**:689–702.

Robertson, D. M., Blight, R., and Lumsden, C. E., 1962, Dialysable peptide as the causative factor in experimental "allergic" encephalomyelitis, *Nature (London)* **196**:1005.

Roboz, E., and Henderson, N., 1959, Preparation and properties of water soluble proteins from bovine cord with "allergic" encephalomyelitis activity, *in Allergic Encephalomyelitis* (M. W. Kies and E. C. Alvord, Jr., eds.), pp. 281–292, Charles C. Thomas, Illinois.

Rodriguez de Lores Arnaiz, G., Aberici de Canal, M., and de Robertis, E., 1971, Turnover of proteins in subcellular fractions of rat cerebral cortex, *Brain Res.* **31**:179–184.

Sammeck, R., 1973, Myelin sheath: Turnover of myelin basic proteins during morphogenesis, *in Abstracts Fourth Meeting International Society for Neurochemistry*, p. 189, Tokyo.

Sammeck, R., and Brady, R. O., 1972, Studies of the catabolism of myelin basic proteins in the rat *in situ* and *in vitro*, *Brain Res.* **42**:441–453.

Sammeck, R., Martenson, R. E., and Brady, R. O., 1971, Studies of the metabolism of myelin basic proteins in various regions of the central nervous system of immature and adult rats, *Brain Res.* **34**:241–254.

Savolainen, H. J., 1972, Proteins and glycoproteins of human myelin and glial cell membrane with special reference to myelin formation, *Tower Int. Technomed. J. Life Sci.* **2**:35–38.

Savolainen, H., and Palo, J., 1972, Proteins of human glial cell membrane, *FEBS Letters* **20**:71–74.

Savolainen, H., Palo, J., Riekkinen, P., Moronen, P., and Brody, L. E., 1972, Maturation of myelin proteins in human brain, *Brain Res.* **37**:253–263.

Scheinberg, L. C., and Korey, S. R., 1958, Studies of white matter, *J. Neuropathol. Exptl. Neurol.* **17**:439–449.

Shapira, R., Chou, F. C-H., McKneally, S. S., Urban, E., and Kibler, R. F., 1971*a*, Biological activity and synthesis of an encephalitogenic determinant, *Science* **173**:736–738.

Shapira, R., McKneally, S. S., Chou, F., and Kibler, R. F., 1971*b*, Encephalitogenic fragment of myelin basic protein, *J. Biol. Chem.* **246**:4630–4640.

Shooter, E. M., and Einstein, E. R., 1971, Proteins of the nervous system, *Ann. Rev. Biochem.* **40**:635–652.

Smith, M., 1968, The turnover of myelin in the adult rat, *Biochim. Biophys. Acta* **164**:285–293.

Smith, M., 1972, The turnover of myelin proteins, *Neurobiology* **2**:35–40.

Smith, M. E., 1973*a*, A regional survey of myelin development: Some compositional and metabolic aspects, *J. Lipid Res.* **14**:541–551.

Smith, M. E., 1973*b*, Studies of the mechanism of demyelination: Triethyl tin induced demyelination, *J. Neurochem.* **21**:357–372.

Smythies, J. R., Benington, F., and Morin, F. D., 1970, Specifications of a possible serotonin receptor site in the brain, *Neurosciences Res. Prog. Bull.* **8**:117–122.

Soto, E. F., 1964, Induction of experimental allergic encephalomyelitis with a myelin fraction obtained from bovine white matter. *Neurology* **14**:938–948.

Steck, A. J., and Appel. S. H., 1974, Phosphorylation of myelin basic protein, *J. Biol. Chem.* **249**:5416–5420.

Sundarraj, N., and Pfeiffer, S. E., 1973, Myelin basic protein arginine methyl transferase: Wide distribution among both neurogenic and non-neurogenic tissues, *Biochem. Biophys. Res. Commun.* **52**:1039–1045.

Tomasi, L., and Kornguth, S. E., 1967, Purification and partial characterization of a basic protein from pig brain, *J. Biol. Chem.* **242**:4933–4938.

Uyemura, K., Tobari, C., and Hirano, S., 1970, Purifications and properties of basic proteins in pig spinal cord and peripheral nerve, *Biochim. Biophys. Acta* **214**:190–197.

Uyemura, K., Tobari, C., Hirano, S., and Tsukada, Y., 1972, Comparative studies on the myelin proteins of bovine peripheral nerve and spinal cord, *J. Neurochem.* **19**:2607–2614.

Uyemura, K., Kitamura, K., and Ogawa, Y., 1975, Studies on the antigenic protein to induce experimental allergic neuritis (EAN), *Acta Neuropathologica* (in press).

Westall, F. C., 1972, Solid phase peptide synthesis as applied to experimental allergic encephalomyelitis, *in Multiple Sclerosis* (E. J. Field, T. M. Bell, and P. R. Carnegie, eds.), pp. 72–79, North-Holland Publ. Co., Amsterdam.

Westall, F. C., 1973, An explanation for the determination of "self" and "non-self" proteins, *J. Theoret. Biol.* **38**:139–141.

Westall, F. C., 1974, Released myelin basic protein: The immunogenic factor? *Immunochemistry.* **11**:513–515.

Westall, F. C., Robinson, A. B., Caccam, J., Jackson, J., and Eylar, E. H., 1971, Essential chemical requirements for induction of allergic encephalomyelitis, *Nature (London)* **229**:22–24.

White, S. R., White, F. P., Barnes, C. D., and Albright, J. F., 1973, Increased shock sensitivity in rats with experimental allergic encephalomyelitis and reversal by 5-hydroxytryptophan, *Brain Res.* **58**:251–254.

Whittingham, S., Bencina, B., Carnegie, P. R., and McPherson, T. A., 1972, Properties of antibodies produced in rabbits to human myelin and myelin basic protein, *Int. Arch. Allergy Appl. Immunol.* **42**:250–263.

Wolman, M., 1971, Distribution of various protein fractions in central and peripheral myelin, *Exptl. Neurol.* **30**:309–323.

Wood, J. G., and Dawson, R. M. C., 1973a, A major myelin glycoprotein of sciatic nerve, *J. Neurochem.* **21**:717–719.

Wood, J. G., and Dawson, R. M. C., 1973b, The effect of trypsin on the proteins and lipids of myelin, *in* "Abstracts Fourth Meeting International Society for Neurochemistry," Tokyo, p. 187.

Wood, J. G., and King, N., 1971, Turnover of basic protein of rat brain, *Nature (London)* **229**:56–58.

CHAPTER 4

BRAIN-SPECIFIC PROTEINS:
S-100 Protein, 14-3-2 Protein,
and Glial Fibrillary Protein

BLAKE W. MOORE

Department of Psychiatry
Washington University School of Medicine
St. Louis, Missouri

1. INTRODUCTION

The differentiated forms and functions of a specialized cell are expressed through the properties of its individual proteins, properties which are determined by their primary structure. Nervous system cells, having extremely specialized functions, are among the most highly differentiated of all types of cells. Therefore, it is important to know which proteins are specific to nervous system cells since these particular proteins would be related to specific functions within the nervous system, such as propagation of action potentials, synaptic transmission involving several chemical transmitters—each with its associated processes of synthesis, inactivation, release, and receptor activity, establishment of specific pathways and connections, action of supportive cells such as various types of glia, and many other functions.

There are, in theory, several possible ways of looking for proteins specific for nervous tissue. One way is to look for a protein responsible for or associated with a particular structure or function specific to the nervous system. This method has been successful, for example, in studying specific proteins of myelin (proteolipid, basic encephalitogenic protein, Wolfgram protein, DM-20), in studying proteins related to synaptic transmission (enzymes of transmitter synthesis, receptors, inactivating enzymes) and less successfully in studying proteins associated with learning and memory.

Another general approach is to screen proteins of the nervous system to find those which are organ specific, that is, present in brain of all species, but absent in other tissues. Organ specific proteins which are related to organ-specific functions have long been known and studied, for example, hemoglobin in red cells and myosin in muscle.

In the last decade, the search for specific proteins in the nervous system has been made feasible by the development of a number of techniques for studying proteins. Fractionation methods have been greatly improved, particularly chromatography of proteins on ion exchange and molecular sieve columns, and zone electrophoresis of proteins on starch or polyacrylamide gels. Methods for fractionating "insoluble" or membrane proteins have also been developed, particularly the use of SDS polyacrylamide gel electrophoresis. Methods for microassay of specific proteins have been improved, particularly the use of immunochemical methods such as complement fixation and radioimmunoassay. Furthermore, better methods of separating the nervous system into component parts have been developed. Batch and single-cell methods for separating neurons from glia have been developed. Methods for preparing reasonably pure nerve-ending particles and synaptic membranes have been worked out (Eichberg *et al.*, 1964; DeLores *et al.*, 1967; Cotman and Matthews, 1971; Morgan *et al.*, 1971). Cell cultures of a number of cloned neuroblastoma and glioma cell types have been grown which retain many of the characteristics of nontumor cells (Benda *et al.*, 1968; Schubert *et al.*, 1974). Current research on specific proteins in nervous systems has relied on all of these techniques, as will be shown later.

2. THE S-100 AND 14-3-2 PROTEINS

2.1. Protein Maps

The "protein map" technique was worked out as a means of looking for specific proteins in the nervous system (Moore and McGregor, 1965). Extracts from brain and other organs (such as liver) were prepared by homogenizing tissue in buffer of low ionic strength and centrifuging at high speed. The soluble proteins in the supernatant fraction were the starting material, which was first chromatographed by salt gradient elution from DEAE–cellulose columns. Chromatographic fractions were then further separated by gel electrophoresis on starch or polyacrylamide giving "two-dimensional protein maps" of the soluble proteins of the extracts. Brain was characterized by having a high proportion of relatively small, acidic proteins compared to liver or other organs. Some of these proteins have been purified from brain, two of which, S-100 and 14-3-2, have been thoroughly studied and shown to be brain specific.

2.2. Preparation and Properties

The general method of preparation of S-100 and 14-3-2 (Moore, 1965; Moore, 1972) is outlined in Figure 1. Approximately 50–100 mg of each protein can be obtained from a kilogram (wet weight) of beef brain. The S-100 protein has a molecular weight of 21,000–24,000 daltons (Moore, 1965; Dannies and Levine, 1971a). There is evidence that it has three subunits of about 7000 daltons each (Dannies and Levine, 1969; 1971a). These cannot be identical since there is a single tryptophan residue per molecule of S-100 (Moore, 1965). The amino acid analysis of S-100 is shown in Table 1. The high content of glutamic and aspartic acid residues is reflected in the high electrophoretic mobility of S-100 on polyacrylamide gel electrophoresis. Both proteins, after preparation from either beef or rabbit brain by the method shown in Figure 1, are pure as judged by gel electrophoresis (SDS

TABLE 1. Amino Acid Analysis of Beef S-100[a]

Glu 36	Tyr 3
Asp 21	Pro 1
Lys 17	Phe 16
His 8	Leu 17
Arg 3	Ileu 6
Ser 10	Val 13
Thr 8	Ala 12
Cys 3	Gly 9
Try 1	Met 4

[a] Values represent numbers of residues per 24,000 daltons to the nearest whole number.

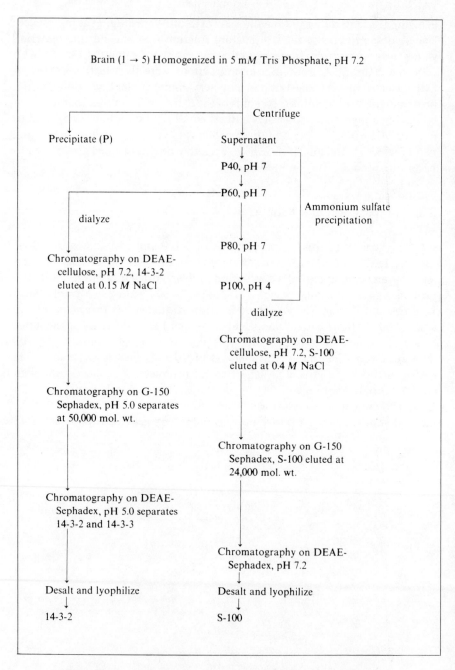

FIGURE 1.   Flow chart for preparation of S-100 and 14-3-2 proteins.

and non-SDS), chromatography, and ultracentrifugation. According to
Kessler *et al.* (1968) the ORD spectrum of native S-100 indicates a helix
content of about 40%. S-100 has also been prepared from human brain
(Uozumi and Ryan, 1973). Aggregation involving disulfide bond formation
tends to occur in S-100. This result can be reversed by heating with 0.01 *M*
2-mercaptoethanol (Dannies and Levine, 1971*b*).

2.3. Immunological Assays for S-100 and 14-3-2

Since the functions of S-100 and 14-3-2 are not known, an assay (such
as enzymatic) based on function is not available. Consequently, immuno-
assays have been developed. Antiserum was first prepared to S-100 (Levine
and Moore, 1965) by conjugating the protein with methylated bovine serum
albumin and injecting the conjugate (with Freund's adjuvant) into rabbits.
Later, antiserum to 14-3-2 was made in the same way. Antisera to both S-100
and 14-3-2 show single precipitin bands by double agar diffusion against

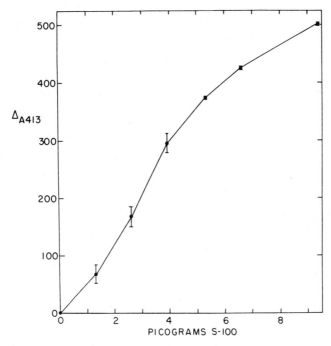

FIGURE 2. Standard curve (beef brain S-100) for micro-complement
fixation assay for S-100 (from Moore and Perez, *J. Immunol.* **96**:101,
Figure 1).

either pure protein or brain extract. No cross-reaction occurs between S-100 and 14-3-2. A complement fixation assay (Moore *et al.*, 1968) based on the method of Wasserman and Levine (1961) was worked out to measure S-100 and 14-3-2 quantitatively with high sensitivity (0.5 to 5 ng) and specificity. The assay was also scaled down to the picogram level (Moore and Perez, 1966) so that assays could be done on single cells or small pieces of nervous tissue such as frozen dried sections of cerebellum (Figure 2). Radioimmunoassay has also been done for S-100 (Uozumi and Ryan, 1973). In this case, the sensitivity was of the order of 1 ng S-100 for the human protein.

2.4. Organ and Species Specificity

2.4.1. *Specificity to Nervous Tissue*

Both S-100 and 14-3-2 are specific to the nervous system (Table 2, Figure 3), that is (by complement fixation assay), brain contains at least 10,000 times more S-100 and 200 times more 14-3-2 than any other organ in the rat (Moore, 1965; Moore and Perez, 1968). Both proteins are also present in optic nerve (Perez *et al.*, 1970) and tibial nerve (Perez and Moore, 1968), as well as in the central nervous system.

TABLE 2. Complement Fixation by Dilutions of Rat Organ Extracts with Anti-Beef S-100 or Anti-Beef 14-3-2

	Dilutions	Brain	Liver	Kidney	Heart	Spleen	Muscle	Intestine
S-100	1	+	+	+	−	−	+	−
	10	+ +	−	−	−	−	±	−
	30	+ +	−	−	−	−	−	−
	100	+ +	−	−	−	−	−	−
	300	+ +	−	−	−	−	−	−
	1,000	+ +	−	−	−	−	−	−
	3,000	+ +	−	−	−	−	−	−
	10,000	±	−	−	−	−	−	−
	30,000	−	−	−	−	−	−	−
14-3-2	3	+	+ +	+ +	+ +	+ +	+ +	+ +
	9	+	+ +	+	+	+	+	+ +
	27	+	+	−	−	−	−	+
	81	+ +	−	−	−	−	−	−
	243	+ +	−	−	−	−	−	−
	729	+ +	−	−	−	−	−	−
	2,187	+	−	−	−	−	−	−

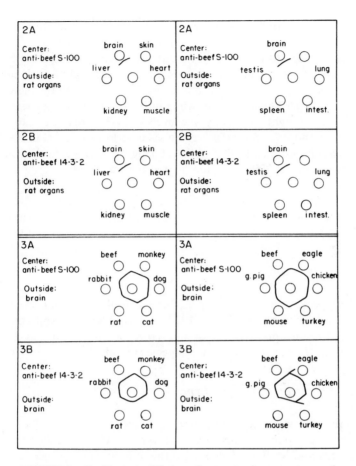

FIGURE 3. Double agar diffusion of extracts of rat organs or of brains of various species against anti-beef S-100 or anti-beef 14-3-2.

2.4.2. Cross-Reactions among Species

A high degree of cross-reactivity by complement fixation assay (using the antiserum to beef brain S-100) is found for S-100 in brains of all vertebrate species tested, including mammals, birds, fish, and reptiles (Moore, 1972; Figure 3). This high degree of cross-reactivity among species suggests a remarkable evolutionary stability for S-100. There is also a high degree of cross-reactivity for 14-3-2 among all mammalian species; there is cross-reactivity for birds, but no detectable amount for fish and reptiles, again using the antiserum to beef brain 14-3-2 in a complement fixation assay. The electrophoretic mobility of S-100 and 14-3-2 also varies only slightly in different species.

There seems to be a great amount of variation in levels of S-100 and 14-3-2 in brain from species to species, even though there is little qualitative variation in the proteins. For example, in the brain of the rat there is about 120 mg S-100 per kg wet weight, while in the brain of the mouse, it is about 20 mg/kg wet weight. Generally, the levels of 14-3-2 are about 2 to 100 times higher than those for S-100 in a given species. For example, in the brain of the rat the amount of 14-3-2 is about 300 mg/kg, whereas in the brain of the chicken, it is about 700 mg/kg (compared to 7 for S-100).

2.5. Distribution in the Nervous System and Localization to Cell Type

2.5.1. *Distribution in Areas*

Both proteins are found in peripheral as well as central nerve tissues. In general, in human brain (Moore, 1972) S-100 is higher in white matter than in gray, while the opposite distribution is true for 14-3-2 (Table 3). Also, S-100 is highest in the cerebellum in every species tested.

2.5.2. *Localization to Cell Type*

Obviously, it is important in understanding the function of a component of the nervous system to localize it to a type of cell, particularly neurons or glia. Hyden and McEwen (1966) used the immunofluorescence technique in an attempt to determine the cellular localization of S-100. They concluded that it was primarily located in glial cytoplasm and to a small extent in neuronal nuclei. More certain localization of S-100 and 14-3-2 was obtained by degeneration studies and direct analysis on cell cultures or single dissected cells. The cloned rat glioma (C-6) cell culture produces S-100 during the stationary phase of its growth cycle (Benda *et al.*, 1968; Herschman, 1971). This glioma culture produces little 14-3-2, whereas a neuroblastoma culture produces large amounts of 14-3-2 and no detectable S-100 (Goldstein and Moore, unpublished data). On the other hand, Schubert *et al.* (1974) have cloned a number of neuroblastoma and glioma cells from brain, some of which produce S-100, some 14-3-2, some both proteins, and some neither, without correlation with cell type. Pfeiffer *et al.* (1972) showed that large amounts of S-100 are made by a human acoustic neurinoma, which is probably a type of Schwannoma.

TABLE 3. S-100 and 14-3-2 Contents of Various Parts of Human Brain

	S-100, μg/g wet weight[a]		14-3-2 μg/g wet weight[a]	
	Mean S.E.M.	N[b]	Mean S.E.M.	N[b]
Frontal gray	45 ± 3	16	191 ± 21	14
Frontal white	177 ± 16	16	181 ± 10	14
Parietal gray	53 ± 4	16	208 ± 20	14
Parietal white	190 ± 22	16	116 ± 11	14
Occipital gray	61 ± 4	16	239 ± 16	14
Occipital white	208 ± 18	16	131 ± 14	14
Temporal gray	49 ± 4	16	170 ± 13	14
Temporal white	134 ± 14	16	101 ± 10	14
Corpus callosum	154 ± 12	16	101 ± 8	14
Globus pallidus	131 ± 13	15	196 ± 12	14
Putamen	59 ± 6	16	271 ± 27	14
Hippocampus	105 ± 8	16	169 ± 11	14
Head of caudate nucleus	61 ± 7	16	237 ± 19	14
Hypothalamus	138 ± 8	16	158 ± 13	14
Thalamus, central nucleus	126 ± 10	16	251 ± 22	14
Thalamus, lateral nucleus	133 ± 10	16	213 ± 16	14
Cingulate gyrus, rostral	54 ± 7	16	186 ± 20	14
Amygdaloid body	68 ± 9	16	201 ± 10	14
Corpus quadrigemina inferior	143 ± 8	12	205 ± 21	11
Cerebellar gray	190 ± 10	16	282 ± 19	14
Cerebellar white	197 ± 16	16	199 ± 10	14

[a] In terms of beef brain equivalents.
[b] Number of brains.

Three types of degeneration studies have been done to localize S-100 and 14-3-2 to cell type. During Wallerian degeneration of rabbit tibial nerve (Perez and Moore, 1968), the S-100 level fell during axonal degeneration (Figure 4). However, during degeneration of rabbit optic nerve (Perez et al., 1970), S-100 rose slightly and 14-3-2 fell to low values, suggesting a glial localization for S-100 and axonal for 14-3-2. It is not known why the S-100 level falls during degeneration of peripheral nerve; one explanation is that it is localized in Schwann cells but its continued synthesis there requires an intact axon. Finally, during retrograde degeneration of the dorsal thalamus (Cicero et al., 1970b) following degeneration of the cortex produced by termination of its blood supply, the S-100 level rose and the level of 14-3-2 fell (Figure 5), in agreement with the optic nerve studies.

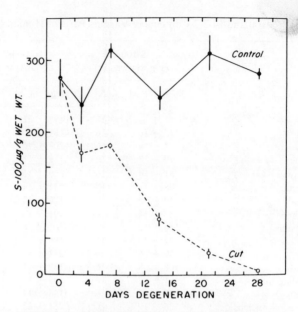

FIGURE 4. Levels of S-100 in cut end of tibial nerve of rabbit during Wallerian degeneration (from Perez and Moore, *J. Neurochem.* **96**:974, Figure 1).

Using the micro-adaptation of the complement fixation assay, S-100 and 14-3-2 were measured in single neurons dissected from frozen-dried sections using Lowry's methods (Perez and Moore, unpublished data; see Table 4). Anterior horn cells or dorsal root ganglion cells contain no S-100, but surrounding neuropil contains large amounts. Both the cell bodies and neuropil contain 14-3-2. Therefore the evidence seems to suggest that S-100 is glial and 14-3-2 primarily neuronal in normal cells of the central nervous system.

2.6.   Developmental Studies

The S-100 level in whole brain of the rat is low from birth until about 10 days postnatally; then it rises rapidly to a stable level at 90–120 days of age (Moore, 1969; Cicero *et al.*, 1972). Zuckerman *et al.* (1970) did a more detailed study of S-100 development in human fetal brains and found that the order of development followed a caudal–rostral pattern, that is, it rose in level in cord, pons, medulla, cerebellum, and midbrain at 10–15 weeks gestational age, but its appearance in frontal cortex was delayed until 30 weeks. Moore and Perez (1968) found that in most areas of human brain there was a consistent rise in level of S-100 from 2 to 80 years of age.

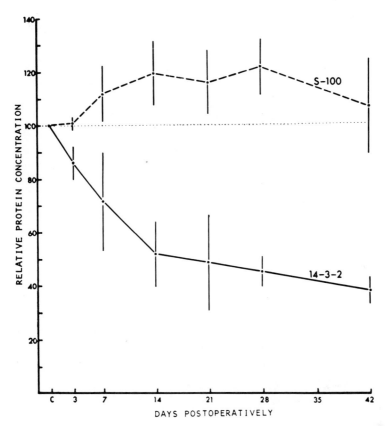

FIGURE 5.   Levels of S-100 and 14-3-2 in degenerating dorsal thalamus (from Cicero, Cowan, Moore, and Suntzeff, *Brain Res.* **18**:28, Figure 1).

TABLE 4.   Contents of S-100 and 14-3-2 in Dissected Nerve Cells and Surrounding Neuropil

	μg protein/g dry tissue		
	Medial neuropil	Dorsal root ganglion cells	Anterior horn cells
Rabbit	874	< 10	< 10
(S-100)	738	< 10	< 10
	792	< 10	< 10
	224	< 10	< 10
	198	< 10	< 10
	307	< 10	< 10
Monkey	2400	210	—
(14-3-2)	1800	170	—

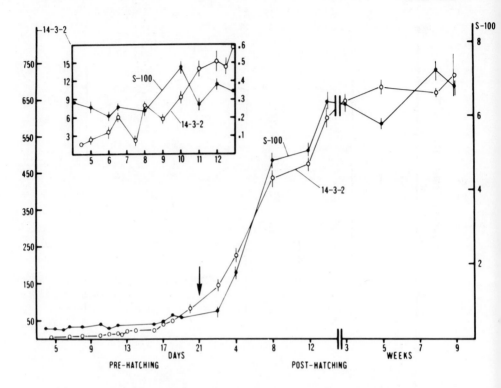

FIGURE 6. Levels of S-100 and 14-3-2 during development of chick optic tectum (from Cicero, Cowan, and Moore, *Brain Res.* **24**:4, Figure 1).

Cicero *et al.* (1970*a*) did a detailed study of S-100 and 14-3-2 in the developing chick optic tectum, a developmental system which has been studied in great detail with regard to time of cell divisions, growth of fibers, cell migrations, and formation of layers (Figure 6). All cell division ceases by 14 days of incubation, but S-100 and 14-3-2 levels remain very low until several days past this period, until at 17 or 18 days the levels of both rise rapidly in unison, and continue to rise particularly around the hatching period, until they reach adult levels at 2 or 3 weeks posthatching. It is significant that some of the differentiated functions of neurons and glia, represented by S-100 and 14-3-2 synthesis, occur relatively late in the process of development of the nervous system. The same phenomenon is present during development of the spinal cord of the chick (Cicero and Provine, 1972), since in this developing system the levels of S-100 and 14-3-2 also start to rise some time after cell division has ceased.

2.7. Turnover Studies of S-100

McEwen and Hyden (1966) attempted to measure the half-life of S-100 protein in rat brain by injecting labeled leucine or lysine and counting the S-100–containing fraction after polyacrylamide gel electrophoresis. They concluded from their data that S-100 turns over extremely rapidly, with a half-life of the order of hours. Cicero and Moore (1970) injected [^{3}H]-leucine, by way of cannulas implanted in the third ventricles of the brains of rats, and then purified the S-100 for counting by a two-step procedure of DEAE–cellulose chromatography of the brain extract followed by polyacrylamide gel electrophoresis. They verified the purity and recovery of the isolated S-100 by complement fixation assay. Their data (Figure 7) indicated a half-life of the order of 12–15 days, which is of the order of magnitude of the proteins of brain that are turning over more slowly. Herschmann (1971) measured the rate of synthesis of S-100 in the C-6 rat glioma cell culture and concluded that his data agree with the 12–15 day value for half-life of S-100. The most likely explanation for the discrepancy between the data of McEwen and Hyden (1966) and that of the other two groups is that in the earlier experiment, the isolated S-100 fraction was contaminated with more rapidly turning-over proteins.

2.8. Chemical Properties of S-100 Possibly Related to Its Function

Under some conditions, S-100 displays multiple forms when electrophoresed on polyacrylamide gels (Gombos et al., 1966; Hyden and McEwen, 1966; Uyemura et al., 1971; Vincendon et al., 1967; Ansborg and Neuhoff, 1971). The appearance of multiple forms on electrophoresis was shown to be dependent on calcium ion (Calissano et al., 1969). In the absence of Ca^{2+}, or even in the presence of Mg^{2+} without Ca^{2+}, only a single band is seen on polyacrylamide gels. The S-100 protein undergoes a conformational change, during Ca^{2+} binding, leading to exposure of the single tryptophan residue (as seen by increase in quantum yield of fluorescence shown in Figure 8), one of the three tyrosine residues (by spectrophotometric titration), and two of the three cysteine residues (as seen by reactivity to Ellman's reagent), all of which are masked in the absence of Ca^{2+}. The dissociation constant for Ca^{2+} (in the presence of 60 mM K^+), as measured by equilibrium dialysis or by increase of tryptophan fluorescence is about 1 mM. There are 8–10 Ca^{2+} binding sites per S-100 molecule. Monovalent cations antagonize the binding, the order of effectiveness being $K^+ > Na^+ > Li^+$ (Figure 8).

Related to the Ca^{2+}-effected conformational change in S-100 is the stimulation, by S-100 and Ca^{2+}, of Rb^+ transport in artificial liposome

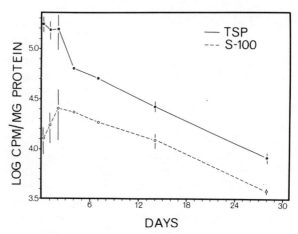

FIGURE 7. Specific activity of total soluble proteins (TSP) and of S-100 protein after intraventricular injection of [³H]-leucine in rats (from Cicero and Moore, *Science* **169**:1334, Figure 2).

membranes (Calissano and Bangham, 1971). The stimulation by either Ca^{2+} or S-100 alone is small, but together they stimulate transport to a great degree.

Apparently, in the absence of Ca^{2+}, there are no hydrophobic sites exposed on the surface of the S-100 molecule since the fluorescent hydrophobic probe, 8-anilinonaphthalene sulfonic acid (ANS), does not bind under those conditions. However, at least one ANS molecule binds to S-100 in the presence of 10 mM Ca^{2+} (Moore, 1972). Furthermore, it has been shown that, in the absence of Ca^{2+}, S-100 does not bind measurably to synaptic membranes, myelin, or red cell ghosts, but in the presence of Ca^{2+}, appreciable amounts of S-100 bind to all three types of membranes (Moore, unpublished data; see Table 5). These data suggest that the relative Ca^{2+}, K^+, and Na^+ concentrations may play a regulating role in determining the amount of S-100 bound to some hydrophobic site such as a membrane.

TABLE 5.   Binding of S-100 to Myelin or Synaptic Membranes

	mM Ca^{2+}	μg S-100 bound
Myelin	0	0
	10	9.2
Synaptic membranes	0	0
	10	7.3

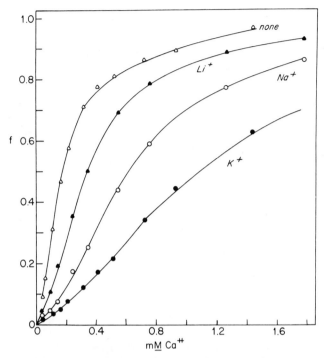

FIGURE 8. Fluorescence titration of S-100 with Ca^{2+} with and without monovalent cations Na^+, K^+, and Li^+ (from Calissano, Moore, and Friesen, *Biochemistry* **8**:4321, Figure 5).

2.9. Chemical Properties of 14-3-2

The 14-3-2 protein was isolated from beef brain by similar procedures used in the preparation of S-100 (Moore and Perez, 1968). The molecular weight of 14-3-2 is about 50,000 daltons (Moore, 1973). It also is a highly acidic protein containing a high proportion of glutamic and aspartic acid residues. Bennet and Edelman (1968) prepared a similar protein antigen from rat brain (antigen alpha). Recently it was shown that 14-3-2 and antigen alpha are immunologically and electrophoretically identical (Schneider, 1973; Bennet, 1974). The 14-3-2 or antigen alpha protein shows a tendency to aggregate (Moore, 1968; Bennet and Edelman, 1968).

2.10. Cell-Free Synthesis of S-100 and 14-3-2

A cell-free polyribosomal system from rat brain was shown to synthesize S-100 (Lerner and Herschmann, 1972). The S-100 was isolated from the reaction mixture for counting by first precipitating with specific antiserum and then purifying the S-100 from the S-100:antibody complex by SDS polyacrylamide gel electrophoresis. Zomzely-Neurath *et al.* (1972) have also used a polyribosomal system to synthesize S-100 in a cell-free system. They showed that S-100 could be synthesized in a reconstituted system containing polysome-derived mRNA and 40 S + 60 S ribosome subunits. A cell-free system containing polyribosomes from rat brain also synthesized 14-3-2 (Zomzely-Neurath *et al.*, 1973). Both S-100 and 14-3-2 were synthesized mainly by free rather than membrane-bound polyribosomes. Liver polyribosomes did not synthesize either protein.

3. THE GLIAL FIBRILLARY PROTEIN

An acidic soluble protein was first isolated (Eng *et al.*, 1971) from tissue rich in fibrous astrocytes obtained from brains with pathological conditions leading to areas of fibrous gliosis (for example, multiple sclerosis). The protein has also been obtained in identical form from normal white matter (Dahl and Bignami, 1973). It is different from other brain-specific proteins in the literature, that is, S-100, 14-3-2, 10B glycoprotein (Bogoch, 1969; Bogoch, 1970), and alpha-2-glycoprotein (Warecka, 1970; Warecka *et al.*, 1972). It has a monomeric molecular weight of 43,000 daltons but tends to aggregate to polymers in excess of 100,000 daltons (Schneider, 1973).

Antiserum has been prepared to the glial fibrillary protein obtained from human brain (Uyeda *et al.*, 1972; Bignami and Dahl, 1973) and cross-reactions were demonstrated in brains of other vertebrates. By immunofluorescence, the protein was localized to the fibrous astrocytes in brain (Bignami *et al.*, 1972).

4. REFERENCES

Ansborg, R., and Neuhoff, V., 1971, Micro-disc electrophoresis of brain proteins. III. Heterogeneity of the nervous specific proteins S-100, *Int. J. Neurosci.* **2**:151–160.

Benda, P., Lightbody, J., Sato, G., Levine, L., and Sweet, W., 1968, Differentiated rat glial cell strain in tissue culture, *Science* **161**:370–371.

Bennet, G., 1974, Immunologic and electrophoretic identity between nervous system specific proteins antigen alpha and 14-3-2, *Brain Res.* **68**:365–369.

Bennet, G. S., and Edelman, G., 1968, Isolation of an acidic protein from rat brain, *J. Biol. Chem.* **243**:6234–6241.

Bignami, A., and Dahl, D., 1973, An immunofluorescence study with antibodies to a protein specific to astrocytes, *Brain Res.* **49**:393–403.

Bignami, A., Eng, L. F., Dahl, D., and Uyeda, C. T., 1972, Localization of the glial fibrillary acidic protein in astrocytes by immunofluorescence, *Brain Res.* **43**:429–435.

Bogoch, S., 1969, Proteins, *in Handbook of Neurochemistry*, Vol. 1, pp. 75–92, Plenum Press, New York.

Bogoch, S., 1970, Glycoproteins of the brain of the training pigeon, *in Protein Metabolism of the Nervous System* (A. Lajtha, ed), pp. 555–569, Plenum Press, New York.

Calissano, P., and Bangham, A. D., 1971, Effect of two brain specific proteins (S-100 and 14-3-2) on cation diffusion across artificial lipid membranes, *Biochem. Biophys. Res. Commun.* **43**:504–509.

Calissano, P., Moore, B. W., and Friesen, A., 1969, Effect of calcium ion on S-100, protein of the nervous system, *Biochemistry* **8**:4318–4326.

Cicero, T. J., and Moore, B. W., 1970, Turnover of the brain specific protein, S-100, *Science* **169**:1333–1334.

Cicero, T. J., and Provine, R. R., 1972, The levels of the brain specific proteins, S-100 and 14-3-2, in the developing chick spinal cord, *Brain Res.* **44**:294–298.

Cicero, T. J., Cowan, W. M., and Moore, B. W., 1970a, Changes in the concentrations of the two brain specific proteins, S-100 and 14-3-2, during the development of the avian optic tectum, *Brain Res.* **24**:1–10.

Cicero, T. J., Cowan, W. M., Moore, B. W., and Suntzeff, V., 1970b, The cellular localization of the two brain specific proteins, S-100 and 14-3-2, *Brain Res.* **18**:25–34.

Cicero, T. J., Ferendelli, J. A., Suntzeff, V., and Moore, B. W., 1972, Regional changes in CNS levels of the S-100 and 14-3-2 proteins during development and aging of the mouse, *J. Neurochem.* **19**:2119–2125.

Cotman, C., and Matthews, D. A., 1971, Synaptic plasma membranes from rat brain synaptosomes: Isolation and partial characterization, *Biochem. Biophys. Acta* **249**:380–394.

Dahl, D., and Bignami, A., 1973, Glial fibrillary protein from normal human brain, purification and properties, *Brain Res.* **57**:343–360.

Dannies, P. S., and Levine, L., 1969, Demonstration of subunits in beef brain acidic protein (S-100), *Biochem. Biophys. Res. Commun.* **37**:587–592.

Dannies, P. S., and Levine, L., 1971a, Structural properties of bovine brain S-100 protein, *J. Biol. Chem.* **246**:6276–6283.

Dannies, P. S., and Levine, L., 1971b, The role of sulfhydryl groups in serological properties of bovine brain S-100 protein, *J. Biol. Chem.* **246**:6284–6287.

DeLores Arnai, R., Aberice, M., and deRobertis, E., 1967, Ultrastructural and enzymic studies of cholinergic and non-cholinergic synaptic membranes isolated from brain cortex, *J. Neurochem.* **14**:215–225.

Eichberg, J., Wittaker, V. P., and Dawson, R. M. C., 1964, Distribution of lipids in subcellular particles of guinea pig brain, *Biochem. J.* **92**:91–100.

Eng, L. T., Vanderhaegen, J. J., Bignami, A., and Gerstl, B., 1971, An acidic protein isolated from fibrous astrocytes, *Brain Res.* **28**:351–354.

Gombos, G., Vincendon, G., Tardy, J., and Mandel, P., 1966, Hétérogénéite électrophorétique et préparation rapide de la fraction protéique S-100, *C.R. Soc. Biol. F.* **D268**:1533–1535.

Herschman, H. R., 1971, Synthesis and degradation of a brain-specific protein (S-100 protein) by clonal cultured human glial cells, *J. Biol. Chem.* **246**:7569–7571.

Hyden, H., and McEwen, B., 1966, A glial protein specific for the nervous system, *Proc. Natl. Acad. Sci. (U.S.)* **55**:354–358.

Kessler, D., Levine, L., and Fasman, G., 1968, Some conformational and immunological properties of a bovine brain acidic protein (S-100), *Biochemistry* **7**:758–764.

Lerner, M. P., and Herschman, H. R., 1972, S-100 protein synthesis by isolated polyribosomes from rat brain, *Science* **178**:995–996.

Levine, L., and Moore, B. W., 1965, Structural relatedness of a vertebrate brain acidic protein as measured immunochemically, *Neurosci. Res. Prog. Bull.* **3**:18–22.

McEwen, B., and Hyden, H., 1966, A study of specific brain proteins on the semi-micro scale, *J. Neurochem.* **13**:823–833.

Moore, B. W., 1965, A soluble protein characteristic of the nervous system, *Biochem. Biophys. Res. Commun.* **19**:739–744.

Moore, B. W., 1969, Acidic proteins, *in Handbook of Neurochemistry*, Vol. 1, pp. 93–99, Plenum Press, New York.

Moore, B. W., 1972, Chemistry and biology of two proteins, S-100 and 14-3-2, specific to the nervous system, *in International Review of Neurobiology*, Vol. 15, pp. 215–225, Academic Press, New York.

Moore, B. W., 1973, Brain specific proteins, *in Proteins of the Nervous System* (D. J. Schneider, ed.), pp. 1–12, Raven Press, New York.

Moore, B. W., and McGregor, D., 1965, Chromatographic and electrophoretic fractionation of soluble proteins of brain and liver, *J. Biol. Chem.* **240**:1647–1653.

Moore, B. W., and Perez, V. J., 1966, Complement fixation for antigens on a picogram level, *J. Immunol.* **96**:1000–1005.

Moore, B. W., and Perez, V. J., 1968, Specific acidic proteins of the nervous system, *in Physiological and Biochemical Aspects of Nervous Integration* (F. D. Carlson, ed.), pp. 343–360, Prentice-Hall, Englewood Cliffs, N.J.

Moore, B. W., Perez, V. J., and Gehring, M., 1968, Assay and regional distribution of a soluble protein characteristic of the nervous system, *J. Neurochem.* **15**:265–272.

Morgan, I. G., Wolfe, L. S., Mandel, P., and Gombos, G., 1971, Isolation of plasma membranes from rat brain, *Biochim. Biophys. Acta* **241**:737–751.

Perez, V. J., and Moore, B. W., 1968, Wallerian degeneration in rabbit tibial nerve: Changes in amounts of the S-100 protein, *J. Neurochem.* **15**:971–977.

Perez, V. J., Olney, J. W., Cicero, T. J., Moore, B. W., and Bahn, B. A., 1970, Wallerian degeneration in rabbit optic nerve: Cellular localization in the central nervous system of the S-100 and 14-3-2 proteins, *J. Neurochem.* **17**:511–519.

Pfeiffer, S. E., Kornblith, P. L., Cares, H. L., Seals, J., and Levine, L., 1972, S-100 protein in human acoustic neurinomas, *Brain Res.* **41**:187–193.

Schneider, D. J., 1973, Studies of nervous system proteins, *in Proteins of the Nervous System*, pp. 67–94, Raven Press, New York.

Schubert, D., Heinemann, S., Carlisle, W., Tarikas, H., Kimes, B., Patrick, J., Steinback, J. H., Culp, W., and Brandt, B. L., 1974, Clonal cell lines from the rat central nervous system, *Nature* **249**:224–227.

Uozumi, T., and Ryan, R. J., 1973, Isolation, amino acid composition and radioimmunoassay of human brain S-100 protein, *Mayo Clin. Proc.* **48**:50–56.

Uyeda, C. T., Eng. L. F., and Bignami, A., 1972, An immunological study of the glial fibrillary acidic protein, *Brain Res.* **37**:81–89.

Uyemura, K., Vincendon, G., Gombos, G., and Mandel, P., 1971, Purification and some properties of S-100 protein fractions from sheep and pig brains, *J. Neurochem.* **18**:429–438.

Vincendon, G., Waksman, A., Uyemura, K., Tardy, J., and Gombos, G., 1967, Ultracentrifugal behavior of beef brain S-100 protein fraction, *Arch. Biochem.* **120**:233–235.

Warecka, K., 1970, Isolation of a brain specific glycoprotein, *J. Neurochem.* **17**:829–830.

Warecka, K., Moller, H. J., Vogel, H.-M., and Tripatzis, I., 1972, Human brain–specific alpha 2-glycoprotein: Purification by affinity chromatography and detection of a new component; Localization in nervous cells, *J. Neurochem.* **19**:719–725.

Wasserman, E., and Levine, L., 1961, Quantitative micro-complement fixation and its use in the study of antigenic structure by specific antigen-antibody inhibition, *J. Immunol.* **87**:290–295.

Zomzely-Neurath, C., York, C., and Moore, B. W., 1972, Synthesis of a brain-specific protein (S-100 protein) in a homologous cell-free system programmed with cerebral polysomal messenger RNA, *Proc. Natl. Acad. Sci. (U.S.)* **69**:2326–2330.

Zomzely-Neurath, C., York, C., and Moore, B. W., 1973, *In vitro* synthesis of two brain-specific proteins (S-100 and 14-3-2) by polyribosomes from rat brain, *Arch. Biochem. Biophys.* **155**:58–69.

Zuckerman, J. E., Herschman, H. R., and Levine, L., 1970, Appearance of a brain specific antigen (the S-100 protein) during human foetal development, *J. Neurochem.* **17**:247–251.

ACTOMYOSIN-LIKE PROTEIN IN BRAIN

S. BERL

Department of Neurology
Mount Sinai School of Medicine
New York, New York

1. INTRODUCTION

Two general categories of ATPases are present in tissue. One group requires Na^+ and K^+ as well as Mg^{2+} for maximum enzyme activity and functions in active transport of Na^+, K^+, and other substances across cell membranes. The second group of ATPases requires Mg^{2+} or Ca^{2+} for activation. The biochemical and physiological significances of the Mg^{2+}–Ca^{2+}-activated enzyme systems are less understood. The one major protein system activated by Mg^{2+} or Ca^{2+} which has received extensive study is the actomyosin complex; in this system the hydrolysis of ATP stimulated by divalent cations plays an essential role in muscle contraction and relaxation.

The question whether there may be present in nervous tissue a contractile actomyosin-like protein was raised by several investigators. Libet (1948) in preliminary studies of Ca^{2+}-activated ATPase activity in squid giant axon suggested that proteins similar to the myosin system in muscle may be associated with the conduction of nerve impulses. Bowler and Duncan (1967, 1968) in their studies of crayfish nerve and frog brain also suggested that actomyosin-like contractile ATPases are probably responsible for the control of excitation in nerve and muscle cells; they felt that these enzymes are responsible for passive permeability of excitable cells and possibly of all cells.

A number of studies have been applied to the description of Mg^{2+}- or Ca^{2+}-stimulated ATPase activity in nervous tissue. Histochemical techniques have been utilized in several of these studies. Naidoo and Pratt (1956) described Mg^{2+}- and Ca^{2+}-stimulated activity in brain tissue as compared with cerebral blood vessels. The intracortical laminar distribution in rat brain was catalogued by Hess and Pope (1959) and Lewin and Hess (1964) and in human frontal cortex by Hess and Pope (1961). The distribution of Ca^{2+}-activated ATPase activity in dorsal root ganglia and peripheral nerve was described by Novikoff (1967). Mg^{2+}–Ca^{2+}-activated ATPase activity has been shown to be present in isolated nerve-ending vesicles of guinea pig brain (Hosie, 1965; Kadota et al., 1967) and rat brain (Germain and Proulx, 1965). The latter investigators suggested that it may function in the storage and release of acetylcholine. Na^+–K^+-stimulated ATPase activity is associated with the synaptic membranes, but not with the vesicles.

Several kinds of movement of glia and nerve endings have been reported that suggest the presence of contractile elements. Speidel (1935) suggested that nerve endings can move. Benitez et al. (1955) described pulsating movements of glia in responses to serotonin. Phase contrast, time-lapse cinematography of brain cultures (Pomerat et al., 1967) has recorded changes in shape and pulsatile activity of glia, movement of nerve endings, neuronal nuclear rotation, and bidirectional flow of particles and vacuoles in the axons.

The isolation of actomyosin-like protein from a variety of cells other than those of striated or smooth muscle offered additional basis for the possibility that similar proteins may also be present in brain cells. Actomyosin-like protein had been described in ascites sarcoma cells (Hoffman–Berling, 1956) and had been isolated from blood platelets (thrombosthenin) (Bettex–Galland and Luscher, 1960); in the latter tissue it is thought to function in clot retraction. Such proteins have also been isolated and well characterized from slime mold plasmodia (Adelman and Taylor, 1969a; 1969b), where it functions in cytoplasmic streaming; from acanthamoeba (Weihing and Korn, 1971; Pollard and Korn, 1973), where it probably functions in movement, from fibroblasts (Yang and Perdue, 1972); and from polymorphonuclear leukocytes (Stossel and Pollard, 1973). Thus, this protein system, which apparently is quite old in the phylogenetic stream of development, has been utilized in many different cells for a variety of functions which require the conversion of chemical to mechanical energy.

To facilitate differentiation between muscle and brain proteins, brain actomyosin has been designated as neurostenin, brain actin as neurin, and brain myosin as stenin (Berl and Puszkin, 1970). It has been suggested that specific names be eliminated and the protein named by the cell of origin, e.g., brain actin (Pollard and Weihing, 1974).

2. BRAIN ACTOMYOSIN (NEUROSTENIN)

The chemical and physical properties that characterize muscle actomyosin, actin, and myosin and which were used to characterize the analogous brain proteins will be described in the course of this chapter.

2.1. Solubility

One of the characteristic properties of muscle actomyosin utilized in the isolation of the brain protein, was its solubility in high ionic strength buffer. It was isolated from brain (Puszkin et al., 1968) by slight modification of the procedure described for the extraction of muscle actomyosin (Szent-Gyorgyi, 1951a). Brains of rat or cat were extracted with 0.6 M KCl in a dilute bicarbonate buffer at pH 8.2. Dilution of the 60,000g supernatant fluid to a KCl concentration of 0.1 M at pH 6.3 yielded a protein precipitate which was again soluble in 0.6 M KCl at neutral pH. The protein can be brought into solution and reprecipitated several times by this procedure. The amount of protein obtained represented approximately 1–2% of the total brain protein. Present studies indicate that, similar to other nonmuscle actomyosins, the brain protein can be extracted with a low ionic strength buffer (Mahendran et al., 1974); the presence of 0.24 M sucrose results in an increased yield and enhanced enzyme activity of the protein. The efficacy of sucrose in the extraction of granulocytes has been reported (Stossel and Pollard, 1973).

2.2. Enzyme Activity

Muscle actomyosin is an ATPase stimulated by either Mg^{2+} or Ca^{2+}, somewhat more by the former cation. The protein isolated from brain also exhibited Mg^{2+}–Ca^{2+}-stimulated ATPase activity (Table 1). Mg^{2+} was better than Ca^{2+} as an activator at 0.03 M KCl, but the reverse was true at 0.6 M KCl. The addition of both was not additive; therefore one enzyme system was probably involved rather than one stimulated by Mg^{2+} and another by Ca^{2+}. The differences in ATPase activity at low and high KCl

TABLE 1. Mg^{2+}–Ca^{2+}-Stimulated ATPase Activity of Protein Isolated from Rat Brain[a]

	μg Pi/mg protein/30 min	
KCl	0.03 M	0.6 M
Mg^{2+}	12.6	2.9
Ca^{2+}	8.2	6.5
Mg^{2+}+ Ca^{2+}	9.6	2.6

[a] The assay mixture contained 0.2 mg protein/ml, $5 \times 10^{-4} M$ ATP, $10^{-3} M$ Mg^{2+}, Ca^{2+}, or both, and 0.05 M imidazole buffer pH 6.8. Incubated for 30 min at 37°C. In the absence of added cations, less than 1 μg Pi was liberated. (From Puszkin *et al.*, 1968.)

concentrations are to be expected from comparison with muscle protein. At low KCl concentration actomyosin predominates; at high KCl concentration the addition of ATP causes dissociation of actomyosin into its component actin and myosin moieties. Actomyosin and myosin both have Ca^{2+}-activated ATPase activity. On the other hand, while the actomyosin complex is activated also by Mg^{2+}, myosin is inhibited by Mg^{2+} (Needham, 1960). Actin has no ATPase activity; its union with myosin results in the development of Mg^{2+}-stimulated enzyme activity. Thus, the brain protein exhibited greater Mg^{2+} activation at low KCl concentrations and greater Ca^{2+} activation at high KCl concentration; in the latter case Mg^{2+} was inhibitory.

The ATPase activity was effectively inhibited (80% or more) by sulfhydryl blocking agents such as mersalyl (2.5×10^{-4}) or *p*-chloromercuribenzoate. Ouabain ($10^{-4} M$), effective against the Na^+–K^+-activated ATPase, was ineffective against the brain protein. The pH optimum for the protein was 6.8–7.2.

The ATPase activity of the brain protein was dependent upon the relative concentrations of Mg^{2+} and ATP (Berl and Puszkin, 1970). Optimum ATPase activity occurred at equimolar concentrations of Mg^{2+} and ATP (Figure 1). When the ATP concentration was either less or more than the Mg^{2+} concentration, the enzyme activity tended to decrease. This relationship was first described for myofibrilar ATPase activity (Perry and Grey, 1956).

Incubation of muscle actomyosin with low concentrations of polyethylene–sulfonate caused inhibition of the Mg^{2+}-stimulated ATPase activity of the protein (Barany and Jaisle, 1960). This result was probably due to dissociation of the actomyosin into actin and myosin, and the drug was designated as an "interaction inhibitor." Polyethylene–sulfonate in

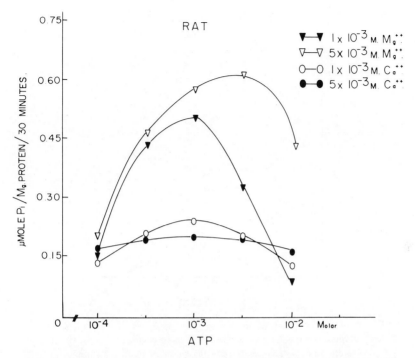

FIGURE 1. Effect of increasing concentrations of ATP with various concentrations of Mg^{2+} and Ca^{2+} on the ATPase activity of the protein isolated from rat brain: imidazole buffer, 0.03 M, pH 6.8, KCl, 0.12 M, final volume 1 ml, 0.1 mg/ml protein, 37°C for 30 min. (From Berl and Puszkin, 1970.)

concentrations as low as 10^{-7} M or greater similarly decreased the Mg^{2+}-activated ATPase activity of brain proteins (Berl and Puszkin, 1970) (Figure 2). The Ca^{2+}-activated hydrolysis of ATP was either unaffected or slightly increased.

2.3. Superprecipitation

Another property of muscle actomyosin which is considered to demonstrate the contractile nature of the protein is the phenomenon of superprecipitation (Szent-Gyorgyi, 1951b). When actomyosin is suspended in 0.1 M KCl at neutral pH and ATP and Mg^{2+} are added, a dense precipitate forms which may undergo syneresis with contraction of the precipitate if sufficient protein is present. The protein isolated from rat brain in dilute suspension did form a flocculant precipitate in the presence of ATP and

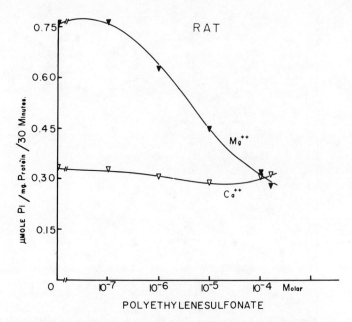

FIGURE 2. Effect of increasing concentrations of polyethylene–sulfonate on the ATPase activity of protein isolated from rat brain. Protein preincubated with polyethylenesulfonate for 10 min prior to addition of the ATP; Mg^{2+} or Ca^{2+} $1 \times 10^{-3} M$, $0.03 M$ imidazole buffer, pH 6.8, $0.05 M$ KCl and $5 \times 10^{-4} M$ ATP; 0.1 mg of protein, final volume 1 ml, 37°C. (From Berl and Puszkin, 1970.)

Mg^{2+} (Puszkin *et al.*, 1968). This result did not occur when either one was omitted or when sulfhydryl inhibitors mersalyl or chloromercuribenzoate were added. Ouabain did not affect the occurrence of superprecipitation.

2.4. Viscosity

The relationship of ATP and Mg^{2+} concentrations and the effect of polyethylene–sulfonate on ATPase activity are considered additional criteria, but not necessarily specific for actomyosin. Probably a more specific criterion for actomyosin is the "sensitivity" of the viscosity of muscle actomyosin to ATP (Portzehl *et al.*, 1950). In solutions at high ionic strength ($0.6 M$ KCl) he addition of small amounts of ATP results in a decrease in viscosity because of dissociation of the actomyosin into actin and myosin. The viscosity rises again as the ATP is hydrolyzed and the concentration of ATP decreased. The protein isolated from brain demonstrated this pheno-

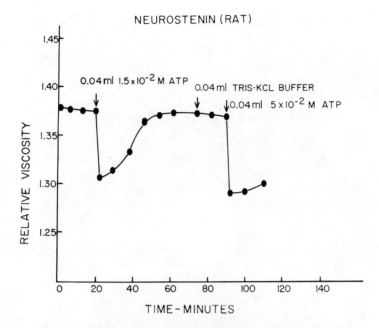

FIGURE 3.   Effect of ATP on the relative viscosity of protein isolated from rat brain. Viscometric determinations were performed in a Cannon–Ubbelohde dilution viscometer, size 50, at 21°C; 6 ml, 2.74 mg/ml protein in 0.6 M KCl–0.05 M Tris, pH 7.2, was used. Neutralized ATP solution was added at indicated points. (From Berl and Puszkin, 1970.)

menon (Berl and Puszkin, 1970). The addition of low concentrations of ATP resulted in a rapid fall in the relative viscosity of the solutions of the protein from brain (Figure 3). The viscosity rose again over a period of 30–50 min. The rate of rise was dependent upon the amount of ATP added; it was slower in the presence of larger amounts of ATP. The response to added ATP could be repeated several times with the same protein solution. This sensitivity of the brain proteins, to ATP, however, was considerably less than that reported for actomyosin of striated muscle.

2.5.   Antisera

Antisera were prepared in the rabbit against actomyosin isolated from rat brain, cat brain, and cat striated muscle (Berl and Puszkin, 1970) and from bovine brain (Puszkin and Berl, 1972). Immunodiffusion studies were carried out by the Ouchterlony technique. Antiserum obtained against the

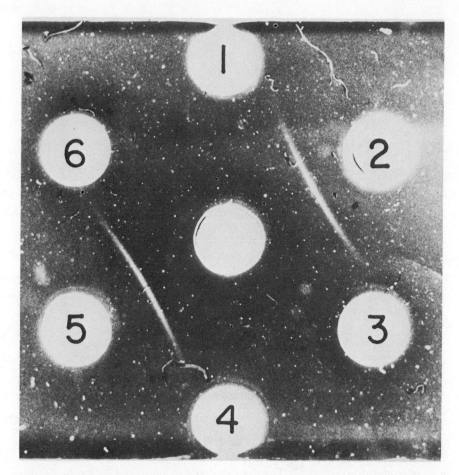

FIGURE 4. Immunodiffusion reactions of rat and cat neurostenin and cat muscle actomyosin with antiserum to the brain protein from rat. Center well contained rabbit antiserum to rat neurostenin. Wells 1 and 4 contained cat neurostenin, wells 2 and 5 contained rat neurostenin, and wells 3 and 6 contained cat muscle actomyosin. Wells 4, 5, and 6 contained twice the protein concentration of wells 1, 2, and 3, respectively. (From Berl and Puszkin, 1970.)

brain protein from rat formed a single precipitation band against the brain antigen from rat, but did not cross-react with the homologous protein isolated from cat brain, nor with striated muscle actomyosin from cat (Figure 4). Similarly, the brain antigen from cat raised antibodies against itself with which it formed a single precipitation band; this antiserum did not cross-react with the brain protein from rat. On the other hand, muscle protein from cat stimulated an antiserum which reacted not only against itself, but also against protein isolated from cat brain; it did not, however, cross-react with protein obtained from rat brain. The actomyosin isolated from bovine brain stimulated antiserum formation which reacted not only against the brain antigen from bovine, but also against antigen isolated from rat or cat brain. This antiserum did not react with muscle actomyosin from cat or with actomyosin isolated from the bovine aorta. Furthermore, although the antiserum to brain actomyosin from bovine did form a band against brain myosin from bovine, it did not form a band against muscle myosin from cat. Whether the above findings are indicative of differences in antigenic properties of the various proteins, or are the result of other factors such as antibody titer of the antisera, requires additional study. However, the indications are that differences in antigenicity among the proteins are probably real. These studies also supported our belief that the vascular smooth muscle component of the brain accounted for little of the various proteins isolated from the brains.

3.   BRAIN ACTIN (NEURIN)

3.1.   Extraction

The presence in brain of actomyosin-like protein was substantiated by the direct isolation from this organ of actin-like and myosin-like protein. The separation from bovine brain of actin-like protein was attempted (Berl and Puszkin, 1970; Puszkin and Berl, 1972) by adaptation of the method described by Carsten and Mommaerts (1963) for the purification of striated muscle actin. Acetone-treated brain tissue was extracted with dilute ATP–ascorbate buffered to pH 7.5. The addition of 0.1 M KCl and 0.1 mM MgCl$_2$ to the 105,000g supernatant resulted in the polymerization of protein which could be centrifuged from solution.

3.2.   Enzyme Activity

This protein had no ATPase activity but did enhance the Mg^{2+}-stimulated ATPase activity of striated muscle myosin tenfold or more (Berl and Puszkin, 1970). Data from representative experiments are shown in Table 2. The Ca^{2+}-stimulated ATPase activity of the muscle myosin was much less affected. The yield by the above procedure was approximately 0.2% of the total brain protein.

TABLE 2. Effect of Actin from Whole Brain on the
ATPase Activity of Muscle Myosin[a]

| | μmol Pi/mg myosin/min | | |
| Muscle myosin | | Muscle myosin + brain actin | |
Mg^{2+}	Ca^{2+}	Mg^{2+}	Ca^{2+}
0.055	0.69	0.49	1.01
0.046	0.33	1.17	0.69
0.026	0.28	0.32	0.26

[a] The incubation medium consisted of 0.03 M imidazole–HCl buffer, pH 6.8, 0.06 M KCl, 5 × 10^{-4} M ATP, 10^{-3} M Mg^{2+}, or Ca^{2+}, 10^{-4} M ouabain, 0.01 mg muscle myosin, and 0.05 mg brain actin in a final volume of 1 ml. Incubation was at 37°C for 30 min. (From Berl and Puszkin, 1970.)

3.3. Viscosity

Measurement of the relative viscosities of the solutions of brain actin and muscle myosin showed that the relative viscosity of the mixture of proteins was considerably higher than that of either one alone. Another distinction was that the combined protein solution developed a "sensitivity" to added ATP which was displayed by neither one alone. The addition of small amounts of ATP resulted in an immediate fall in the relative viscosity of the combined protein solution; the relative viscosity then rose again over a period of approximately 1 hr (Figure 5).

3.4. ATP Content and Exchange

Muscle actin in its depolymerized, globular state (G-actin) contains approximately 1 mol of ATP per mol of protein (Gergely, 1964); this ATP should exchange completely with added [^{14}C]ATP, (Martonosi et al., 1960; Kuehl and Gergely, 1969). The protein isolated directly from brain did contain ATP which did exchange with [^{14}C]ATP. Assuming, however, a similar molecular weight for both the muscle and brain proteins, 47,000 daltons (Rees and Young, 1967), the latter contained and exchanged approximately 0.5 mol per mol of protein. Although considerable variation has been reported for the nucleotide content of the muscle protein (Martonosi and Gouvea, 1961; Barany et al., 1961; Strohman and Samorodin, 1962; Kuehl and Gergely, 1969), the data suggest that the brain protein contained de-

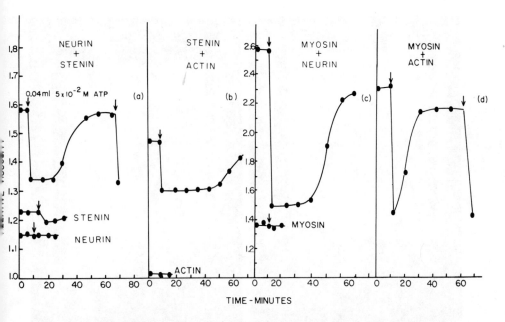

FIGURE 5. Effect of ATP on the relative viscosities of brain actinlike protein (neurin), brain myosin-like protein (stenin), striated muscle actin, and myosin, and their mixtures. Neurin and stenin were isolated from bovine brain and actin and myosin from the long back muscles of the cat. The protein concentrations were: neurin 1.62 mg/ml, stenin 2.0 mg/ml, actin 1.62 mg/ml, and myosin 2.1 mg/ml. See Figure 3 for additional details. (From Berl and Puszkin, 1970.)

natured protein, protein which did not bind nucleotide, or protein which contained nonexchangeable nucleotide. This property of the protein to contain and to exchange ATP is a rather labile one and is easily lost.

The bovine brain actin separated from brain actomyosin by zone sedimentation on sucrose gradients (see below) contained bound ATP which could be released from the protein by addition of perchloric acid. The highest value obtained was 0.98 mol of nucleotide per 50,000 g of protein. In muscle, the ratio of nucleotide to protein is probably on a one mole to one mole basis (Gergely, 1964). This neurin exchanged its bound ATP with free [^{14}C]ATP. The values of the three most active preparations were again in the range of 0.5 mol of nucleotide per 50,000 g protein.

Boundary sedimentation velocity of brain actin isolated from whole bovine brain was determined in a Spinco Model E analytical ultracentrifuge. The analysis showed a single, major, symmetrical boundary with a sedimentation coefficient, $S_{20,w} = 2.8$ (Figure 6), (Puszkin and Berl, 1972).

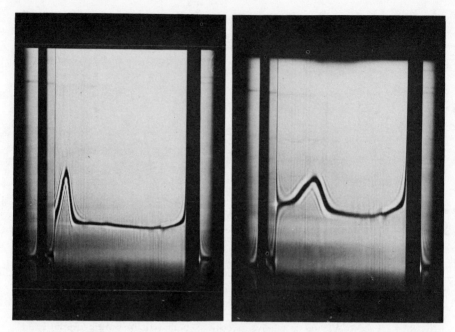

FIGURE 6. Boundary sedimentation of bovine brain neurin. The protein was depolymerized in 0.2 mM ascorbate–0.2 mM ATP and aggregated protein removed by centrifugation at 105,000 × g for 20 min. The protein concentration was 4 mg/ml. Pictures were taken at 8 min (left) and at 152 min (right). Taken by Dr. H. S. Rosenkrantz, Columbia University. (From Puszkin and Berl, 1972.)

3.5. Separation from Brain Actomyosin

It is also possible to isolate the actin-like moiety directly from the brain actomyosin-like complex by chromatography on a column of Sephadex G-200 or by ultracentrifugation on 3–30% sucrose gradients (Puszkin and Berl, 1972). This extraction is facilitated by the substitution of 0.6 M KI for the KCl in the separation medium. Although in the presence of 0.6 M KCl and 1 mM ATP, actomyosin dissociates into actin and myosin, the actin retains its polymerized state, and there remains the problem of the separation of two proteins of high molecular weight. When 0.6 M KI replaces the KCl, the actin depolymerizes without loss of its ability to repolymerize (A. G. Szent-Gyorgyi, 1951a). The problem is now one of separating a protein of approximately 47,000 mol wt actin, from one of approximately 500,000 mol wt myosin. KI has been used by A. G. Szent-Gyorgyi (1951b) to purify actin from striated muscle as well as from actomyosin.

TABLE 3. Activation of Muscle Myosin Mg^{2+}-
ATPase by Actin Isolated from Brain
Actomyosin[a]

Mg^{2+}-Activated ATPase

	μmol Pi/min/mg myosin ($\pm$S.D.)		
	Myosin	Myosin + brain actin	n^b
1.	23 ± 8	100 ± 9	5
2.	20 ± 6	100 ± 15	4

[a] See Table 2 for assay conditions. Brain actin separated from brain actomyosin: (1) by gel filtration on Sephadex G-200, and (2) by centrifugation on sucrose gradients. (From Puszkin and Berl, 1972.)
[b] n = number of preparations.

Thus, when bovine brain actomyosin was centrifuged on a linear sucrose gradient containing KI and ATP, two bands were obtained, a heavier one with a peak calculated to be at $0.35\ M$ sucrose and a lighter one equilibrating at $0.15\ M$ sucrose. The lighter band protein proved to have several properties characteristic of actin. Whether separated from brain actomyosin by chromatography either on Sephadex G-200 or on sucrose gradients, the protein did stimulate the Mg^{2+}-activated ATPase of muscle myosin approximately four- to fivefold (Table 3). The Ca^{2+}-activated ATPase of the myosin was either slightly increased or remained unchanged.

Brain actin isolated directly from brain or from brain actomyosin stimulates the Mg^{2+}-ATPase activity of muscle myosin. However, the brain protein is less effective than muscle actin in activating myosin. Studies reveal that an excess of brain actin over muscle myosin, approximately fivefold, may be required for maximal activation (Table 4). For the muscle proteins the reverse is true. The approximate ratio of actin to myosin is 1:4 on a weight basis (A. G. Szent-Gyorgyi, 1951b; Tonomura et al., 1962). In general, the actin-to-myosin ratio for maximal activation is greater for nonmuscle actins than for muscle actin (Pollard and Weihing, 1974).

The brain actin separated on sucrose gradients could be polymerized by diluting the KI concentration from $0.6\ M$ to $0.1\ M$. It can then be depolymerized in $0.2\ mM$ ATP–$0.2\ mM$ ascorbate and repolymerized by the addition of $0.1\ M$ KCl and $1\ mM$ Mg^{2+}; repolymerization was established by the release of Pi from bound ATP. During the conversion Globular (G) actin $\rightarrow$ fibrous (F) actin, ATP in the G-actin is hydrolyzed:

$$G\text{-actin} - ATP \rightarrow F\text{-actin} - ADP + Pi$$

The amount of Pi released ranged from 0.81–1.06 mol per 50,000 g protein

TABLE 4.   Activation of Muscle Myosin ATPase
Activity by Increasing Concentrations of Brain
Actin[a]

Brain actin (mg/ml)	μmol Pi/min/mg myosin	
	Mg^{2+}-ATPase	Ca^{2+}-ATPase
0.1	12.5	157
0.5	35	190
1.0	62	253
2.5	40	237
5.0	127	249
7.5	157	257
10.0	175	275

[a] See Table 2 for incubation conditions. (From Puszkin and
Berl, 1972.)

from four preparations. During repolymerization the relative viscosity of
the protein solution also increased.

Disc electrophoresis on 7.5% polyacrylamide gel containing 8 M
urea revealed a single major band with brain actin separated directly from
acetone-treated brain, from brain actomyosin on a sucrose gradient or on
Sephadex G-200 (Figure 7).

3.6.   Chick Nerve and Neuroblastoma

The presence of actin in the nerve cells of growing cultures of chick
sympathetic ganglia and chick embryo brain was recently shown by Fine
and Bray (1971). These authors compared the radioactively labeled peptide
maps of the nervous tissue actin with that isolated from chick breast muscle
and found extensive similarities which warranted the conclusion that actin
was present in the nervous tissue. It has also been shown that chick embryonic nerve cells contain actin-like fibers which interact with heavy
meromyosin to form characteristic arrowheads (Ishikowa et al., 1969).
However, the cell morphology was disrupted during the process and exact
localization of the actin-heavy meromyosin complexes could not be determined. A similar kind of study with neuroblastoma cells in culture suggested
that a network of actin-like protein is distributed from the cell body to the
nerve endings (Chang and Goldman, 1973).

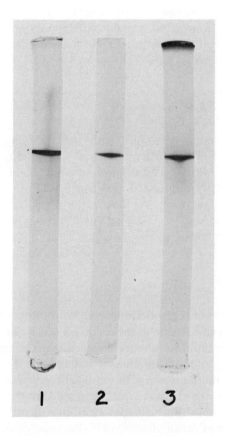

FIGURE 7. Acrylamide gel electrophoresis of neurin. Electrophoresis was performed on 7.5 % single acrylamide gels containing 8 M urea. 75–100 μg protein in 10 % sucrose was applied to the top of each gel. A current of 1 mA/gel was applied for 45 min followed by a current of 4–5 mA/gel; the total time was 115 min at 4°C. Gel 1, neurin separated from whole brain by the acetone procedure; Gel 2, neurin separated from neurostenin on a sucrose gradient; Gel 3, neurin separated from neurostenin on Sephadex G-200. (From Puszkin and Berl, 1972.)

4. BRAIN MYOSIN (STENIN)

4.1. Extraction

Myosin-like protein was prepared from bovine brain by a modification of the procedure of Richards et al. (1967) for the preparation of muscle myosin. The protein was extracted directly from fresh brain cleansed of superficial blood vessels and meninges (Berl and Puszkin, 1970). The method calls for rapid extraction of the protein with approximately 0.3 M KCl in the presence of ATP. It is then further purified by differential precipitation at lower ionic strengths.

4.2. Enzyme Activity

Two representative studies with the brain myosin-like protein are shown in Table 5. The ATPase activity of the protein is stimulated far more by Ca^{2+} than by Mg^{2+}. The addition of either brain actin or muscle actin, however, markedly stimulated the Mg^{2+}-ATPase activity of the brain myosin whereas the Ca^{2+}-ATPase activity was far less stimulated. The stimulation of the Mg^{2+}-ATPase activity by actin protein is quite characteristic of myosin proteins.

4.3. Viscosity

The interaction of the brain myosin with brain actin or muscle actin is also reflected in an increase in the relative viscosity of the mixture over that of either protein solution alone and an increase in the sensitivity of the relative viscosity of the proteins in mixtures to that of either protein alone (Figure 5). The mixture of brain myosin with brain actin or muscle actin demonstrated an increased relative viscosity which responded to the addition of ATP with a rapid fall in viscosity which rose again over a period of 30–60 min. Calculated as percent sensitivity to ATP (Portzehl *et al.*, 1950), the mixtures were considerably increased over that of the individual solutions (Table 6). The specific viscosity, which considered also the protein concentration, also

TABLE 5.   Effect of Brain Actin and Muscle Actin on the ATPase Activity of Brain Myosin[a]

μmol Pi/mg myosin/min					
Brain myosin		Brain myosin + brain actin		Brain myosin + muscle actin	
Mg^{2+}	Ca^{2+}	Mg^{2+}	Ca^{2+}	Mg^{2+}	Ca^{2+}
0.071	0.34	0.55	0.39		
0.025	0.13	0.23	0.17	0.15	0.14

[a] See Table 2 for assay conditions. (From Berl and Puszkin, 1970.)

TABLE 6. Sensitivity to ATP and Specific Viscosity of Brain Proteins and Their Mixture with Each Other and with Muscle Proteins[a]

	Sensitivity to ATP, Percent		Specific viscosity	
MA[b]	0		0.010	
BA	0	0	0.085	0.097
MM	3.4	0	0.15	0.17
BM	16.8	0	0.10	0.12
MA + MM	113.6		0.22	
MA + BA	49.9		0.11	
BA + MM	133.6	59.5	0.26	0.23
BA + BM	52.4	73.0	0.12	0.18
BAM (rat)	18.9	25.0		
BAM (cat)	38.4	45.9		

[a] Data from two sets of experiments. (From Berl and Puszkin, 1970.)
[b] MA and MM—striated muscle actin and myosin from cat; BA and BM—brain actin and myosin from bovine; BAM—brain actomyosin from rat or cat.

tended to be higher in the mixed solutions. With the exception of the mixtures of brain actin or muscle actin with muscle myosin, the values for the sensitivity to ATP were lower than have been reported for striated muscle (Portzehl et al., 1950) or for some smooth muscles (Barany et al., 1966; Filo et al., 1963; Needham and Williams, 1963). They were similar to the values reported for the actomyosin-like protein isolated from slime mold (Adelman and Taylor, 1969a,b).

5. SUBCELLULAR DISTRIBUTION IN BRAIN

The subcellular locations of Mg^{2+}–Ca^{2+}-activated ATPases have been described by several workers (Hosie, 1965; Germain and Proulx, 1965; Kadota et al., 1967). Such ATPase activity with varying characteristics was found to be present in all fractions examined. Since the enzyme activity evidently represented a variety of different enzymes, it was essential to isolate the protein and to establish its characteristics to determine whether any of the activity present in the various fractions was contributed by an actomyosin-like protein.

Subcellular fractions of rat and bovine brain were prepared by modification of established methods as described by Abdel-Latif (1966) and Clark and Nicklas (1970) and modified by Puszkin et al. (1972). A brain tissue homogenate in 0.25 M sucrose, 0.01 M Tris, 0.5 mM-EDTA, pH 7.4 was used for the preparation of the crude mitochondrial pellet. A fairly pure microsomal pellet was obtained from the supernatant. The mitochondrial pellet, suspended in 3 % Ficoll, 0.24 M mannitol, 0.06 M sucrose, and 50 mM Tris-EDTA (pH 7.4), was layered onto the same medium containing 6 % Ficoll. Centrifugation (11,500g, 30 min) pelleted the bulk of the mitochondria leaving the synaptosomes in suspension. The synaptosomal fraction was then diluted and pelleted. This enriched synaptosomal pellet could be further separated from myelin by centrifugation on a discontinuous gradient of 4, 8, and 12 % Ficoll or separated into synaptic vesicle and synaptosomal membrane fractions by the osmotic shock technique of De Robertis et al. (1966), or Whittaker and Sheridan (1965).

With the method used for the extraction of actomyosin, proteins exhibiting Mg^{2+}–Ca^{2+}-stimulated ATPase activity were extracted from the crude nuclear subcellular fraction, the microsomal fraction and the synaptosomal enriched fraction of bovine cerebral cortex. No protein could be extracted from a purified mitochondrial fraction or from a myelin fraction by this technique.

Since much of the tissue remained in the crude nuclear fraction in the form of cellular debris and unbroken cells, it is not surprising that actomyosin-like protein could be isolated from this fraction. Indeed, the ATPase extracted from this fraction did show superprecipitation and viscometric sensitivity to ATP. On the other hand, the small amount of protein isolated from the microsomal fraction, although it did exhibit Mg^{2+}–Ca^{2+}-stimulated ATPase activity, had no other actomyosin-like properties. It did not show superprecipitation or viscometric sensitivity to ATP, it could not be split into actin-like and myosin-like proteins, nor did the protein show an immunodiffusion reaction to antibody prepared against actomyosin-like protein prepared from whole brain (Puszkin et al., 1972).

The relative yield of actomyosin-like protein was greater from the synaptosome-enriched fractions of bovine or rat brain than from the whole brain; from the former, 8–10 % of the total protein was extracted as neurostenin, while from the latter, 1–2 % of the total protein was extracted as this protein. In addition, the ATPase activity of the synaptosomal protein was four to five times greater than that from either the whole brain or the nuclear fraction (Table 7).

The presence of contractile protein in mitochondria for control of mitochondrial swelling has been subject to controversy. The isolation of such a protein from liver mitochondria (Ohnishi and Ohnishi, 1962; Neifakh and Kazakova, 1963; Arcos et al., 1967) and from brain mitochondria preparations (Poglazov, 1966) have been reported. Conover and Barany (1966), however, could not obtain myosin from liver mitochondria. In our studies we could not extract contractile protein from purified preparations of brain

TABLE 7. ATPase Activity of Actomyosin-like Protein
Isolated from Bovine Brain[a]

	ATPase activity (μmol/mg protein/30 min $\pm$ S.D.)	
	Mg^{2+}	Ca^{2+}
Whole Brain	0.24 $\pm$ 0.08 (6)[b]	0.14 $\pm$ 0.04 (6)
Nuclear fraction	0.28 $\pm$ 0.05 (6)	0.17 $\pm$ 0.04 (6)
Synaptosomal fraction	1.07 $\pm$ 0.10 (5)	0.41 $\pm$ 0.15 (5)

[a] See Table 2 for assay conditions. (From Puszkin et al., 1972.)
[b] ( ) = number of preparations.

or liver mitochondria. The mitochondria of Poglazov (1966) may have
been contaminated with other subcellular structures, such as synaptosomes.

6. SYNAPTOSOMAL PROTEIN

By the criteria of Mg^{2+}–Ca^{2+}-stimulated ATPase activity, ratio of
Mg^{2+}/Ca^{2+} activation, sensitivity of its viscosity to ATP, and superprecipitation, the protein isolated from the synaptosomal fraction had actomyosin-like properties similar to those of the protein isolated from whole
brain.

Zonal centrifugation in 3–30% (w/v) sucrose gradients containing
0.6 M KI had been used to separate actomyosin-like protein from whole
brain into its two major components, actin-like and myosin-like protein.
The application of this procedure to the synaptosomal protein again yielded
two major protein bands. The heavier of the two, the myosin-like protein,
equilibrated at 0.35 M sucrose and the lighter band, the actin-like protein,
centered at 0.15 M sucrose. The ratio of the recovered proteins myosin/actin
was approximately 1.3–1.4. This ratio is lower than that found in striated
muscle where it is approximately 2.5. It suggests that in brain the proportion
of actin to myosin is higher than in muscle. This relationship appears to be
generally true for all nonmuscle actomyosin-like systems (Pollard and
Weihing, 1974).

The ATPase activity of several representative preparations of the two
proteins and their mixtures are described in Table 8. The heavier protein,
similar to myosin, was essentially a Ca^{2+}-activated ATPase. The lighter
protein, similar to actin, exhibited little or only very small Mg^{2+}–Ca^{2+}-
stimulated ATPase activity. Upon recombination of the two proteins,

TABLE 8.   ATPase Activity of the Myosin-like and Actin-like Proteins Separated from Synaptosomal Actomyosin-like Protein (Rat)[a]

		μmol Pi/mg protein/30 min			
(1) Myosin-like protein		(2) Actin-like protein		Combination (1) + (2)	
Ca^{2+}	Mg^{2+}	Ca^{2+}	Mg^{2+}	Ca^{2+}	Mg^{2+}
10.3	0.31	1.4	0.44	16.2	10.7
10.5	0.45	0.04	0.35	17.9	11.6
6.9	2.45	0.03	0.02	6.9	10.1
4.2	0.10	0.76	0.32	7.5	5.3
22.9	0.93	0.55	1.50	10.5	8.0

[a] See Table 2 for incubation conditions. (From Puszkin *et al.*, 1972.)

however, there resulted a marked increase in the Mg^{2+}-stimulated activity and a considerably smaller effect on the Ca^{2+}-stimulated activity. The variations in the enzymatic activities of the different preparations probably are the result of incomplete separation of one protein from the other. Incomplete separation would also result in varying ratios of one to the other in the combination experiments with less than optimum ratios of the two proteins. In general the Ca^{2+}-stimulated activity of the isolated myosin-like protein and the Mg^{2+}-stimulated ATPase activity of recombined complex are greater than those of the "native" synaptosomal protein. These differences may indicate the loss of an inhibiting factor by the isolation procedure on the sucrose gradient. It is probably not due to severalfold purification of the proteins since 70–100% of the protein placed on the sucrose gradient is recovered in the bands of actin-like and myosin-like proteins. In present studies the presence of sucrose during isolation enhances enzyme activity.

The synaptosomal actin and myosin were also combined with striated muscle myosin and actin, respectively, and their ATPase activity was measured (Table 9). Similar to the recombination studies of the two brain proteins, the Mg^{2+}-stimulated ATPase activity of muscle myosin was greatly enhanced by the addition of the synaptosomal actin and that of the synaptosomal myosin by the addition of the muscle actin. The stimulation was of the same order of magnitude as that observed when muscle actin and myosin were combined.

Viscosity studies and sensitivity to added ATP were also performed as with the proteins isolated from whole brain. The relative viscosity of the synaptosomal myosin or actin was not affected by the addition of ATP. However, the addition of synaptosomal actin or muscle actin to synaptosomal myosin resulted in an elevation of the relative viscosity. Addition of ATP

TABLE 9. ATPase Activity of Synaptosomal Actin and Myosin with Striated Muscle Myosin and Actin, Respectively[a]

				μmol Pi/mg protein/30 min					
MM[b]		MM + SA		MA		SM		SM + MA	
Ca^{2+}	Mg^{2+}	Ca^{2+}	Mg^{2+}	Ca^{2+}	Mg^{2+}	Ca^{2+}	Mg^{2+}	Ca^{2+}	Mg^{2+}
22.6	1.35	22.6	13.4	0.71	0.26	13.7	0.48	19.7	13.2
12.3	0.48	11.7	4.6	0.20	0.17	22.9	0.93	14.9	5.8
8.6	0.71	11.4	10.0						
24.5	1.99	22.6	17.9						

[a] See Table 2 for incubation conditions. (From Puszkin et al., 1972.)
[b] MM—muscle myosin; MA—muscle actin; SM—synaptosomal myosin; SA—sypaptosomal actin.

caused a decrease to approximately the relative viscosity of the synaptosomal myosin, and the viscosity then increased again with time. Similarly, when synaptosomal actin was added to muscle myosin, the relative viscosity of the mixture increased. Upon addition of ATP the relative viscosity declined but increased again within 15–20 min. The results obtained from the cross-reaction of the synaptosomal protein with muscle proteins correlate with the data obtained from similar studies with whole brain actomyosin-like protein and support the contention that the brain proteins are similar to the muscle proteins.

It has also been established that 3-methylhistidine is a constituent of actin from muscle as well as from nonmuscle sources (Asatoor and Armstrong, 1967; Johnson and Perry, 1970; Elzinga, 1970; Weihing and Korn, 1972). In muscle actin, 3-methylhistidine is present in an amount representing 1 mol per 47,000 daltons of protein. The amino acid analysis of hydrolyzed protein previously purified on a Sephadex G-200 column was approximately 0.85 mol per molecular weight of 47,000 daltons. The ratio of 3-methyl-histidine:histidine was approximately 1:10, this also is similar to the reported ratio of these two amino acids in muscle actin. Muscle myosin also contains 3-methylhistidine as well as N-ε-methyllysine. These two amino acids were also found to be present in the synaptosomal myosin. Mobility on SDS polyamylamide gel electrophoresis indicated that the molecular weight of synaptosomal actin was approximately 47,000 and that of the major unit of synaptosomal myosin was approximately 220,000–240,000. These values are similar to those reported for muscle actin and myosin, respectively.

7. SYNAPTOSOMAL MEMBRANE AND VESICULAR PROTEIN

In further studies of the distribution of these proteins within the synaptosomes, the fraction obtained from rat brain was partially purified on a discontinuous Ficoll gradient (Puszkin *et al.*, 1972). It was then subjected to osmotic shock to obtain the presynaptic vesicle and membrane fractions (De Robertis *et al.*, 1966). The tissue pellets thus obtained were extracted for the isolation of actomyosin-like protein (Berl *et al.*, 1973). The extracted protein was then subjected to zonal centrifugation in sucrose gradients containing 0.6 M KI and 1 mM ATP. The centrifuged vesicular protein concentrated in one major band which centered at 0.35 M sucrose. In contrast, the centrifuged sucrose gradient of membrane protein showed one major band centered at 0.15 M sucrose. The vesicle protein was similar to the myosin-like protein isolated from either whole brain or synaptosomal

TABLE 10. ATPase Activity of Protein Isolated from Rat Synaptosomal Vesicle and Membrane Fractions

	μmol Pi/mg protein/30 min[a]					
Vesicle protein		Membrane protein		Vesicle + membrane protein	
Ca^{2+}	Mg^{2+}	Ca^{2+}	Mg^{2+}	Ca^{2+}	Mg^{2+}
7.8	0.9	0.09	0.03	7.8	5.4
8.4	0.9	0.06	0.06	8.1	4.8
16.5	0.9	2.25	1.65	12.7	6.9

[a] See Table 2 for incubation conditions.
(From Berl et al., 1973.)

actomyosin in that it exhibited Ca^{2+}-stimulated ATPase activity and little Mg^{2+}-stimulated enzyme activity (Table 10). The membrane protein was similar to the actin-like protein isolated from either whole brain or from synaptosomal actomyosin in that it demonstrated little enzyme activity alone but enhanced the Mg^{2+}-stimulated ATPase activity of the vesicle protein approximately five- to eightfold. The Mg^{2+}-stimulated ATPase activity of the vesicle protein was also enhanced by muscle actin and the membrane protein enhanced the Mg^{2+}-stimulated ATPase activity of muscle myosin (Table 11). The protein isolated from the vesicle preparation contained 3-methylhistidine and N-ε-methyllysine residues, similar to the myosin-like protein isolated from whole brain or synaptosomal preparations.

Because little myosin-like protein was obtained from the membrane fractions and little actin-like protein was extracted from the vesicle fraction,

TABLE 11. ATPase Activity of Vesicle Myosin and Membrane Actin with Striated Muscle Actin and Myosin, Respectively[a]

	μmol Pi/mg protein/30 min	
	Ca^{2+}	Mg^{2+}
Vesicle myosin	14.9	1.11
Muscle actin	0.06	0.03
Vesicle myosin + muscle actin	14.5	3.30
Membrane actin	0.18	0.21
Muscle myosin	7.5	0.81
Membrane actin + muscle myosin	9.9	3.60

[a] See Table 2 for incubation conditions.
(From Berl et al., 1973.)

the results were interpreted as indicating that myosin-like protein may be associated with presynaptic vesicles, and actin-like protein with presynaptic membranes. However, these conclusions, drawn from studies on the distribution of the proteins in subcellular fractions, are tempered by the realization that the fractions were not pure. The contribution of the subcellular fragments that might have been present, such as glial cells or postsynaptic elements, cannot be evaluated. For a definitive answer to the problem of the distribution of these proteins, other approaches are required.

8. Ca^{2+}-SENSITIVE COMPONENT

Another important protein complex associated with striated and smooth muscle is the tropomyosin–troponin system. Without going into details about the composition and structural relationships of this system in muscle, it may suffice for the purpose of this chapter to point out that this complex, in its interaction with Ca^{2+}, controls the interaction of actin with myosin and thus the contraction of actomyosin. Its presence in the actomyosin-like system of brain would add to the understanding of the function of this protein system in brain as well as to the understanding of at least one of the mechanisms by which Ca^{2+} may function in brain.

Attention was drawn by Douglas (1968) to the parallelism between excitation–contraction in muscles and stimulus–secretion in secretory tissues and nerve endings. This relationship was based in part on the absolute requirement for Ca^{2+} for stimulus–secretion as well as for acetylcholine release at the neuromuscular junction (Douglas, 1965, 1968; Katz and Miledi, 1967). The release of norepinephrine and dopamine β-hydroxylase from sympathetic nerve endings has also been shown to be activated by Ca^{2+} (Boullin, 1967; Kirpekar and Misu, 1967; Smith et al., 1970). Ca^{2+} is required for the stimulated release of transmitter agents as well as release of secretory products in general. Thus the hypothesis suggested by Berl et al. (1973), involving actomyosin-like protein in exocytosis, for the release of neurotransmitters at nerve endings would be strengthened by a Ca^{2+}-sensitive component.

Indeed a Ca^{2+}-sensitive component in the actomyosin-like protein isolated from synaptosomal preparations of bovine brain has been substantiated (Mahendran et al., 1974). This fact is demonstrated by the finding that the addition of the Ca^{2+} chelator ethylene glycol-bis-(β-aminoethyl ether)-N,N'-tetracetate (EGTA) to the assay medium reduces the Mg^{2+}-stimulated ATPase activity by approximately 40–50% (Table 12). In the brain system, as in muscle, it is assumed that the EGTA chelates endogenous

TABLE 12. Reconstruction of Ca^{2+} Sensitivity of Synaptosomal Actomyosin and Its Dependence on —SH Groups[a]

Preparations	Additions	Percent activity
Native protein	Mg^{2+}	100
	Mg^{2+}, EGTA	55
	Mg^{2+}, 10^{-5} M Ca^{2+}, EGTA	105
Desensitized protein[b]	Mg^{2+}	100 (95)
(+DTT)	Mg^{2+}, EGTA	91 (87)
	Mg^{2+}, 10^{-5} M Ca^{2+}, EGTA	102 (97)
Desensitized protein[b]	Mg^{2+}	100 (56)
(−DTT)	Mg^{2+}, EGTA	103 (58)
	Mg^{2+}, 10^{-5} M Ca^{2+}, EGTA	114 (65)
70,000g supernatant	Mg^{2+}	0
(+DTT)	Mg^{2+}, EGTA	0
	Mg^{2+}, 10^{-5} M Ca^{2+}, EGTA	0
70,000g supernatant	Mg^{2+}	0
(−DTT)	Mg^{2+}, EGTA	0
	Mg^{2+}, 10^{-5} M Ca^{2+}, EGTA	0
Reconstituted protein[c]	Mg^{2+}	100 (94)
(+DTT)	Mg^{2+}, EGTA	58 (55)
	Mg^{2+}, 10^{-5} M Ca^{2+}, EGTA	104 (98)
Reconstituted protein[c]	Mg^{2+}	100 (63)
(−DTT)	Mg^{2+}, EGTA	103 (65)
	Mg^{2+}, 10^{-5} M Ca^{2+}, EGTA	116 (72)

[a] The Mg^{2+} stimulated ATPase activity of each preparation is considered to be 100%. The values in parentheses represent activity as a percentage of the MgATPase activity of the native actomyosin. (From Mahendran et al., 1974.) Desensitized actomyosin and its reconstitution was carried out in the presence or absence of DDT.
[b] Desensitized by dialysis against 2 mM Tris-HCl pH 7.6.
[c] Reconstituted by reprecipitation from 0.6 M KCl in the presence of the supernatant.

Ca^{2+}. The inhibition induced by the EGTA can be overcome by the addition of Ca^{2+} sufficient to yield a free Ca^{2+} concentration of 10^{-6} M (Mahendran et al., 1974). The EGTA inhibition of the Mg^{2+}-stimulated ATPase activity of the brain protein is considerably less than the near 100% inhibition observed with skeletal actomyosin (Weber and Winicur, 1961). However, it is comparable to the values that have been reported for actomyosin-like complexes from nonstriated muscle sources such as uterine smooth muscle (Carsten, 1971), blood platelets (Hanson et al., 1972), and leukocytes (Shibata et al., 1972).

In striated muscle, Ca^{2+} sensitivity can be separated from the protein complex by dialysis of a suspension of the protein complex in a low ionic strength buffer (2 mM Tris-HCl, pH 7.6) against the same buffer (Hartshorne and Mueller, 1967). This Ca^{2+} sensitivity can be restored to the protein complex by reprecipitation of the complex from solution in 0.6 M KCl in the presence of the supernatant from the original protein suspension. This procedure was also used to demonstrate the presence of a Ca^{2+}-sensitive component in the synaptosomal actomyosin-like protein (Table 12). However, the reconstitution of the Ca^{2+} sensitivity can be demonstrated only if dithiothreitol (DTT) is present during both desensitization and reconstitution procedures. In addition, in the absence of DTT, the Mg^{2+}-stimulated ATPase activity of the desensitized synaptosomal actomyosin is considerably lower than the corresponding preparation in the presence of DTT. It is apparent that the integrity of the sulfhydryl groups needs to be maintained in the brain protein as it is in the muscle protein (Stewart and Levy, 1970).

Recently, proteins very similar to muscle tropomyosin have been isolated and characterized from human blood platelets (Cohen and Cohen, 1972), from the electric organs of the torpedo and electric eel (Kaminer and Szonyi, 1972) and from chick embryo brain (Fine *et al.*, 1973). Substitution of the brain protein for muscle tropomyosin in a calcium-regulated actomyosin ATPase system showed that the brain tropomyosin can interact with muscle troponin to confer calcium sensitivity to the Mg^{2+}-activated actomyosin ATPase of muscle (Fine *et al.*, 1973). The brain tropomyosin is similar but not identical to the muscle protein; it binds to muscle actin but the binding is weaker. It is smaller molecular weight (30,000 vs 35,000) paracrystals are formed with $MgCl_2$ but are of shorter periodicity. Amino acid composition, although similar, is somewhat different; peptide maps show eight similar peptides, but there are also some differences.

Thus, three contractile proteins which are similar to those in muscle actomyosin—actin, myosin, and tropomyosin—are present in brain. However, there is no direct evidence that troponinlike elements are also present. Molluscan muscle does not contain troponin; the Ca^{2+}-sensitive sites are not on the tropomyosin but are associated with the myosin molecule (Kendrick-Jones *et al.*, 1970). Since the factor responsible for Ca^{2+} sensitivity can be removed from and restored to the brain actomyosin complex, it is more likely that the Ca^{2+}-sensitive system in brain is similar to that of striated muscle rather than that of molluscan muscle.

9. STUDIES WITH COLCHICINE, VINBLASTINE, AND CYTOCHALASIN B

9.1. Colchicine and Vinblastine

It has been reported that colchicine and vinca alkaloids, such as vinblastine can inhibit the stimulated release of substances from several organs.

Malaisse et al. (1971) showed that these alkaloids inhibited the glucose-induced secretion of insulin from pancreas slices. Similarly, colchicine and vinblastine inhibited the acetylcholine or nicotine-induced release of catecholamines from the perfused adrenal medulla (Poisner and Bernstein, 1971). More recently, the inhibition of the electrically stimulated release of dopamine-β-hydroxylase and norepinephrine from sympathetic nerves by these agents has been demonstrated (Thoa et al., 1972). These effects have been interpreted as evidence that microtubules are involved in the stimulus–secretion coupling process, since the above agents are known to interact with microtubular protein. However, vinblastine can also precipitate a variety of acidic proteins including muscle actin (Wilson et al., 1970) as well as actin from neuronal cultures of chick embryo (Fine and Bray, 1971).

When crude synaptosomal preparations were preincubated with increasing concentrations of colchicine, [^{3}H]-dopamine uptake was inhibited in a dose-dependent manner (Nicklas et al., 1973). With 1 mM colchicine there was an approximately 50% decrease in dopamine uptake, whereas glutamate uptake was only 20% inhibited. Vinblastine proved to be a far more potent inhibitor of the uptake of putative transmitters (Table 13). Vinblastine (10^{-4} M) decreased the uptake of GABA, dopamine and norepinephrine by 65–75%; glutamate uptake was only slightly affected. Studies on the kinetics of inhibition by vinblastine on norepinephrine uptake indicated that it was noncompetitive in nature with a K_i of approximately 10^{-4} M, whereas the K_m for norepinephrine uptake was approximately 1.4×10^{-7} M. The data are consistent with the interpretation that vinblastine does not compete with catecholamines for transport sites but rather may have a direct effect on membrane components.

TABLE 13.   Effect of Vinblastine on Uptake of Putative Transmitters by a Crude Synaptosomal Preparation from Rat Brain[a]

	Percentage of control uptake $\pm$ S.E.M.		
	0.05 mM vinblastine	0.10 mM vinblastine	0.25 mM vinblastine
L-[^{14}C]-glutamate	103 $\pm$ 4	90 $\pm$ 5	43 $\pm$ 2
[^{14}C]-GABA	50 $\pm$ 0.5	27 $\pm$ 1	8 $\pm$ 1
[^{3}H]-dopamine	68 $\pm$ 1	29 $\pm$ 1	11 $\pm$ 0.5
L-[^{3}H]-norepinephrine	66 $\pm$ 2	36 $\pm$ 1	18 $\pm$ 2[b]

[a] Vinblastine was preincubated with the preparation for 20 min at 37°C prior to addition of the labeled compound. (From Nicklas et al., 1973.)
[b] 0.15 mM vinblastine instead of 0.25 mM.

When the synaptosomal preparation was preloaded with radioactive glutamate, GABA, dopamine, or norepinephrine and then the external $[K^+]$ increased from 5 to 30 mM, radioactivity was rapidly released from the tissue into the medium (Nicklas *et al.*, 1973). Vinblastine also inhibited the ability of the preparation to maintain the levels of these substances. Adding vinblastine after preloading with either $[^{14}C]$GABA or $[^3H]$norepinephrine caused a leakage of radioactivity into the medium which was dependent on the concentration of the drug. The amount of radioactivity released by K^+ was decreased although there appeared to be little effect on the relative efflux of radioactivity caused by the elevated concentration of K^+, i.e., the percentage of accumulated radioactivity released by vinblastine was unchanged.

The effect of vinblastine and colchicine on the enzymatic activity of the synaptosomal actomyosin-like protein was also studied. These drugs, particularly the former, inhibited the Mg^{2+}-stimulated ATPase activity of the protein (Table 14). The inhibition by vinblastine was greater at sub-maximal concentrations of ATP indicating that the nucleotide offered some protection to the enzyme. The Ca^{2+}-stimulated ATPase activity was not significantly affected by either drug. These results suggest that the inhibition of uptake and release by vinblastine may result from an effect on membrane components—one of which may be the brain actinlike protein—rather than on the microtubules.

TABLE 14. Effect of Vinblastine and Colchicine on Mg^{2+}-ATPase Activity of Synaptosomal Actomyosin-like Protein (Neurostenin)

ATP (mM)	Percentage of control activity of ATPase[a] ± S.E.M.			
	0.1 mM vinblastine	0.2 mM vinblastine	0.55 mM vinblastine	1 mM colchicine
0.50	$71^b \pm 8$ (10)	$65^b \pm 6$ (6)	23 (1)	65 ± 12 (2)
0.25	$48^b \pm 16$ (5)	$44^b \pm 10$ (6)		

[a] Activity was measured as μmoles of Pi released $\cdot$ (mg of protein)$^{-1} \cdot$ (30 min)$^{-1}$. The numbers of duplicate determinations of different preparations are given in parentheses. Duplicates differed by <10% from each other. Combined controls averaged $100 \pm 8\%$ for 14 preparations. (From Nicklas *et al.*, 1973.)
[b] $p < 0.01$ from control values.

9.2. Cytochalasin B

The mold metabolite cytochalasin B (Aldridge *et al.*, 1967) disrupts a large variety of contractile cellular functions such as cytokinesis, cell locomotion, cytoplasmic streaming, blood clot retraction, and neuronal and glial movements associated with growth and development; these diverse processes may be associated with microfilamentous processes (Wessels *et al.*, 1971; Lin *et al.*, 1974). This drug has also been reported to inhibit stimulated release of secretory products, e.g., thyroid secretion (Williams and Wolff, 1971), growth hormone (Schofield, 1971), posterior pituitary and adrenal medullary hormones (Douglas and Sorimachi, 1972), as well as norepinephrine and dopamine–β-hydroxylase from sympathetic nerve endings (Thoa *et al.*, 1972) and norepinephrine from guinea pig atria (Sorimachi *et al.*, 1973). In addition, it has been shown to cause a decrease in the intrinsic viscosity of muscle actin (Spudich and Lin, 1972; Lin *et al.*, 1974), to alter the morphology of actin filaments isolated from muscle and blood platelets (Spudich, 1972), and to disrupt the cardiac myofibrils of chick embryo (Manasek *et al.*, 1972).

We have studied the effect of cytochalasin B on the uptake and K^+-stimulated release of norepinephrine, dopamine, glutamic acid, and GABA by rat brain synaptosomal preparations (Nicklas and Berl, 1974). We have also studied the effect of this drug on the ATPase activity of myosin-like and actin-like proteins, isolated from synaptosomal vesicular and membrane preparations, as they interact with each other or with the analogous muscle proteins (Nicklas and Berl, 1974).

Cytocholasin B had a small but significant inhibitory effect ($p < 0.01$) on the uptake of norepinephrine (20%) and dopamine (30%). Its major effect was on the K^+-stimulated release of norepinephrine (60–90%). The release of dopamine was also significantly affected but to a lesser extent (22–32%). Neither the uptake nor the release of glutamic acid or GABA was affected. It would appear that the mechanisms for uptake and release of glutamic acid and GABA may be different than those for the catecholamines.

Preincubation for 10 min in 0.1 mM cytochalasin B of the actomyosin-like protein isolated from rat brain synaptosomal preparations resulted in approximately 50% inhibition of the Mg^{2+}-stimulated ATPase activity. The Ca^{2+}-stimulated ATPase activity was not affected. Similarly, in recombination studies of the actin-like and myosin-like brain proteins with each other and with their counterparts from striated muscle, 0.1 mM cytochalasin inhibited the Mg^{2+}-stimulated ATPase activity by approximately 50% (Nicklas and Berl, 1974). The fact that the effect is on the Mg^{2+}- but not on the Ca^{2+}-stimulated enzyme activity suggests that the action of the drug is on the interaction between actin and myosin; the Mg^{2+}-stimulated ATPase activity is dependent upon this interaction. Studies with cytochalasin D indicate that this drug binds to myosin (Puszkin et al., 1973). Although it is probable that both cytochalasins bind to the same site, this fact has not been established.

10. FUNCTION IN BRAIN

In considering the function or functions of these protein systems we have to bear in mind that there is no direct experimental proof of their action in any of the nonmuscle systems, in part, because there exists no adequate picture of the structural relationships of the actin to the myosin; these relationships are only well understood in the striated systems. (For an extensive review of actin and myosin in cell movement, see Pollard and Weihing, 1974.) By analogy with their actions in the muscle system and based on a great deal of circumstantial evidence, we assume that the nonmuscle proteins are capable of converting chemical to mechanical energy and of providing some mobile or contractile force, as in muscle. In blood platelets they are thought to function in clot retraction, but they may also function in serotonin release, since the latter is in high concentration in vesicular structures in blood platelets. In dividing cells (newt, HeLa, echinoderm), the contractile ring formed during cytokinesis is thought to involve actin-like protein. In the slime mold actin-like protein probably functions in cyto-plasmic streaming; in fibroblasts, polymorphonuclear leukocytes, and amoeba it probably functions in motility and also in phagocytosis in the latter two. It may function in all mobile cells, and in the immature nervous system it may provide the mechanism for cell migration.

In the axon, the association of the myosin-like protein with the vesicle would place it in the appropriate position for sultatory movement of vesicles down the axon, perhaps associated with the microtubules as suggested by Schmitt (1968).

Examining the subcellular distribution of these proteins in the mature brain, we have focused on the suggestion that this protein system functions in exocytosis for the quantal release of neurotransmitter substances at nerve endings (Berl et al., 1973). We suggest that actin is associated with the pre-synaptic membrane, perhaps as the microfilaments, and myosin with the vesicles. The synaptic vesicles come to be in intimate contact with the pre-synaptic membrane. The entrance of Ca^{2+} in response to stimulation, or the release of Ca^{2+} from the membrane, triggers the interaction between actin and myosin as it does in muscle. Conformational changes in the membranes result in opening of the vesicular and synaptosomal membranes. Transmitter is released into the synaptic cleft or replaces transmitter in the membrane. The action is terminated by the release or binding of Ca^{2+}. This singular role of Ca^{2+} is in line with the hypothesis of Katz and Miledi (1967b) that depolarization at the presynaptic terminal causes an increase in the permeability of the terminal to Ca^{2+}, which enters and functions in quantal release of transmitter from vesicles. Whether the vesicle is used again or remains fused with the membrane depends upon the system studied and the experimental condition (Clark et al., 1972). Some studies indicate that the vesicles fuse with the membrane. On the other hand, other studies support the contention that, even with extensive stimulation, vesicles may not deplete but may be reused. Whether fusion is a primary or secondary process is yet to be established.

Recently, Bray (1973) has put forth the formulation that in the growth cone of the growing neurite the contractile proteins are responsible for movement and elongation of the filopodia. In the growth cone there are present numerous tubular vesicles. These may arrive along the microtubules propelled from their site of synthesis in the cell body to the neurite tip. In the filopodia the actomyosin proteins associated with the vesicles and membranes orient and move the vesicle toward the tip. The vesicle fuses with the membrane and results in extension and growth of the neurite.

No doubt other functions can be assigned to the actomyosin-like protein system in nervous tissue. Which of these will eventually prove to be true is part of the wonder of research.

11. REFERENCES

Abdel-Latif, A. A., 1966, A simple method for isolation of nerve-ending particles from rat brain, Biochim. Biophys. Acta 121:403–406.

Adelman, M. R., and Taylor, E. W., 1969a, Isolation of an actomyosin-like protein complex from slime mold plasmodium and the separation of the complex into actin- and myosin-like fractions, Biochemistry 8:4964–4975.

Adelman, M. R., and Taylor, E. W., 1969b, Further purification and characterization of slime mold myosin and slime mold actin, Biochemistry 8:4976–4988.

Aldridge, D. C., Armstrong, J. J., Speake, R. N., and Turner, W. B., 1967, The structure of cytochalasins A and B, J. Chem. Soc. 1967(C):1667–1676.

Arcos, J. C., Stacey, R. E., Mathison, J. B., and Argus, M. F., 1967, Kinetic parameters of mitochondria swelling, Exp. Cell Research 48:448–460.

Asatoor, A. M., and Armstrong, M. D., 1967, 3-methylhistidine, a component of actin, Biochem. Biophys. Res. Comm. 26:168–174.

Bárány, M., and Jaisle, F., 1960, Kontraktioniszklus und interaktion zwischen aktin und L-myosin unter der wirkung spezifische interaktions—inhibitoren, Biochim. Biophys. Acta 41:192–203.

Bárány, M., Bárány, K., Gaetjens, E., and Bailin, G., 1966, Chicken gizzard myosin, *Arch. Biochem. Biophys.* **113**:205–221.

Bárány, M., Nagy, B., Finkelman, F., and Chrambach, A., 1961, Studies on the removal of the bound nucleotide of actin, *J. Biol. Chem.* **236**:2917–2925.

Benitez, H. H., Murray, M. R., and Wooley, D. W., 1955, Effects of serotonin and certain of its antagonists upon oligodendroglial cells *in vitro*, *Proceedings Second International Congress Neuropathology*, Pt II, 423–428, Exerpta Medica Foundation.

Berl, S., and Puszkin, S., 1970, $Mg^{2+}-Ca^{2+}$-activated adenosine triphosphatase system isolated from mammalian brain, *Biochemistry* **9**:2058–2067.

Berl, S., Puszkin, S., and Nicklas, W. J., 1973, Actomyosin-like protein in brain, *Science* **179**:441–446.

Bettex-Galland, M., and Luscher, E. F., 1960, Thrombosthenin, the contractile protein from blood platelets and its relation to other contractile proteins, *Adv. Protein Chem.* **20**:1–35.

Boullin, D. J., 1967, The action of extracellular cations on the release of the sympathetic transmitter from peripheral nerves, *J. Physiol. (London)* **189**:85–99.

Bowler, K., and Duncan, C., 1967, Studies on the actomyosinlike membranes preparation from crayfish nerve cord, *Comp. Biochem. Physiol.* **20**:543–551.

Bowler, K., and Duncan, C., 1968, The temperature characteristics of the ATPases from a frog brain microsomal preparation, *Comp. Biochem. Physiol.* **24**:223–227.

Bray, D., 1973, Model for membrane movements in the neural growth cone, *Nature* **244**:93–96.

Carsten, M. E., 1971, Uterine smooth muscle: Troponin, *Arch. Biochem. Biophys.* **147**:353–357.

Carsten, M. E., and Mommaerts, W. F. H. M., 1963, A study of actin by means of starch gel electrophoresis, *Biochemistry* **2**:28–32.

Chang, C-M., and Goldman, R. D., 1973, The localization of actinlike fibers in cultured neuroblastoma cells as revealed by heavy meromyosin binding, *J. Cell Biol.* **57**: 867–874.

Clark, J. B., and Nicklas, W. J., 1970, The preparation of rat brain mitochondria. Preparation and characterization, *J. Biol. Chem.* **245**:4724–4731.

Clark, A. W., Hurlbut, W. P., and Mauro, A., 1972, Changes in the fine structure of the neuromuscular junction of the frog caused by black widow spider venom, *J. Cell. Biol.* **52**:1–14.

Cohen, I., and Cohen, C. J., 1972, A tropomyosinlike protein from human platelets, *J. Mol. Biol.* **68**:383–387.

Conover, T. E., and Bárány, M., 1966, The absence of a myosin-like protein in liver mitochondria, *Biochim. Biophys. Acta* **127**:235–238.

De Robertis, E., Alberici, M., Rodriguez De Lores Arnaiz, G., and Azcurra, J. M., 1966, Isolation of different types of synaptic membranes from the brain cortex, *Life Sci.* **5**:577–582.

Douglas, W. W., 1965, Calcium dependent links in stimulus-secretion coupling in the adrenal medulla and neurohypophysis, *Int. Wenner-Gren Symposium*, Stockholm, pp. 267–290, Pergamon Press, London.

Douglas, W. W., 1968, The First Gaddum Memorial Lecture. Stimulus-secretion coupling. The concept and clues from chromaffin and other cells, *Brit. J. Pharmacol.* **34**:451–474.

Douglass, W. W., and Sorimachi, M., 1972, Affects of cytochalasin B and colchicine on secretion of posterior pituitary and adrenal medullary hormones, *Brit. J. Pharmacol.* **45**:143–144P.

Elzinga, M., 1970, Amino acid sequence studies on rabbit skeletal muscle actin. Cyanogen bromide cleavage of the protein and determination of the sequence of seven of the resulting peptides, *Biochemistry* **9**:1365–1374.

Filo, R. S., Ruegg, J. C., and Bohr, D. F., 1963, Actomyosin-like protein of arterial wall, *Amer. J. Physiol.* **205**:1247–1252.

Fine, R. E., and Bray, D., 1971, Actin in growing nerve cells, *Nature New Biol.* **234**:115–118.

Fine, R. E., Blitz, A. L., Hitchcock, S. E., and Kaminer, B., 1973, Tropomyosin in brain and growing neurones, *Nature New Biol.* **245**:182–186.

Gergely, J., 1964, *in Biochemistry of Muscle Contraction* (J. Gergely, ed.), p. 119, Little, Brown and Co., Boston, Mass.

Germain, M., and Proulx, P., 1965, Adenosine triphosphatase activity in synaptic vesicles of rat brain, *Biochem. Pharm.* **14**:1815–1819.

Hanson, J. P., Repke, D. I., Katz, A. M., and Aledort, L. M., 1972, A troponin–tropomyosin-like Ca^{++}-sensitizing system in human platelets, *Int. Soc. Thrombosis and Haemostasis.* IIIrd Congress, Washington, D.C. (Abstracts), p. 200.

Hartshorne, D. J., and Mueller, H., 1967, Separation and recombination of the ethylene glycol bis (β-aminoethyl ether)-N, N^1-tetraacetic acid–sensitizing factor obtained from a low ionic strength extract of natural actomyosin, *J. Biol. Chem.* **242**:3089–3092.

Hess, H. H., and Pope, A., 1959, Intralaminar distribution of adenosine triphosphatase activity in rat cerebral cortex, *J. Neurochem.*, **3**:287–299.

Hess, H. H., and Pope, A., 1961, Intralaminar distribution of adenosine triphosphatase activity in human frontal isocortex, *J. Neurochem.*, **8**:299–309.

Hoffman-Berling, H., 1956, Das kontraktile eiweiss undifferenzierter zellen, *Biochim. Biophys. Acta* **19**:453–463.

Hosie, R. J., 1965, The localization of adenosine triphosphatase in morphologically characterized subcellular fractions of guinea-pig brain, *Biochem. J.* **96**:404–412.

Ishikawa, H., Bischoff, R., and Holtzer, H., 1969, Formation of arrowhead complexes with heavy meromyosin in a variety of cell types, *J. Cell. Biol.* **43**:312–328.

Johnson, P., and Perry, S. V., 1970, Biological activity and 3-methylhistidine content of actin and myosin, *Biochem. J.* **119**:293–298.

Kadota, K., Mori, S., and Imaizumi, R., 1967, The properties of ATPase of synaptic vesicle fraction, *J. Biochem.* **61**:424–432.

Kaminer, B., and Szonyi, E., 1972, Tropomyosin in electric organ of eel and torpedo, *J. Cell Biol.* **55**:129a.

Katz, B., and Miledi, R., 1967*a*, The timing of calcium action during neuromuscular transmission, *J. Physiol. (London)* **189**:535–544.

Katz, B., and Miledi, R., 1967*b*, The release of acetylcholine from nerve endings by graded electric pulses, *Proc. Roy. Soc.* **B167**:23–38.

Kendrick-Jones, J., Lehman, W., and Szent-Gyorgyi, A. G., 1970, Regulation in molluscan muscles, *J. Mol. Biol.* **54**:313–326.

Kirpekar, S. M., and Misu, Y., 1967, Release of noradrenaline by splenic nerve stimulation and its dependence on calcium, *J. Physiol. (London)* **189**:219–234.

Kuehl, W. M., and Gergely, J., 1969, The kinetics of exchange of adenosine triphosphate and calcium with G-Actin, *J. Biol. Chem.* **244**:4720–4729.

Lewin, E., and Hess, H. H., 1964, Intralaminar distribution of Na–K ATPase in rat cortex, *J. Neurochem.* **11**:473–481.

Libet, B., 1948, Adenosinetriphosphatase (ATPase) in nerve, *Fed. Proc.* **7**:72.

Lin, S., Santi, D. V., and Spudich, J. A., 1974, Biochemical studies on the mode of action of cytochalasin B, *J. Biol. Chem.* **249**:2268–2274.

Mahendran, C., Nicklas, W. J., and Berl, S., 1974, Evidence for calcium-sensitive component in brain actomyosin-like protein (neurostenin), *J. Neurochem.* **23**:497–501.

Malaisse, W. J., Malaisse-Lagae, F., Walker, M. O., and Lacy, P. E., 1971, The stimulus-secretion coupling of glucose-induced insulin release, *Diabetes* **20**:257–265.

Manasek, F. J., Burnside, B., Stroman, J., 1972, The sensitivity of developing cardiac myofibrils to cytochalasin B, *Proc. Nat. Acad. Sci. (U.S.)* **69**:302–312.

Martonosi, A., and Gouvea, M. A., 1961, Studies on actin. VI. The interaction of nucleoside triphosphates with actin, *J. Biol. Chem.* **236**:1345–1352.

Martonosi, A., Gouvea, M. A., and Gergely, J., 1960, Studies on actin. I. The interaction of [C^{14}]-labeled adenosine nucleotide with actin, *J. Biol. Chem.* **235**:1700–1706.

Naidoo, D., and Pratt, O. E., 1956, The effect of magnesium and calcium ions on adenosine triphosphatase in the nervous and vascular tissues of the brain, *Biochem. J.* **62**:465–469.

Needham, D., 1960, *in Structure and Function of Muscle* (G. H. Bourne, ed.), Vol. 2, p. 72, Academic Press, New York.

Needham, D., and Williams, J. M., 1963, Proteins of the uterine contractile mechanism, *Biochem. J.* **89**:552–560.

Neifakh, S. A., and Kazakova, T. B., 1963, Actomyosin-like protein in mitochondria of the mouse liver, *Nature* **197**:1106–1107.

Nicklas, W. J., and Berl, S., 1974, Effects of cytochalasin B on uptake and release of putative transmitters by synaptosomes and on brain actomyosin-like protein, *Nature* **247**:471–473.

Nicklas, W. J., Puszkin, S., and Berl, S., 1973, Effect of vinblastine and colchicine on uptake and release of putative transmitters by synaptosomes and on brain actomyosinlike protein, *J. Neurochem.* **20**:109–121.

Novakoff, A. B., 1967, Enzyme localization and ultrastructure of neurones, *in The Neurone* (H. Hyden, ed.), pp. 255–318, Elsevier, Amsterdam.

Ohnishi, T., and Ohnishi, T., 1962, Extraction of contractile protein from liver mitochondria, *J. Biochem. (Tokyo)* **51**:380–381.

Perry, S. V., and Grey, T. C., 1956, A study of the effects of substrate concentration and certain relaxing factors on the magnesium-activated myofibrillar adenosine triphosphatase, *Biochem. J.* **64**:184–192.

Poglazov, B. F., 1966, *Structure and Functions of Contractile Proteins* (Poglazov, B. F., ed.), p. 69, Academic Press, New York.

Poisner, A. M., and Bernstein, J., 1971, A possible role of microtubules in catecholamine release from the adrenal medulla: Effect of colchicine, vinca alkaloids and deuterium oxide, *J. Pharm. Exptl. Ther.* **177**:102–108.

Pollard, T. D., and Korn, E., 1972, The "contractile" proteins of *Acanthamoeba castellanii, in Cold Spring Harbor Symposia on Quantitative Biology*, Vol. XXXVII, pp. 573–583.

Pollard, T. D., and Weihing, R. R., 1974, Actin and myosin and cell movement, *CRC Critical Reviews in Biochemistry*, January, 1–65.

Pomerat, C. M., Handelman, W. J., and Raiborn, C. W., Jr., 1967, Dynamic activities of nervous tissue *in vitro, in The Neurone* (H. Hyden, ed.), pp. 119–178, Elsevier, Amsterdam.

Portzehl, H., Schramm, G., and Weber, H. H., 1950, Aktomyosin und seine komponenten, I. Mitt., *Z. Naturforsch.* **5B**:61–74.

Puszkin, S., and Berl, S., 1972, Actomyosin-like protein from brain: Separation and characterization of the actin-like component, *Biochim. Biophys. Acta* **256**:695–709.

Puszkin, S., Berl, S., Puszkin, E., and Clarke, D. C., 1968, Actomyosin-like protein isolated from mammalian brain, *Science* **161**:170–171.

Puszkin, S., Nicklas, W. J., and Berl, S., 1972, Actomyosin-like protein in brain: Subcellular distribution, *J. Neurochem.* **19**:1319–1333.

Puszkin, E., Puszkin, S., Lo, L. W., and Tanenbaum, S. W., 1973, Binding of cytochalasin D to platelet and muscle myosin, *J. Biol. Chem.* **248**:7754–7761.

Rees, M. K., and Young, M., 1967, Studies on the isolation and molecular properties of homogeneous globular actin, *J. Biol. Chem.* **242**:4449–4458.

Richards, E. G., Chung, C. S., Menzel, D. B., and Olcott, H. S., 1967, Chromatography of myosin on diethylaminoethylsephadex A-50, *Biochemistry* **6**:528–540.

Schmitt, F. O., 1968, The molecular biology of neuronal fibrous proteins, *Neurosciences Res. Prog. Bull.*, Vol. 6, No. 2, pp. 119–144.

Schofield, J. G., 1971, Cytochalasin B and release of growth hormone, *Nature New Biol.* **234**:215–216.

Shibata, N., Tatsumi, N., Tanaka, K., Okamura, Y., and Senda, N., 1972, A contractile protein possessing Ca^{2+}-sensitivity (natural actomyosin) from leucocytes, *Biochim. Biophys. Acta* **256**: 565–576.

Smith, A. D., DePotter, W. P., Moerman, E. J., and De Schaedryver, A. F., 1970, Release of dopamine β-hydroxylase and chromogranin A upon stimulation of the splenic nerve, *Tissue Cell* **2**: 547–568.

Sorimachi, M., Oesch, F., and Thoenen, H., 1973, Effects of colchicine and cytochalasin B on the release of ³H-norepinephrine from guinea-pig atria evoked by high potassium, nicotine and tyramine, *Naunyn-Schmiederberg's Arch. Pharmacol.* **276**: 1–12.

Speidel, C. C., 1935, Studies of living nerves; phenomena of nerve irritation and recovery, degeneration and repair, *J. Comp. Neurol.* **61**: 1–80.

Spudich, J. A., 1972, Effects of cytochalasin B on actin filaments, *Cold Spring Harbor Symposium on Quantitative Biology*, Vol. XXXVII, pp. 585–593.

Spudich, J. A., and Lin, S., 1972, Cytochalasin B, its interaction with actin and actomyosin from muscle, *Proc. Nat. Acad. Sci. (U.S.)* **69**: 442–446.

Stewart, J. M., and Levy, H. M., 1970, The role of the calcium–troponin–tropomyosin complex in the activation of contraction, *J. Biol. Chem.* **245**: 5764–5772.

Stossel, T. P., and Pollard, T. D., 1973, Myosin in polymorphonuclear leukocytes, *J. Biol. Chem.* **248**: 8288–8294.

Strohman, R. C., and Samorodin, J., 1962, The requirements for adenosine triphosphate binding to globular actin, *J. Biol. Chem.* **237**: 363–370.

Szent-Gyorgyi, A., 1951a, *Chemistry of Muscle Contraction*, p. 151, Academic Press, New York.

Szent-Gyorgyi, A., 1951b, *Chemistry of Muscle Contraction*, p. 34, Academic Press, New York.

Szent-Gyorgyi, A. G., 1951a, The reversible depolymerization of actin by potassium iodide, *Arch. Biochem. Biophys.* **31**: 97–103.

Szent-Gyorgyi, A. G., 1951b, A new method for the preparation of actin, *J. Biol. Chem.* **192**: 361–369.

Thoa, N. B., Wooten, G. F., Axelrod, J., and Kopin, I. J., 1972, Inhibition of release of dopamine-β-hydroxylase and norepinephrine from sympathetic nerves by colchicine, vinblastine, or cytochalasin-B, *Proc. Nat. Acad. Sci. (U.S.)* **69**: 520–522.

Tonomura, Y., Tokura, S., and Sekiya, K., 1962, Binding of myosin A to F-actin, *J. Biol. Chem.* **237**: 1074–1081.

Weber, A., and Winicur, S., 1961, The role of calcium in the superprecipitation of actomyosin, *J. Biol. Chem.* **236**: 3198–3202.

Weihing, R. R., and Korn, E. D., 1971, Acanthamoeba actin: Isolation and properties, *Biochemistry* **10**: 590–600.

Weihing, R. R., and Korn, E. D., 1972, Acanthamoeba actin. Composition of the peptide that contains 3-methylhistidine and a peptide that contains *N*-methyllysine, *Biochemistry* **11**: 1538–1543.

Wessels, N. K., Spooner, B. S., Ash, J. F., Bradley, M. O., Ludena, M. A., Taylor, E. L., Wrenn, J. T., and Yamada, K. M., 1971, Microfilaments in cellular and developmental processes, *Science* **171**: 135–143.

Whittaker, V. P., and Sheridan, M. N., 1965, The morphology and acetylcholine content of isolated cerebral cortical synaptic vesicles, *J. Neurochem.* **12**: 363–372.

Williams, J. A., and Wolff, J., 1971, Cytochalasin B inhibits thyroid secretion, *Biochem. Biophys. Res. Comm.* **44**: 422–425.

Wilson, L., Bryan, J., Ruby, A., and Mazia, D., 1970, Precipitation of proteins by vinblastine and calcium ions, *Proc. Nat. Acad. Sci. (U.S.)* **66**: 807–814.

Yang, Y., and Perdue, J. R., 1972, Contractile proteins of cultured cells, *J. Biol. Chem.* **247**: 4503–4509.

BIOCHEMICAL MARKERS OF THE PRIMARY OLFACTORY PATHWAY:
A Model Neural System

FRANK L. MARGOLIS

Roche Institute of Molecular Biology
Nutley, New Jersey

> "Give me a man with a good allowance of nose . . .
> I always choose a man, if suitable otherwise, with a long nose."
>
> NAPOLEON BONAPARTE

> "Thus, the task is, not so much to see what no one has yet seen;
> but to think what nobody has yet thought, about what everybody sees."
>
> ARTHUR SCHOPENHAUER

1. INTRODUCTION

The purpose of biochemistry is to try to explain biology at the molecular level. Thus, by analogy, the role of neurochemistry is to try to explain the biology of neural tissue and then, ultimately, to integrate biochemical correlates of neural activity with associated behavioral events. The brain of a mammal is perhaps its most complex organ with regard to both structure and function. To the naked eye it is composed of several morphologically distinct subsections apparently randomly joined together. As one proceeds to finer and finer levels of resolution, it rapidly becomes apparent that this tissue is composed of billions of cells which interact with each other in ways which are extremely complex, morphologically variable, and yet extremely specific. Nevertheless, the usual biochemical approach to this tissue is to treat it quite cavalierly and to convert it into a homogeneous "thin soup." This results in total destruction of structure and renders virtually impossible any attempts to understand structure–function relationships at supra-molecular levels. Intercellular relationships in neural tissue *in vivo*, occur largely between dissimilar groups of cells. An approach to a study of these relationships by means of biochemical markers will permit the evaluation of the physiological state of a selected cell in the presence of various other cell types.

Detailed studies of structure–function relationships and of the regulation of genetic expression in organisms as "simple" as viruses and prokaryotes become feasible only with the accumulation of sufficient numbers of specific biochemical markers. Yet, in nervous systems only a relatively few examples of cell-specific genetic expression are known (Gainer and Wollberg, 1974; Schneider, 1973; Moore, 1975). The vast majority of known biochemical markers are localized in neuroendocrine areas of the vertebrate brain. Thus, there are the releasing hormones of the hypothalamus (Reiss, 1970), the hormones of the anterior and posterior pituitary (Reiss, 1970), and hydroxy-indole O-methyl transferase in the pineal (Wurtman, 1970). However, these neuroendocrine regions represent only a small percentage of the entire brain mass. In the balance of the vertebrate brain, although several proteins have been isolated that occur exclusively in nervous tissue (Shooter and Einstein, 1971; Schneider, 1973; Moore, this volume), few region-specific or cell-specific proteins have been studied (Davies, 1970; Margolis, 1972*b*; Bignami *et al.*, 1972; Cuenod *et al.*, 1973).

We have searched for examples of specific genetic expression by individual kinds of neurons in mammalian brain which could then enable us to study the physiological functioning of a given neuron in a complex mass of interacting neurons and glia. Two examples of neural systems where such markers have been exploited to study the functioning of a single-cell type in the midst of a complex heterogeneous system are (1) the studies of Sachs and collaborators (1974) on the neurohypophysis in organ culture using neurophysin and vasopressin as markers, and (2) the studies of Moscona and collaborators (Moscona, 1971) using the developing retina and the influence of the steroid-mediated elevations in glutamine synthetase as a biochemical marker. In certain other systems, neurotransmitter-metabolizing enzymes have been used as markers.

Correlations of biochemical changes in the vertebrate brain with changes in behavior are among the ultimate goals in evaluating the molecular basis of cerebral function. In general such studies have tended to concentrate on cerebral areas that might be considered to be involved in major integrative functions and to deemphasize the importance of variable sensory responsiveness of the subject on the subsequent behavioral and biochemical events. Thus, for example, in an intriguing study of the influence of variations of genotype on learning ability (Bovet *et al.*, 1969) it was eventually realized that several strains of mice in one behavioral category were homozygous for the gene *rd* which causes postnatal retinal degeneration (Henry *et al.*, 1969; Wahlsten, 1972). The influence of this sensory deficit on learning ability is not understood but presumably modifies visually mediated behavior. In addition, the question of whether other sensory deficiences were present as well is unknown. The existence of this general problem, while undoubtedly widespread, is largely ignored. In other cases, the possibility that specific drug effects on learning, memory, and performance in behavioral tasks may be to cause primary alterations in sensory function or integration is rarely considered. For reasons such as these, the emphasis of my laboratory for several years (Bondy and Margolis, 1971) has been to concentrate on biochemical changes in primary sensory systems (rather than deeper integrative centers) as a function of alterations of input to these systems.

In initiating a search for biochemical markers as examples of cell-specific genetic expression to be used as probes of function, it was essential to make certain strategic decisions. Before describing our experimental results it will be helpful to consider what alternatives were available in order to understand our plan of attack and to consider other potentially profitable approaches that might be pursued in the future or that are currently being employed in our own and other laboratories.

Elegant studies have been carried out with the relatively simpler nervous systems of invertebrates, particularly molluscs (Gainer, 1972*a,b,c*; Gainer and Wollberg, 1974; Wilson, 1974), nematodes (Dusenbery, 1973; Ward, 1973), and drosophila (Woolf, 1972; Levine and Wyman, 1973). In invertebrates, particularly molluscan species, there has been some success in detecting examples of cell specific gene expression since one can more easily identify specific neurons morphologically or electrophysiologically, separate them by microdissection, and thus evaluate them for biochemical difference by microanalytical techniques. However, studies of molluscan systems suffer from the disadvantages of the lack of examples of known genetic variants and the difficulty in generating and studying alterations in behavior and learning. In the nematode and drosophila systems, where both genetics and certain kinds of behavior can be studied, there are potential problems in obtaining sufficient quantities of nervous tissue for biochemical studies although some progress has been reported (Ostroy and Pak, 1973). However, in order to study a system perhaps more relevant to man and for reasons of personal partiality, we chose to deal with mammalian vertebrates. This decision, coupled with the realization of the extreme power of genetics in helping to elucidate other systems, indicated that the mouse would be the species of choice for us. There is more known about the influence of genetics on the biochemistry, behavior, morphology, and development of the mouse (Green, 1967) than of any other mammal with the possible exception of man.

Our earlier studies concerned the visual system, where we utilized a denervation procedure in the hope that synaptic degeneration in the avian visual tectum, after sectioning of the optic nerve, would enable us to detect large, specific, selective alterations in the large- and/or small-molecule populations. Although these studies were rewarding, our efforts to discover markers by this approach were largely unsuccessful (Bondy and Margolis, 1971; Margolis and Bondy, unpublished observations). However, a recent report (Cuenod *et al.*, 1973) using the visual system of the adult pigeon rather than of the immature chicken indicates that a membrane protein found only in the optic tectum is lost following optic nerve section.

Thus, denervation techniques which classically have been used to trace neural pathways can be coupled to biochemical techniques to discover local macromolecular biochemical markers in sensory pathways. The search for micromolecular markers associated with specific cells has also been pursued intensively but generally within the context of the attempt to identify specific neurotransmitters of specific cells. Denervation has played a prominent role in these studies also. In general these studies have utilized microchemical methods of quantitating changes in contents of amino compounds (Aprison and Werman, 1968; Fonnum, 1972; Roberts *et al.*, 1973) or alterations in ability of tissue to concentrate radiolabeled materials thought to be potential neurotransmitters (Kuhar, 1973; Snyder *et al.*, 1973a,b).

The search for brain-specific macromolecular markers has relied primarily on immunological and electrophoretic procedures as applied to proteins of membrane or cytosol origin. Much of the work on specific proteins of the nervous system has recently been reviewed (Schneider, 1973; Moore, 1975). The approach has generally been to attempt to identify proteins specific to nervous tissue and less often to attempt to identify proteins which are localized to selected brain areas or cell types. One of the few efforts to characterize the proteins in a specific sensory pathway has been the studies of Davies (1970) on the auditory pathway. He was able to show discrete reproducible differences in gel electrophoretic patterns in extracts of different portions of the central areas of the auditory pathway. The concept that knowledge of the occurrence and function of proteins restricted to specific pathways or cells will be important in understanding information processing in the nervous system has been a major determinant of the direction of our work in the primary olfactory pathway.

Our interest in the olfactory pathway arose initially from a chance juxtaposition of logic, serendipity, and an experimental observation. The olfactory bulb is a region of high cell density (Altman, 1969), manifesting postnatal neurogenesis (Altman, 1969), and is the site of the primary synapse from the olfactory chemoreceptor neurons (Siefert and Ule, 1967; Ottoson, 1963; Moulton and Beidler, 1967; Shepherd, 1972). The bulb, which is a laminated structure, has been proposed as a model cortical system for neurophysiological studies (Shepherd, 1970) because various inputs and outputs are independently accessible. The primary olfactory pathway manifests anatomical similarities across wide phylogenetic distances (Nieuwenhuys, 1967), and, indeed, chemoreception is ubiquitous—occurring in prokaryotes (Adler, 1972) as well as eukaryotes. This neural pathway manifests unique aspects of ontogeny and anatomy relative to other sensory pathways (Sinclair, 1971; Waterman and Meller, 1973). Olfaction is the only primary sensory pathway which does not pass through a thalamic relay on its way to cortical integrative centers. The receptor cells derive embryologically from an epithelial placode and invade the central nervous system during development rather than being an evagination of the central nervous system as is the retina. These olfactory chemoreceptor cells are primary sensory neurons, unlike the gustatory chemoreceptor cells in the tongue which are not neurons but rather specialized epithelial cells innervated by neurons (Moulton and Beidler, 1967). Extensive morphological studies have been performed on this brain region at the light-microscopic level since Cajal (Pinching and Powell, 1972; Hinds, 1972a), as well as at the electron-microscopic (Pinching and Powell, 1971, 1972; Berger, 1971a,b, 1973; Graziadei and Metcalf, 1971) and scanning electron-microscopic (Graziadei, 1971) levels. It has been a site of extensive neurophysiological investigations (Shepherd, 1970).

In addition, surgical manipulation of this brain region has been reported to modify physiological parameters as diverse as serum protein levels (Loyber et al., 1972), cerebral catecholamine metabolism (Pohorecky et al., 1969), heart rate (Phillips and Martin, 1972), and sexual maturation (Whitten, 1956; Winans and Powers, 1974). Even in man, anomalies of olfaction or the olfactory apparatus have been associated with trisomy 13–15, Patau's syndrome (Taylor, 1968), hereditary hypogonadism (Labhart, 1974), and other endocrine (Hamilton et al., 1973; Marshall and Henkin, 1971) and nonendocrine states (Singh et al., 1970; Henkin et al., 1972; Schechter et al., 1972). In other species extensive evidence has accumulated for the importance of olfaction, or the so-called olfactoendocrine axis in modulating or mediating many behavioral parameters related to inter- and intragroup societal activities such as exploration, aggression, territoriality, sexual and maternal behavior, nutrition, navigation, and so forth in species as diverse as moths, mackeral, mice, and men (Cheal and Sprott, 1971; Beidler, 1971; Alberts, 1974). In spite of all the work from other disciplines on this neural pathway, it has been virtually ignored biochemically until very recently (Getchell and Gesteland, 1972; Gross, 1973; Rappoport and Daginwala, 1968; Weiss and Holland, 1967; Kurihara and Koyama, 1972; Neidle *et al.*, 1973; Villet, 1974).

Therefore, we chose to concentrate our efforts on biochemical studies of the primary olfactory pathway utilizing the mouse as our experimental animal and began with a search for examples of specific macromolecular gene expression. It is our hope that such markers will eventually help in elucidating molecular mechanisms of function in the area of the nervous system which we have used as a model.

2. STUDIES WITH THE OLFACTORY PATHWAY MARKER PROTEIN

Brain tissue tends to be richer in low-molecular-weight soluble acidic proteins than are other tissues (Moore and MacGregor, 1965; Griffith *et al.*, 1970). This fraction and the membrane-rich fraction have yielded several nervous tissue-specific, species-nonspecific proteins (Schneider, 1973; Moore, 1975). Our initial approach in the search for cell-specific markers was to study the cytosol fraction from various anatomical regions of the adult mouse brain to see if intratissue variations could be detected. As an analytical tool, we chose polyacrylamide gel electrophoresis at alkaline pH and 14% gel concentration to focus on the class of low-molecular-weight acidic proteins. It rapidly became evident that, in addition to the intertissue variations described by Moore and others, extensive intratissue variation existed in the mouse brain (Margolis, 1972b). Reproducible quantitative and qualitative differences in acrylamide gel patterns were seen to exist among regions of the mouse brain (Figure 1), much like a set of chemical fingerprints. In particular a major band was seen to be present in extracts of mouse olfactory bulb which was apparently absent from extracts of other mouse brain regions.

The presence of the major protein band, apparently localized in an area of the mouse brain which is involved in processing a major portion of the mouse sensory input, was very exciting to us. For several years our approach had been to emphasize the study of biochemical changes occurring in those brain regions associated with processing initial sensory input as a function of alterations of input. Here at last was a potential biochemical marker

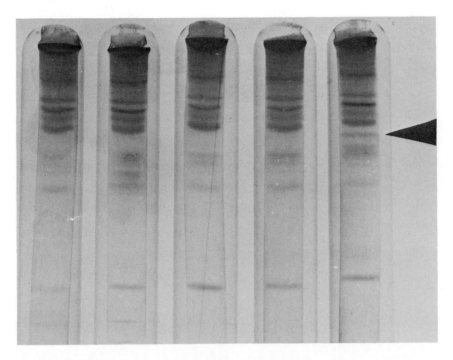

FIGURE 1. Polyacrylamide gel patterns of extracts of regions of the mouse brain. From right to left: olfactory bulb, colliculi, cerebral cortex, cerebellum, brain stem. Electrophoretic migration was from top to bottom. Gel was fixed and stained with Coomassie Blue. The arrow indicates the specific protein band. (From Margolis, 1972b.)

which gave entree to the problem of biochemistry and behavior at the level of a primary information processing site.

Since a protein marker unique to this brain region could be of great value as a probe of the molecular mechanisms of neural function, we proceeded to isolate and characterize the protein corresponding to the unique band seen on acrylamide gel electrophoresis. The protein was purified to homogeneity from pooled mouse olfactory bulbs by ammonium sulfate precipitation, DEAE–cellulose column chromatography, and isoelectric focusing using acrylamide gel electrophoresis as the analytical tool (Margolis, 1972b). The purified protein was homogeneous by electrophoresis in SDS gels, Ornstein–Davis gels, and isoelectric focusing gels (Figure 2). This material was then used to induce the formation of specific antibody in a goat (Margolis, 1972b). The antiserum thus produced was used to develop specific immunoprecipitin and radioimmunoassays to study the properties of this protein and to establish whether or not it is in fact a marker protein for this region.

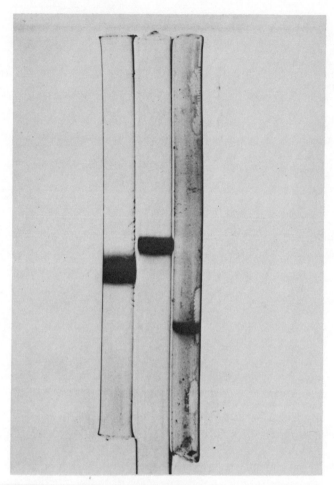

FIGURE 2. Polyacrylamide–gel electrophoresis patterns of the specific protein purified from mouse olfactory bulb. On the left, electrophoresis in the presence of sodium dodecyl sulfate; in the center, in the discontinuous Ornstein–Davis system; on the right, by isoelectric focusing. Coomassie Blue was the stain.

2.1. Distribution of the Marker Protein

One of the primary questions to consider is whether the marker protein is in fact specifically localized in the brain region from which it was isolated. To evaluate this, various immunological tests were applied. Preliminary results from Ouchterlony double diffusion analysis indicated that a single

immunoprecipitin band was formed between the goat antiserum and extracts of mouse olfactory bulb but not against extracts of cerebral hemispheres, cerebellum, liver, adrenal, or harderian gland (Figure 3). This
result was only a qualitative indication of the unique localization of the
protein. Additional evidence was sought from quantitative immunoprecipitin
titrations as well as from the effect of preabsorption of the antiserum with
various tissue extracts on the quantitative immunoprecipitin titrations.
Direct immunoprecipitin titrations indicated that the purified protein and
the olfactory bulb extract gave superimposable titration curves (Figure 4). The

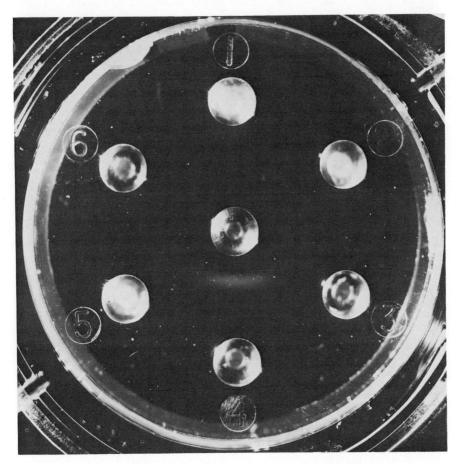

FIGURE 3. Immunodiffusion analysis of extracts of mouse tissues. Specific goat antiserum
is in the center. The peripheral wells contain, in clockwise order starting from the top: supernatant extracts of liver (1), adrenal (2), cerebellum (3), olfactory bulb (4), cerebral hemispheres
(5), and harderian gland (6). (From Margolis, 1972b.)

antiserum did not react with extracts of cerebellum, nor did the presence of cerebellar extracts alter the titration curve of the olfactory protein. Quantitative immunoprecipitin titrations thus permitted us to estimate that the purified protein represented about 0.5–1% of the total soluble protein in the mouse brain region. This result agrees with the fact that homogeneous protein results following 100- to 150-fold purification from supernatant extracts of mouse olfactory bulbs (Margolis, 1972*b*).

Antisera absorbed with bovine serum albumin, liver extracts, or extract of whole brain lacking olfactory bulbs all gave virtually identical quantitative immunoprecipitation titration curves against mouse olfactory bulb extracts (Figure 5). In contrast, preincubation of antiserum with extracts of whole brain, including olfactory bulbs, completely eliminated the ability of the antiserum to react with olfactory bulb extracts (Margolis and Tarnoff, 1973). These results were consistent with the hypothesis that this isolated protein was uniquely localized to the olfactory bulb. To evaluate this important question further these observations were extended using a much more sensitive radioimmunoassay utilizing the purified olfactory protein

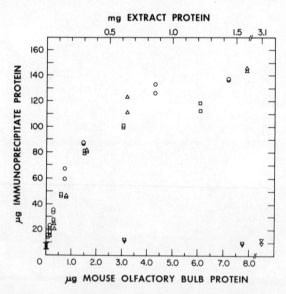

FIGURE 4. Quantitative immunoprecipitin titrations of the purified protein and extracts of mouse tissue by goat antiserum to the mouse olfactory protein. All titrations were done with 50 μl antiserum or preimmune serum. Titration of olfactory bulb (□) and cerebellum (▽) extracts are plotted on the upper abscissa, while titration of the purified protein in the presence (○) and absence (△) of cerebellum extract are plotted on the lower abscissa. Various control incubations all gave values of 5–10 μg protein, as indicated on the ordinate. (From Margolis, 1972*b*.)

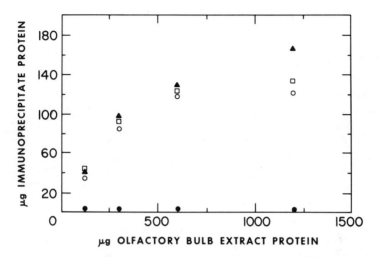

FIGURE 5. Effect of preabsorption of mouse olfactory protein antiserum with various mouse tissue extracts on the immunoprecipitation titration against mouse olfactory bulb extracts. Antiserum (1.5 ml) preabsorbed with 150 mg of lyophilized soluble extract of: whole brain including olfactory bulb (●), whole brain following removal of olfactory bulb (□), liver (○), and bovine serum albumin (▲). (From Margolis and Tarnoff, 1973.)

(tritium labeled) as tracer (Margolis, 1972a) and the specific antibody bound either to activated Sepharose (Margolis, 1972a) or to polystyrene latex beads (Rush et al., 1975; Keller and Margolis, 1975). The latter procedure gives nearly ten times the sensitivity of the former.

It is appropriate at this point to consider briefly the anatomy and ontogeny of this area of the brain. The olfactory bulb is a region of high cell density which manifests postnatal neurogenesis (Altman, 1969) and has been proposed as a neurophysiological model system (Shepherd, 1970). In addition to the cells which make all their synaptic connections within the bulbs themselves or send axons out to the rest of the brain (Heimer 1972), there are several inputs from nonbulb regions. One of these is the catecholaminergic input from brain stem (Dahlstrom et al., 1965). A major source of synaptic input to the bulb derives from the primary chemoreceptor cells in the nasal mucosa (Figure 6). The perikarya of these neurons lie in the nasal mucosa and their unmyelinated axons join in bundles to form the first cranial nerve which passes through the cribriform plate to synapse directly in the olfactory bulb (Ottoson, 1963; Shepherd, 1972; Moulton and Beidler, 1967). This represents, therefore, the only sensory pathway which does not pass through a thalamic relay but synapses directly into cortical tissue with major secondary inputs into neuroendocrine and limbic areas (Heimer,

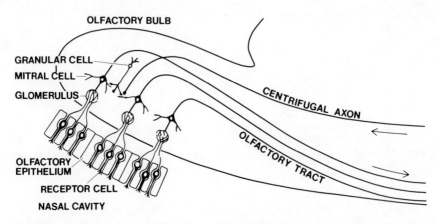

FIGURE 6. Olfactory system of the rat has receptor cells in the nasal cavity that are stimulated by odorous substances and transmit messages to mitral cells in the olfactory bulb. Mitral cell axons go to the olfactory cortex, which includes the olfactory tubercle. Incoming centrifugal pathways may modify olfactory responses. (Modified from Heimer, 1971.)

1968; Scott and Pfaffman, 1972). It was therefore desirable to extend our studies of specificity of localization of this protein to include other neural tissues as well. Extracts of various mouse tissues were evaluated by the radioimmunoassay and, as can be seen in Figure 7, extracts of the olfactory epithelium and bulb gave essentially superimposable titration curves indicating similar amounts of the marker protein in these two sites. Jacob-

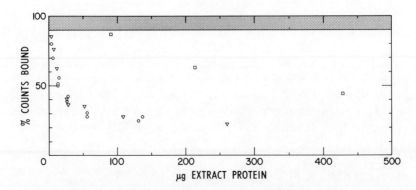

FIGURE 7. Radioimmunoassay of various mouse tissue high-speed supernatant extracts for mouse olfactory marker protein content. Olfactory bulb (○), olfactory epithelium (▽), and Jacobson's vomeronasal organ (□). In the hatched area are all data for retina, lung, muscle, spleen, adrenal, tongue, cerebral cortex, cerebellum and balance of brain. The goat antibody to the mouse olfactory protein was bound to Sepharose. (From Margolis, 1972*a*.)

son's vomeronasal organ, which has about 4–5 % of the number of chemo-receptor cells as are present in the olfactory epithelium (Moulton and Beidler, 1967), gave a curve consistent with this reduced level of chemorecep-tor cells indicating the presence of the marker protein in the chemoreceptor cells of that tissue as well. In contrast, under conditions where microgram quantities of soluble protein from extracts of olfactory bulb or epithelium had potent reactivity, extracts of cerebellum, cortex, balance of the brain, spinal cord, adrenal, spleen, retina, tongue, and lung all fell within the hatched area (Figure 7) even when as much as 2000 μg of extract protein was added to the assay mixture, indicating the absence of this protein in other brain areas, in other sensory receptors, or in respiratory epithelium. Thus it seemed quite probable that this protein was in fact a marker for the primary olfactory pathway where it was present in at least 500–1000 times higher content than in any other site studied.

2.2. Physiological and Genetic Influences on the Marker Protein

We next began to look for evidence of physiological and genetic modula-tion or manipulation of this protein in the hope of learning something of its function. As we had done earlier for the S-100 protein (Margolis, 1971), we began a search for mutants which might exhibit deficiencies of this protein or structural polymorphisms indicated by variation in electrophoretic mobility (Table 1). Although some quantitative interstrain variability in specific activity of this protein was observed by immunoprecipitin titrations, no strains were found which lacked the protein nor were any electrophoretic polymorphisms of this protein detected (Table 1). These data suggest that the presence of the protein is very important for the function of this brain region and furthermore that possibly its absence cannot be tolerated. These possibilities are intriguing in view of the importance of olfaction to rodent behavior (Cheal and Sprott, 1971; Alberts, 1974).

The reports of decreased gonadal function following olfactory bulbec-tomy in rodents (Whitten, 1956), and the correlation of hereditary anosmia and hypogonadism in man (Labhart, 1974), suggested that the effect of hormones on the level of the marker protein would be a useful aspect to consider. Thus a variety of mouse strains were evaluated by immunoprecipitin titrations with regard to the effect of gender on intrastrain level of the marker protein (Table 2). In the eight strains tested, there did not seem to be any influence of sex on the protein level. In addition, castration, oophorectomy, adrenalectomy, hypophysectomy, lactation, or pregnancy had no significant effect on the level of the protein in the olfactory bulbs (Margolis, unpublished observations).

TABLE 1. Strain Survey of the Level of Olfactory Marker Protein
in Female Mouse Olfactory Bulbs

μg immunoprecipitate protein ――――――――――――――――― mg extract protein	Strain
0–200	
200–400	SEA/GnJ, DBA/2J, LP/J, 129/J, C3H/HeJ, DBA/1J,[a] C3HeB/FeJ[a]
400–600	BUB/BnJ, PL/J, Au/SsJ, C58/J,[a] Ttf/t[6],[a] SM/J, AKR/J, C57L/J, TP/R1, ot[1],[a] RF/J, RIII/2J, C57BL/6J, C57BL/KsJ,[a] CBA/CaJ,[a] LB/J, P/J,[a] DBA/2DeJ,[a] C57BL/6J-c[J],[a] CF-1, C57BL/6J-T[2J],[a] MWT[a]
600–800	BALB/cJ, C57BL/10J, CBA/J, SJL/J, MA/J,[a] C57Br/cdJ, A/J, A/HeJ, SWR/J, DBP/J,[a] I/LnJ,[a] ST/bJ[a]
800–1000	CE/J, SEC/1ReJ

[a] Not tested for electrophoretic variant. Assays were performed by quantitative immuno-precipitin titrations.

The level of the protein thus does not seem to be responsive to alteration in the endocrine state of adult mice. Comparison of the level of this protein in the olfactory epithelium and bulb as a function of ontogeny (Figure 8) demonstrated the protein to be present at birth at low content in both locations. The content of the protein rose slowly during postnatal develop-

TABLE 2. Effects of Sex and Strain Differences on the Level
of Olfactory Marker Protein in Mouse Olfactory Bulbs

Strain	μg immunoprecipitate protein ―――――――――――――――――― mg extract protein	
	Female	Male
AKR/J	432; 380	491; 511
AU/SsJ	560; 600; 581	567; 653
CF-1	551; 533	484; 504
C57L/J	508; 613	544; 524
MWT	575; 704	639; 638
PL/J	572; 510; 521	451; 564
C57BL/6J-T[2J]	606; 623	545; 531
Ttf/t[6] +	682; 742	480; 611

Assays were performed by quantitative immunoprecipitin titrations.

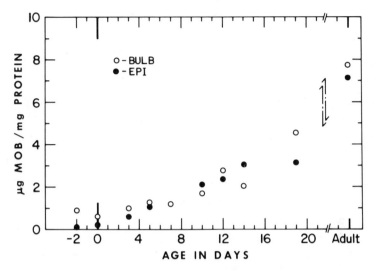

FIGURE 8. Age-dependent increase of the olfactory marker protein in supernatant extracts of mouse olfactory bulb (○) and olfactory epithelium (●).

ment to reach adult levels in several weeks—similar to many other brain enzymes and proteins. It would be of interest to evaluate the content of the protein prenatally in the bulb and epithelium in order to correlate it with the neuroembryology of this pathway (Hinds, 1972; Filogamo and Marchisio, 1971).

To ascertain the phylogenetic distribution of the protein, the radioimmunoassay was used to assay olfactory areas of several species for their content of the marker protein. When antiserum prepared against the mouse olfactory protein was used for this purpose (Figure 9), only certain species seemed to possess the protein (Margolis, 1972b). Thus, although the mouse, rat, and hamster evidenced similar levels of the protein, extracts prepared from rabbit, guinea pig, chicken, frog, or garfish were apparently devoid of it. To determine whether this result was due to an antiserum of very high specificity or was due, in fact, to a very restricted distribution of the protein among species was our next problem. Therefore, a program was begun with A. Keller to purify the equivalent protein from the rat (which was known to differ physicochemically from the mouse protein) and to evaluate the species specificity of antisera to the rat olfactory protein raised in both rabbit and goat. When the goat antiserum to the rat olfactory protein was tested by a variety of immunological techniques, it rapidly became evident that the olfactory marker protein was in fact present in virtually all vertebrates tested, from garfish to man (Keller and Margolis, 1975).

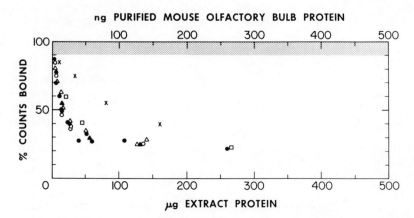

FIGURE 9. Species distribution of the olfactory marker protein by radioimmunoassay using the goat antiserum to the mouse olfactory protein coupled to Sepharose.
Olfactory epithelium of mouse (●) and rat (□). Olfactory bulb of mouse (▲), rat (○),
and hamster (△). Purified mouse olfactory marker protein (×) which is indicated
on the upper abscissa. In the hatched area are all the data for olfactory bulb and
cerebellum of rabbit, guinea pig, and chicken; cerebellum of rat and hamster; brain
and olfactory nerve of garfish.

A positive and specific reaction was observed in Ouchterlony plates
(Figure 10) with boosted sera from both goat and rabbit against extracts
of olfactory bulbs or olfactory epithelia from all the mammalian species
tested, except goat and human (Table 3). A single sharp immunoprecipitin
band of identify appeared against both antisera. In contrast, when extracts
of cerebellum or other parts of the brain of these mammals were used, no

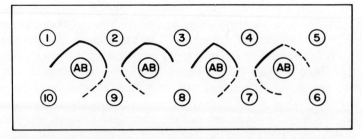

FIGURE 10. Immunodiffusion analysis of extracts from olfactory tissue
of several species. The specific antiserum was placed in the central row of
wells. The top and bottom rows of wells contain the olfactory tissue extracts
from : (1) rat epithelium ; (2) rat bulbs ; (3) mouse epithelium ; (4) mouse bulbs ;
(5) pig epithelium ; (6) pig bulbs ; (7) sheep bulbs ; (8) goat bulbs ; (9) guinea pig
bulbs ; (10) mouse cerebellum. (From Keller and Margolis, 1975.)

TABLE 3. Cross-Reactivity of Olfactory Tissue Extracts by Ouchterlony Immuno-diffusion Against Rabbit and Goat Antisera to the Purified Rat Olfactory Protein

Species	Olfactory tissue	Goat antiserum	Rabbit antiserum
Rat, mouse, hamster, guinea pig	Epithelium and bulbs	Strong positive	Strong positive
Dog	Bulbs	Strong positive	Strong positive
Rabbit, sheep, beef, pig	Bulbs	Weak positive	Weak positive
Goat, human, frog, chicken	Bulbs	Negative	Negative
Garfish	Nerve	Negative	Negative
Rat, rabbit, pig, mouse	Cerebellum	Negative	Negative

cross-reaction was visible. No precipitate was observed when the antiserum was replaced by preimmune serum. No cross-reaction was seen by im-munodiffusion with olfactory tissue extracts from the nonmammalian species tested, i.e., chicken, frog, garfish (Table 3). Extending these studies by the use of the quantitative immunoprecipitin titration we were able to observe that, in general, phylogenetically more distant species gave smaller protein precipitates at equivalence (Table 4). Although dog olfactory bulb extracts did not cross-react with antibody to the mouse protein, in these immuno-precipitin tests using antibody to the rat olfactory protein, extracts of dog

TABLE 4. Quantitative Immunoprecipitin Titrations of Olfactory Bulb Extracts from Various Species with Goat Antiserum to the Rat Olfactory Protein[a]

Species	μg extract protein to reach equivalence	μg immunoprecipitate protein per 100 μl antiserum at equivalence
Rat	400	65
Mouse	200	70
Hamster	500	75
Guinea pig	600	75
Sheep	250	30
Dog	1000	65
Rabbit	300	50
Cow (total bulb)	800	35
Cow (cortex of bulb)	100	25
Frog	>2000	0
Man	>2000	0
Garfish	>2000	0
Rat cerebellum	>2000	0

[a] From Keller and Margolis. 1975.

olfactory bulb did cross-react and gave 65 μg of protein in the immunoprecipitate at equivalence similar to that given by the rodents (rat, mouse, hamster, guinea pig). The maximal amount of protein precipitated with 100 μl of goat antiserum was the same for the olfactory epithelium and olfactory bulbs of the same species, a result indicating a probable identity of the protein in both locations.

The olfactory marker protein appears to be present in variable contents in olfactory bulbs of different species. Thus, for the mouse, 200 μg of extract protein was required to reach the equivalence point, whereas 400 μg of rat extract protein, 600 μg of guinea pig extract protein, and about 500 μg of hamster extract protein were required. In the case of the cow, it was possible to dissect the olfactory bulbs into a gray cortical fraction and a white subcortical fraction. The olfactory protein was present primarily in extracts from the cortical portion as shown by the immunoprecipitin test. In these immunoprecipitin titrations about 800 μg of extract protein was needed to reach the equivalence zone of the curve when whole cow olfactory bulbs were used, but only 100 μg of extract protein was necessary when the cortical region of the bulb was used. This preferential content of the protein in the periphery of the bulb agrees with its probable origin from the chemoreceptor neurons, which synapse in the glomerular layer at the periphery of the olfactory bulb (Figure 6). Human olfactory bulb extracts, assayed by the immunoprecipitin reaction, showed no precipitates which were significantly different from those obtained with extracts of nonolfactory areas.

In order to test the olfactory tissue extracts of those species which did not cross-react with the goat antiserum by the previous two methods, we

TABLE 5. Species and Tissue Distribution of the Olfactory Marker Protein[a]

Species	Tissue	Extract protein, μg	Binding inhibition, %
Rat	Olfactory bulbs	18	40
Hamster	Olfactory epithelium	10	41
Rabbit	Olfactory bulbs	54	40
Human	Olfactory bulbs	750	41
Garfish	Olfactory nerve	725	40
Frog	Olfactory bulbs	4700	16
Rat	Cerebellum	3425	0
Rat	Liver	2535	0
Rat	Lung	3035	0
Rat	Muscle	2929	0

[a] High-speed supernatant extracts were assayed in duplicate by the competitive-binding radioimmunoassay using antibody-coated polystyrene latex beads and [^{3}H]-labeled rat olfactory marker protein. The protein contents of the extracts were assayed with fluorescamine. (From Keller and Margolis, 1975.)

used the much more sensitive radioimmunoassay. As expected, species which had previously been shown to cross-react with the goat antibody to the pure rat olfactory marker protein, competed with the labeled rat olfactory protein for binding to the specific antiserum. More interestingly, previously unreactive extracts of olfactory tissues of man and garfish inhibited homogeneous rat olfactory protein binding (Table 5). Also, when sufficient frog olfactory bulb extract was used (4700 μg), a reproducible inhibition of labeled rat olfactory protein binding was observed. No inhibition was ever observed for the chicken olfactory bulb extracts. No olfactory marker protein could be detected by this radioimmunoassay (Table 5) in the rat cerebellum (as an example of a nonolfactory brain region), lung (as an example of respiratory epithelium), muscle (as an example of another excitable tissue), or liver, even when more than 2000 μg of extract protein was tested (Keller and Margolis, 1975). The binding inhibition curve obtained with varying amounts of garfish olfactory nerve extract (Figure 11) is parallel to that obtained with the pure rat olfactory protein, a fact indicating that the antigenic sites involved in binding to the antibody are quite similar in these two phylogenetically distant species (Keller and Margolis, 1975).

The apparent restriction of the olfactory protein exclusively to rodent species as seen initially was therefore due to the specificity of the anti-mouse olfactory bulb protein antiserum. Using antisera produced by goat and

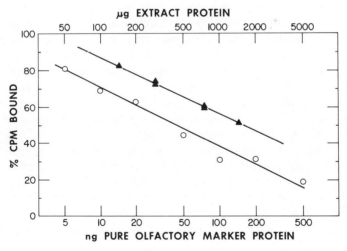

FIGURE 11. Radioimmunoassay for cross-reactivity of garfish olfactory nerve extracts with antibody directed against the rat olfactory marker protein : (○) pure rat olfactory marker protein ; (▲) garfish olfactory nerve extract. These assays were performed with the antibody bound to polystyrene latex beads. (From Keller and Margolis, 1975.)

rabbit against the rat olfactory marker protein, it has been possible to extend the species distribution of this protein to include olfactory tissue from representative rodentia, cavidae, lagomorpha, artiodactyla, carnivora, primates, amphibia, and teleosts. Of all the species tested, only the avians have not given a positive result. Clearly this protein is very widely distributed phylogenetically and has been present in an immunologically related form for many millions of years in the primary olfactory pathway. We would therefore expect to find this protein or an analog of it in all vertebrate groups and perhaps in olfactory chemoreceptor tissue of nonvertebrates as well. Presumably its persistence during evolution is an indication that it performs some critical function in this pathway. Furthermore, the unique localization of this protein within the olfactory pathway demonstrates that it is distinct from any of the other nervous tissue–specific antigens previously described (Moore, 1975; Schneider, 1973).

2.3. Cellular Localization of the Marker Protein

The nasal olfactory epithelium and Jacobson's vomeronasal organ both contain bipolar chemoreceptor neurons which form their primary synapses within the glomeruli of the olfactory bulbs. The unique presence of the olfactory marker protein in these three sites, but nowhere else in the brain or in any other tissue studied, strongly implies, but does not prove, that it is a marker for the primary olfactory chemoreceptor cells. The marker protein could be synthesized by the chemoreceptor cell perikarya and transported to the synapses by anterograde axoplasmic flow, or it could be synthesized by cells in the olfactory bulb and transported to the olfactory epithelium by retrograde axoplasmic flow. To answer this question we attempted to determine the site of biosynthesis of this protein, as well as to evaluate the effects of central denervation and peripheral deafferentation procedures on the level of this protein in this neural pathway.

To study the biosynthesis of the marker protein, tissues were incubated with a mixture of [^{3}H]-aminoacids, and the labeled marker protein was isolated by precipitation with specific antiserum in the presence of carrier olfactory marker protein (Margolis and Tarnoff, 1973). Because immunoprecipitates can nonspecifically adsorb or occlude small amounts of labeled proteins, the presence of counts in the specific immunoprecipitate is not necessarily proof of the incorporation of precursor into the specific protein under study. Thus, it is essential to demonstrate that the specific protein is, in fact, responsible for the isotope associated with the immunoprecipitate. To accomplish this, the washed immunoprecipitates were lyophilized and dissociated, and the resultant solubilized proteins were then subjected to electrophoresis

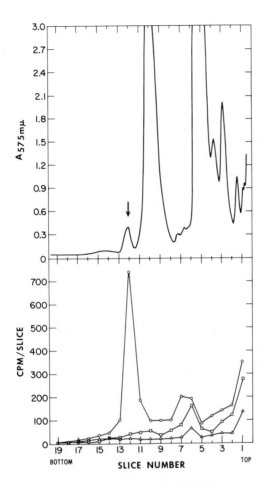

FIGURE 12. Sodium dodecyl sulfate–polyacrylamide gel electrophoresis patterns of the immunoprecipitate from extracts of cerebellum (△), olfactory bulb (□), and olfactory epithelium (○) incubated with [³H]-amino acids. Nonradioactive olfactory bulb extract was added to the cerebellum extract as carrier. The upper half represents the band pattern in the stained gel and the arrow indicates the position of the mouse olfactory bulb protein. The distribution of radioactivity on the gels is represented in the lower half. The olfactory epithelium was incubated in the presence of 10 μCi [³H]-amino acids and the others in the presence of 100 μCi [³H]-amino acids (Margolis and Tarnoff, 1973).

in sodium dodecyl sulfate–polyacrylamide gels. The Coomassie blue-stained gels contained two major bands (Figure 12), corresponding to the light and heavy chain of γ-globulin at slices 10 and 5, respectively. A band slightly in advance of the light antibody chain corresponds to the position of the mouse olfactory marker protein run as a standard in identical gels.

This band, at slice 12 (Figure 12), was heavily labeled in extracts derived from epithelium, but essentially unlabeled in extracts from cerebellum or olfactory bulbs. The counts co-migrating with the authentic mouse olfactory marker protein band constitute 20–30% of the total counts observed in gels of olfactory epithelium, 3–5% of the total counts in gels of olfactory bulbs, and 3–4% of the total counts in gels of cerebellum. The nature of the counts remaining in the top of the gel and at slices 6–7 is unknown, although similar phenomena have been reported for other systems (Herschman, 1971).

In addition to the olfactory epithelium, synthesis of the mouse olfactory marker protein was also seen in the vomeronasal organ (Figure 13). In contrast, neither lung (a source of respiratory epithelium) nor tongue (another site of chemoreception) seemed capable of synthesizing this protein (Figure 13), nor did they contain detectable levels of the marker protein (Figure 7) (Margolis, 1972).

The synthesis of the mouse olfactory marker protein in the olfactory epithelium and vomeronasal organ, but not in the bulb or in the cerebellum, tongue, or lung, supported the idea that the primary olfactory chemoreceptor cells were carrying out the synthesis. The occurrence of the mouse olfactory marker protein in the olfactory bulb suggests that it is transported by axoplasmic flow from the apparent cellular site of synthesis in the bipolar

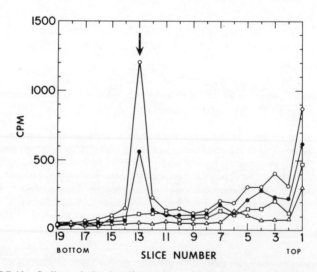

FIGURE 13. Sodium dodecyl sulfate–polyacrylamide gel electrophoresis patterns of the [³H]-labeled immunoprecipitates from extracts of olfactory epithelium (○), Jacobson's vomeronasal organ (●), lung (□), and tongue (△) following incubation with [³H]-amino acids *in vitro*. Carrier nonradioactive bulb extract was added to the lung and tongue extracts. The arrow indicates the location of the olfactory marker protein. (From Margolis and Tarnoff, 1973.)

neurons to the site of the first synapses in the bulbs. Preliminary immuno-fluorescent studies in collaboration with Dr. Boyd Hartman are consistent with this idea. In the bulb a positive immunofluorescent reaction was seen only in the area of the synaptic glomeruli and in cross-sections of incoming nerve bundles from the olfactory epithelium and not elsewhere in the olfac-tory bulb. These results are consistent with arrival of the protein in the bulb by axoplasmic flow from the chemoreceptor cells, with the immunological observations in the cow olfactory bulb (Table 4), and also with our bio-synthetic studies. These data do not rule out the unlikely possibility that the mouse olfactory marker protein is synthesized by the epithelial sustentacular cells in the olfactory mucosa and then is transferred to the chemoreceptor neurons for transport. However, the denervation studies, to be considered next, render this possibility extremely improbable.

As an approach to this last question it was decided to evaluate the effect of removal of the olfactory bulb on the level of the marker protein in the olfactory epithelium. It is known that bulbectomy results in the rapid, specific destruction of the receptor cells in the olfactory epithelium by retrograde degeneration (Clark, 1957; Takagi, 1971; Alberts, 1974). This would enable us to evaluate whether selective loss of the neurons resulted in a change in the level of the protein. At the same time we chose to take advantage of the anatomy of this pathway and to perform in a reciprocal set of experiments a peripheral deafferentation procedure using stringent intranasal irrigation with $0.17\ M\ ZnSO_4$ to destroy the olfactory mucosa and then to evaluate the effect of this treatment on the marker protein content of the olfactory bulbs (Margolis et al., 1974).

Olfactory bulbectomy is reported (Clark, 1957; Metcalf, 1973) to cause rapid selective retrograde degeneration of the olfactory receptor cells within 24–48 hr after operation. The effect of this treatment on the marker protein (Table 6) content in the nasal olfactory mucosa is also very rapid, falling dramatically with a half time of about 2 days, in reasonable agreement

TABLE 6. Effect of Olfactory Bulbectomy on the Level of the Olfactory Marker Protein in Mouse Olfactory Epithelium[a]

Days after surgery	ng olfactory marker protein/μg extract protein	
	Bulbectomized	Sham
Unoperated	7.96 ± 1.7 (6)	
2	3.75 ± 2.1 (6)	7.72 ± 2.0 (6)
7	0.73 ± 0.2 (6)	8.30 ± 1.25 (6)
15	0.5 ± 0.2 (5)	—

[a] Data are presented as means ± S.D. for the number of mice indicated in parentheses.

with the reported morphological changes. This result gives additional confirmation of the localization of this marker protein.

In the reciprocal experiment when we studied the effect of peripheral denervation by intranasal irrigation with $ZnSO_4$ solution, both morphological and biochemical studies were performed. In many cases intranasal $ZnSO_4$ administration has been reported to produce only a temporary impairment in olfactory function followed by a complete return of function as monitored behaviorally, electrophysiologically, and morphologically (Alberts, 1974). Evidence for permanent impairment in olfactory function following intranasal $ZnSO_4$ has recently appeared (Van den Bergh, 1973). Nevertheless, there seem not to have been any detailed studies of the effect of intranasal irrigation with zinc sulfate on the morphology or biochemistry of the olfactory bulbs. We therefore began such a study to evaluate whether irreversible bulbar effects can occur following intranasal zinc sulfate treatment (Margolis et al., 1974).

There is a 20% decrease in the weight of the bulbs at 1 week following the zinc sulfate treatment (Table 7) with a progressive continued decrease reaching a plateau at 3–4 weeks. This weight loss is consistent with that to be expected from postdenervation atrophy. A major change was observed in the microscopic morphology of the olfactory bulbs, particularly in the glomerular layer (Figure 14), similar to that reported following surgical removal of the epithelium (Berger, 1971a,b; Pinching and Powell, 1972; Estable–Puig and Estable, 1969). It can be seen from the sections stained with NAFT stain (Figure 14) that rapid progressive changes occur following the $ZnSO_4$ treatment. The glomeruli are grossly shrunken and the overall thickness of the glomerular layer is reduced while the periglomerular cells become compacted. Similar findings have been noted by other workers following surgical destruction of the olfactory muscosa. The INT stain is reported

TABLE 7. Effect of Intranasal Irrigation with 0.17 M $ZnSO_4$ on Olfactory Bulb Weight[a]

Days after treatment	mg wet weight/pair bulbs[b]
Control	26.0 (34)
7	21.3 (6)
19	18.9 (7)
24	17.1 (12)
26	14.8 (6)
51	13.2 (6)
87	14.7 (6)

[a] Margolis et al., 1974.
[b] Average weight with number of mice pooled together in parentheses.

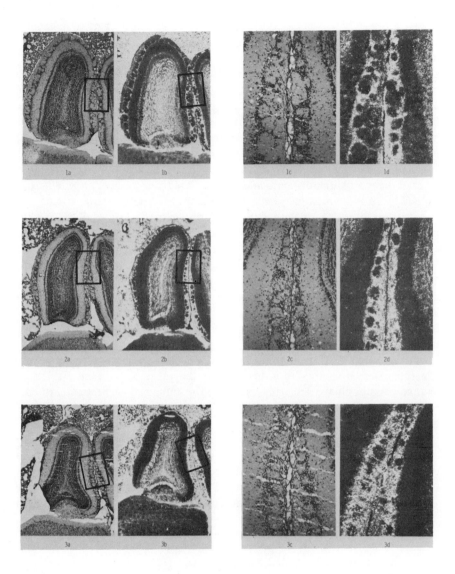

FIGURE 14. The effect of intranasal irrigation with 0.17 M zinc sulfate on microscopic morphology of mouse olfactory bulbs. Adjacent cryostat sections were stained with the NAFT stain (columns a and c) or with the iodonitrotetrazolium violet stain (columns b and d). Olfactory bulb tissue from control mice (top row) and from mice 5 days (middle row) and 28 days (bottom row) after zinc sulfate treatment is presented. Columns a and b are at a magnification of 32 ×, the areas within the rectangles have been further magnified to 125 × as presented in columns c and d. (From Margolis et al., 1974.)

to give a heavy blue-black deposit at the sites of synaptic terminal degeneration (Steward *et al.*, 1973). In our hands, however, it functions essentially as a stain for succinic dehydrogenase activity. The glomerular region is seen (Figure 14) to stain intensely in the control sections in agreement with reports of high succinic dehydrogenase activity in the glomeruli (Ortmann, 1957; Nandy and Bourne, 1966). In agreement with the results from the NAFT-stained sections the succinic dehydrogenase staining intensity is progressively lost following the $ZnSO_4$ irrigation. Evidence of morphological changes were seen as early as 3 days following the $ZnSO_4$ treatment. The morphological changes seen appeared to be restricted to the glomerular layer of the main olfactory bulb and to be absent from the accessory olfactory bulb (Figure 14), which receives synapses from the vomeronasal organ.

Intranasal irrigation with $ZnSO_4$ solution caused the level of the marker protein in the bulb to decrease with a half-time of about 4–5 days (Table 8). This result was slower than the fall in the epithelium after bulbectomy but was in agreement with the morphological changes seen in the bulb (Figure 4). Thus interference with either end of the primary olfactory pathway results in rapid effects on the content of marker protein and morphological appearance in the reciprocal portion of the pathway, consistent with the exclusive localization of this protein in the primary olfactory neurons which make up the first cranial nerve.

A question arising at this junction was that of the specificity of the effects; that is, does the fall in level of marker protein represent a selective change as though we are truly marking the influence of these treatments on a single-cell type in a complex mass of cells, or is it merely a reflection of general tissue damage in this region? To test this question, the activities of three neurotransmitter-metabolizing enzymes were measured in order to see if they were altered along with the morphological and marker protein changes (Margolis *et al.*, 1974). It is evident from Table 9 that no significant alterations in the activities of glutamic decarboxylase, cholineacetyltransferase or acetylcholinesterase were seen in epithelium or bulb at a time when

TABLE 8. Effect of Intranasal Irrigation on the Level of the Olfactory Marker Protein in Mouse Olfactory Bulbs[a]

Days after treatment	Treatment	Marker protein, ng/extract protein, μg
6	0.17 M $ZnSO_4$	1.12 $\pm$ 0.6 (6)
15	0.17 M $ZnSO_4$	0.67 $\pm$ 0.1 (5)
21	0.17 M $ZnSO_4$	N.D. (6)
6–21	0.15 M NaCl	3.72 $\pm$ 2.0 (16)

[a] Data are presented as mean $\pm$ S.D. for the number of mice indicated in parentheses. N.D. indicates marker protein was not detectable.

TABLE 9. Several Enzyme Levels in Olfactory Tissues at Three Weeks After Denervation

Olfactory tissue	Treatment	Acetyl-cholinesterase[a]	Cholineacetyl-transferase[b]	Glutamic acid decarboxylase[c]	
				−AOAA	+AOAA
Epithelium	BULBX	5.6 ± 2.5	—	1.2 ± 0.2	1.4 ± 0.2
Epithelium	SHAM	5.6 ± 3.3	0.6	1.3 ± 0.2	1.4 ± 0.2
Bulbs	ZnSO$_4$	62.4 ± 5.3	344 ± 65	36.0 ± 1.9	1.4 ± 0.2
Bulbs	Saline	53.3 ± 3.9	379 ± 142	35.4 ± 1.3	1.1 ± 0.2

[a] nmol/min/μg protein ± S.D. for four mice.
[b] pmol/min/mg protein ± S.D. for six mice.
[c] nmol/hr/mg tissue ± S.D. in presence (+) and absence (−) of 10^{-3} M aminooxyacetic acid (AOAA), for five mice. (From Margolis et al., 1974.)

the marker protein level was essentially absent. Thus this protein does, in fact, function as a marker for the state of a specific cell type in the presence of a variety of other cells and therefore fulfills certain of the roles postulated for such biochemical markers. The low levels of acetylcholinesterase in the epithelium are consistent with the reports of Filogamo and Marchisio (1971) and of Baradi and Bourne (1959). A recent study of GABA and glutamic acid decarboxylase activity in various layers of the olfactory bulb (Graham, 1973) reports the lowest content of these two components in the olfactory nerve layer, consistent with our findings in the olfactory epithelium. The very low levels of these enzyme activities in the epithelium suggest that neither acetylcholine nor GABA is involved in the intimate functioning of these chemoreceptor neurons. This possibility raises the question as to what the actual neurotransmitter in these cells might be.

Corroborative biochemical evidence that the intranasal zinc sulfate treatment does in fact selectively alter neuronal synaptic function in the bulb has recently been reported by Meisami and Manoochehri (1974). These authors observed that, after intranasal zinc sulfate application to the olfactory epithelium of young rats, there was a reduction of Na^+-K^+-ATPase activity but not of Mg^{2+}-ATPase activity in the olfactory bulbs. They suggest that these results indicate that destruction of the receptor cells interferes with neuronal synaptic function in the olfactory bulb.

2.4. Characterization of the Olfactory Marker Protein

In addition to studying biological aspects of the marker protein, we have also begun to characterize it physiochemically. The olfactory marker

TABLE 10.   Amino Acid Composition of Purified
Olfactory Marker Proteins from Rat and Mouse

Amino acid[a]	Mol %	
	Mouse	Rat
Lysine	8.1	8.1
Histidine	0.9	0.7
Arginine	5.2	5.7
Aspartic acid	12.4	13.6
Threonine	4.9	4.9
Serine	5.8	3.9
Glutamic acid	16.9	16.6
Proline	4.6	4.8
Glycine	7.6	5.7
Alanine	7.4	6.7
Half cystine	0	0
Valine	4.9	5.7
Methionine	1.9	2.4
Isoleucine	3.2	3.1
Leucine	11.2	12.9
Tyrosine	1.3	1.2
Phenylalanine	3.9	4.1
Tryptophan[b]	1.3	4.2

[a] Amino acid analyses were performed on samples of the electrophoretically homogeneous proteins after 22-hr hydrolysis in constant boiling
HCl at 110°C.
[b] Determined spectrophotometrically.

protein has been purified to homogeneity from the cytosol of olfactory bulbs
of both the mouse (Margolis, 1972b) and the rat (Keller and Margolis, unpublished observations), by conventional procedures as described earlier
(Margolis, 1972b). The amino acid analyses of both these proteins indicate
that the sum of the acidic amino acid residues (glutamic and aspartic acids)
is nearly twice the sum of the basic residues (lysine, arginine, and histidine)
(Table 10). The analyses for the proteins in mouse and rat are very similar
and are unusual only in the apparent absence of cystine. The amino acid
analyses are consistent with the view that these proteins are acidic brain
proteins as determined by isoelectric focusing. The protein in mouse has an
isoelectric point of 4.7 and the protein in rat an isoelectric point of 5.0
(Figure 15). This difference in isoelectric points is consistent with the slightly
faster mobility of the mouse protein observed in Ornstein-Davis polyacrylamide gels as compared to the rat protein. In addition these two proteins
straddle the location of bovine serum albumin (pI 4.9) in isoelectric-focusing
acrylamide gels. To test whether the marker protein contained any significant

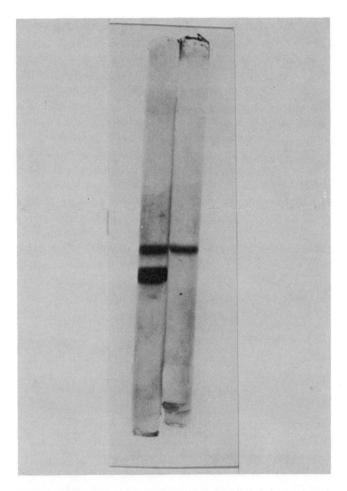

FIGURE 15. Isoelectric focusing polyacrylamide–gel electrophoresis of purified olfactory marker proteins. On the right purified olfactory marker protein from the mouse. On the left a mixture of the purified olfactory marker protein from the mouse and the rat (Keller and Margolis, unpublished observation).

content of carbohydrate, gel-electrophoresis was performed on the purified mouse protein and comparative staining was carried out with periodic acid–Schiff reagent and Coomassie blue. No evidence for any carbohydrate could be obtained by this technique. Additionally, under conditions in which the glycoprotein dopamine-β-hydroxylase binds to Concanavalin-A Sepharose, there was no evidence of any binding of the mouse olfactory protein to this material, arguing for the absence of any terminal mannose or glucose residues (Margolis and Blume, unpublished observations).

The rapid mobility of the purified olfactory marker protein from rat and mouse in 14% acrylamide gels indicated these proteins were probably relatively small. Apparent molecular weight was estimated by several different techniques. Filtration on a column of Biogel-P-60 indicated that the molecular weight of the native mouse olfactory protein was about 27,000 daltons. On filtration through Sephadex G-75 (Figure 16) the marker proteins of the pure tritium–labeled rat and mouse both have apparent native molecular weights of about $30–35 \times 10^3$ daltons. The marker protein of fresh cytosol extracts of rat olfactory bulb and olfactory epithelium manifested identical elution profiles from Sephadex G-75 indicating no major size or shape difference in the protein from these two anatomical sites. The purified homogeneous protein is slightly delayed in elution position on the Sephadex column, relative to the position of the immunoreactive peak of the cytosol extracts. This shift, an increase of perhaps 20% in apparent molecular weight, may be due to small conformational changes occurring in the course of purifying the protein. Extracts of the olfactory nerve

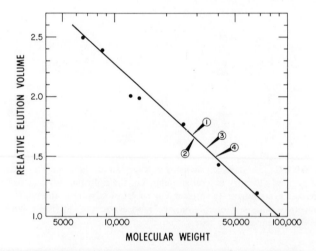

FIGURE 16. Elution pattern of the olfactory marker protein from Sephadex G-75. Elution volumes were calculated relative to Dextran Blue and for standard proteins are represented by the full circles. The standards used and their molecular weights are: egg-white trypsin inhibitor (6500); pancreatic trypsin inhibitor (8500); cytochrome-c (12,300); ribonuclease (13,700); chymotrypsinogen (25,700); ovalbumin (45,000); bovine serum albumin (67,000). Extract of garfish olfactory nerve at 1; extract of rat olfactory bulb and olfactory epithelium at 2; [^{3}H]-labeled purified mouse and rat olfactory proteins at 3; purified rat olfactory protein before and after ^{3}H-labeling at 4. (From Keller and Margolis, unpublished observations.)

of the garfish also show an immunoreactive elution profile very similar to that seen for the mouse and rat, a result indicating conservation of size and shape of this protein during evolution as well as of immunological reactivity and presumably of function (Keller and Margolis, unpublished observations).

On polyacrylamide electrophoresis in the presence of SDS, the purified olfactory bulb marker protein isolated from the rat and the mouse have identical mobilities indicating identical subunit molecular weights of about $15–18 \times 10^3$ daltons (Figure 17). When the elution of the $[^3H]$-labeled mouse

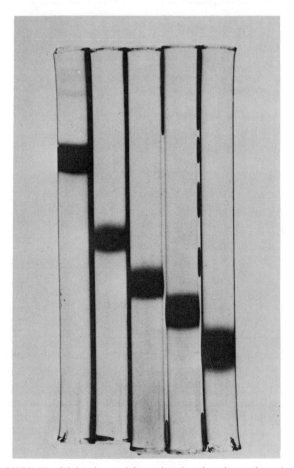

FIGURE 17. Molecular weight estimation by electrophoresis on polyacrylamide gels in the presence of sodium dodecyl sulfate. From left to right: ovalbumin, chymotrypsinogen, purified mouse olfactory marker protein, myoglobin, ribonuclease.

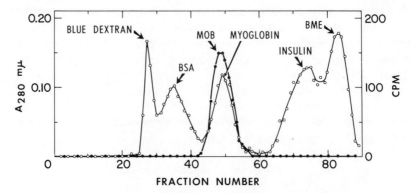

FIGURE 18. Molecular weight estimation by elution from Sepharose-2B in the presence of 6 M guanidinehydrochloride. Absorbance profile (O—O) of Blue Dextran, bovine serum albumin (BSA), myoglobin, insulin and β-mercaptoethanol (BME). Radioactivity profile (●—●) of [³H]-labeled, purified mouse olfactory marker protein (MOB).

protein (Margolis, 1972) was studied on Sepharose 2B in the presence of 6 M guanidine HCl (Fish et al., 1969), it essentially co-eluted with myoglobin—indicating a subunit molecular weight of about 18,000 daltons by this technique as well. These data suggest that the native protein may be a dimer composed of two subunits of 15,000–20,000 daltons each. Attempts to demonstrate the existence of dimers by the use of the cross-linking reagent dimethylsuberimidate were unsuccessful, however, and this aspect of the structure of the olfactory marker proteins is under investigation.

2.5. Possible Approaches to Function and Utility of the Marker Protein

The marker protein represents nearly 1% of the total soluble protein of the mouse olfactory bulb and epithelium. Since this protein is a marker for the primary receptor neurons which synapse in the bulb, the actual content of this protein in these specific neurons and their specific nerve endings within the bulb must be much higher than 1%. Thus, this protein, which has been conserved during evolution, appears to be a major component of a single-cell type and should have an important function in the neurons. What is that function? The marker protein may be involved in maintaining the structural integrity of these cells or function in some kind of transport system for either ions, metabolites, or neurotransmitters. Conceivably it could be an enzyme involved in a unique metabolic pathway in these neurons.

In view of the morphogenetic influence of the invading olfactory receptor cells on the developing olfactory bulb (Hinds, 1972), perhaps the marker protein serves a trophic or information-transfer function.

In order to attempt to study these questions, we could pursue various approaches. If this protein is involved in some aspect of olfactory transduction, we might expect alterations in its turnover rate and/or axoplasmic transport rate as a function of olfactory stimulation. The long, unmyelinated C-fibers of the garfish olfactory nerve offer an admirable system for such a study (Easton, 1965; Gross, 1973). The possible function of this protein as a carrier would best be tested at this time by a trial-and-error method of evaluating its binding activity against various metals, ions, and transmitter candidates. One approach to the question in another system has been the study of the influence of ions on the conformation of the S-100 protein (Calissano et al., 1969; Dannies and Levine, 1971) and the demonstration of its affinity for Ca^{2+}, an important ion in neural processes.

It has been observed that morphogenetic events in the developing olfactory bulb are strongly influenced by the invading axons of the olfactory receptor neuron (Hinds, 1972). It would be of great interest to study the quantity of the marker protein as a function of cellular development and synapse formation during early neuroembryology of this area. In addition, the ability to maintain explants of neonatal olfactory bulb in organ culture (Kim, 1972) and of olfactory epithelium as well (A. I. Farbman and R. C. Gesteland, personal communication) suggests several interesting experiments utilizing the marker protein and its antibody to explore questions relating to cellular recognition during ontogeny of this neural pathway.

Several authors have studied the influence of brain-specific antisera on electrophysiological activity of selected brain areas in an attempt to learn something about the function of specific nervous tissue antigens (Jankovic et al., 1968; MacPherson and Chinerman, 1971). Clearly such an approach is indicated here both at the electrophysiological level as well as at the level of modifying sensory reception and subsequently, perhaps behavior. The ability of the olfactory receptor cells to take up exogenously administered proteins (Kristensson and Olsson, 1971) and viruses (Sabin and Olitsky, 1937; Nir et al., 1965) suggests that it may be possible to introduce the specific antibody into the receptor cells. Conceivably the resultant antigen–antibody reaction could damage or destroy the chemosensory cells. If all the chemosensory neurons were thus killed, we would have performed an immunoepitheliectomy analogous to the use of antibody to NGF to produce an immunosympathectomy (Steiner and Schonbaum, 1972). This procedure would be very useful since it would eliminate surgical side effects. When immunized with rat protein, the rabbit produced antibodies to the protein of the rat which cross-reacted against its own olfactory marker protein *in vitro*.

Since γ-globulin can cross the placenta (Ralph et al., 1973), it would be theoretically possible to obtain an immunized pregnant rabbit producing antibodies against the olfactory receptor cells of its own offspring which would then be congenitally anosmic and serve as a model for behavioral and biochemical studies.

The isolation of specific neurons for study has been primarily based on microdissection techniques (Giacobini, 1968). An attempt to achieve the separation of chemosensory neurons by differential centrifugation has been reported by Ash et al. (1966). One of the major problems with this approach is the rapid loss of characteristic morphology and the difficulty in identifying the specific cell type of the isolated material. Similarly, preparations of nerve ending particles, synaptosomes, from cerebral tissue have consisted of a heterogeneous population deriving from many different cell types. Clearly, for various biochemical studies it would be useful to be able to isolate a preparation of synaptosomes deriving primarily or exclusively from a single neuron type. The availability of the marker protein described in this chapter encourages us to think that it may facilitate the isolation of the olfactory chemoreceptor neurons and of their synaptic endings as homogeneous populations for further biochemical studies.

The existence of rare human olfactory neuroblastomas (Jakumheit, 1971) and the ability to induce such tumors in hamsters (Herrold, 1964) suggest that it may prove feasible to clone olfactory neurons in cell culture as has been done for neuroblastoma (McMorris et al., 1973). This procedure seems particularly promising in view of the apparent normal turnover of the olfactory receptor cells and their replacement from undifferentiated staminal cells in the olfactory mucosa (Graziadei and DeHan, 1973; Metcalf, 1973; Moulton, 1974; Andres, 1966; Moulton and Fink, 1972).

3. SEARCH FOR TRANSMITTER CANDIDATES AND MICROMOLECULAR MARKERS OF THE PRIMARY OLFACTORY PATHWAY: CARNOSINE

3.1. Introduction

Peripheral denervation by intranasal irrigation with zinc sulfate solution resulted in a specific decrease in the level of the olfactory marker protein without any major changes in the levels of three neurotransmitter-metabolizing enzymes (Table 9). These observations, coupled with the very low levels of the three enzymes observed in the olfactory epithelium, encouraged us to try to determine the nature of the neurotransmitter utilized by the olfactory receptor neurons at their synapses in the olfactory bulb glomeruli. Electron microscopic studies have demonstrated that these synapses do contain what appear to be synaptic vesicles (Shepherd, 1972), but whether these vesicles contain a functional neurotransmitter is unknown. Since we can monitor the state of these synapses by monitoring the marker protein level in the bulb, it became feasible to attempt biochemical studies of putative transmitters in these synapses.

3.2. Putative Transmitter Uptake Studies

High, but not low, affinity uptake systems for various compounds have been implicated as indicating the presence of specific sites where these compounds function as neurotransmitters (Kuhar, 1973; Snyder et al., 1973b). However, the localization and function of these high affinity uptake systems are not absolutely defined since they have been demonstrated to exist in synaptosomal fractions (Snyder et al., 1973) as well as in glial cells (Shrier and Thompson, 1974). Nevertheless, it has been shown that choline level and uptake decrease after denervation of a cholinergic tract (Kuhar et al., 1973), and that glycine level and uptake is reduced following hypoxic loss of interneurons in the spinal cord (Davidoff et al., 1967; Aprison and Werman, 1968).

We studied the effect of peripheral deafferentation and the attendant synaptic degeneration on various high-affinity uptake systems for neuro-transmitter candidates by means of uptake of labeled compounds from a physiological buffer medium (Bradford, 1972) into tissue slices (Iversen and Neal, 1968) prepared from control or deafferented mouse olfactory bulbs. Data for sixteen neuroactive compounds are presented in Table 11; for half of these, the affinity constant of the uptake system was measured. The rate of uptake for control and deafferented olfactory bulbs computed as tissue: medium ratios was studied in the nanomolar concentration range to ensure minimal contribution from any low-affinity uptake system present in the tissue. It can be seen that the intranasal irrigation with zinc sulfate had no effect on the uptake into slices of olfactory bulb of any of the compounds studied, despite the wide range of uptake activities evidenced by tissue: medium ratios from 0 to 30, of exogenous transmitter concentrations varying from 4 to 287 nM, or of observed K_m values varying from 0.27–132 μM. The affinity constants we measured for neurotransmitter uptake in the olfactory bulb are, with the exception of glycine, all in excellent agreement with literature values for the high-affinity uptake systems in other brain regions (Iversen and Neal, 1968; Shaskan and Snyder, 1970; Balcar and Johnston, 1973; Snyder et al., 1973b). Glycine has an affinity constant in

TABLE 11. Effect of Peripheral Denervation by ZnSO₄ Irrigation on Putative Neurotransmitter Uptake Systems in the Olfactory Bulbs[a]

Compound	K_m control, μM	Tissue: medium ratio		Exogenous transmitter, nM
		Control	3 Weeks after ZnSO₄	
Adenosine	2.6	2.0	2.4	28.2
β-Alanine	—	0.5	0.6	6.0
γ-Aminobutyric acid	14.0	24.0	30.0	52.7
Aspartic acid	19.0	27.6	26.9	7.4
Arginine	—	0.9	0.7	40.0
Choline	3.3	2.9	3.2	159.0
Dopamine	—	4.0	5.2	65.0
Histamine	—	0	0	66.7
Histidine	—	4.2	3.8	4.0
Glutamic acid	25	16.0	15.0	58.6
Glycine	132	0.9	0.9	42.3
Norepinephrine	0.5	1.6	1.7	36.7
Proline	—	3.6	3.6	43.9
Tyramine	0.27	1.8	2.1	60.8
Tyrosine	—	6.3	6.4	8.1
Tryptophan	—	6.4	5.8	287.0

[a] From Margolis et al., 1974.

the olfactory bulb which is similar to the low-affinity constants seen in cortex and is distinctly different from the high-affinity constant seen in spinal cord (Balcar and Johnston, 1973; Snyder et al., 1973a,b). Neidle et al. (1973) reported a study of low-affinity amino acid uptake in olfactory bulbs. Although high-affinity uptake systems for catecholamines exist in the bulb (Table 11) as do catecholaminergic endings (Dahlstrom et al., 1965), they are apparently in deep layers and not in the glomerular layers where the primary afferent synapse takes place. It is possible that the transmitter used by the receptor cells is also used by other cells in the olfactory bulb and that loss of the receptor cell uptake system might represent only a small percentage of the total uptake capacity of the bulb. Nevertheless, these data do suggest that none of the compounds function as the synaptic neurotransmitter from the chemoreceptor neurons to their synapses in the glomeruli. The virtual absence of glutamic decarboxylase and choline acetylase activities in the epithelium, and the absence of any denervation effect on their levels in the bulbs, corroborates that viewpoint for GABA and acetylcholine as do the anatomical data (Dahlstrom et al., 1965) for the catecholamines. What then might be a transmitter candidate for this pathway? Are there any specific denervation effects on other small molecules or transmitter candidates in the primary olfactory pathway?

3.3. Studies of Small Molecule Content in the Primary Olfactory Pathway

To study small molecule content we chose a very sensitive but relatively nonspecific reagent, dimethylaminonaphthalene sulfonylchloride (dansyl-Cl). Dansyl-Cl will react with primary and secondary amines, imidazoles without ring substitutions, and phenols. This list includes reactive groups associated with all the known and postulated neurotransmitters except for acetylcholine, which, based on the data already presented, seems to be an unlikely transmitter candidate for this pathway. Procedures for preparation of tissue extracts, reaction with dansyl-Cl, and separation by thin-layer chromatography in two dimensions have been described (Neuhoff et al., 1971; Roberts et al., 1973; Airhart et al., 1973). On comparison of tissue extracts from mouse olfactory bulbs before and after peripheral deafferentation with extracts of whole brain–lacking olfactory bulbs, it became evident that an orange fluorescent dansyl derivative was present in olfactory bulb extracts which disappeared following peripheral deafferentation and was missing from extracts of whole brain–lacking olfactory bulbs. Thus, there did seem to exist a compound which might potentially fulfill our hopes of a micromolecular marker and possibly a transmitter candidate. It was then necessary to identify and to quantitate this unknown compound. The use of [H^3]-dansyl-Cl enabled us to use scintillation counting and radio-autography to increase the sensitivity of our detection system. The new compound was demonstrated to be present in both olfactory epithelium and bulb (Figure 19) and to be essentially undetectable in extracts of whole brain–lacking bulbs. Following peripheral deafferentation or olfactory bulbectomy, the compound seemed to decrease selectively (Figure 19) in the reciprocal portion of the primary olfactory pathway.

The restricted regional distribution of the compound and its decrease subsequent to denervation were the same qualitative pattern we had observed for the olfactory marker protein; this encouraged us to think we might have a micromolecular marker for the primary olfactory pathway. Identification of the compound was approached by several methods. The orange fluorescence of the dansyl derivative was distinct from the yellow-green fluorescence of most amino acids except histidine and tyrosine and suggested that we might be dealing with an aromatic compound. We observed that many of the dansyl derivatives of a variety of indoleamines and catecholamines migrated to the same quadrant of the TLC plate as did the unknown compound (Figure 19). Finally, the dansyl derivatives of the dipeptide carnosine (β-ala-l-his) and homocarnosine (GABA-l-his) were found to comigrate with that of the unknown compound on TLC. Since homocarnosine has been considered to be the major histidine dipeptide in nervous tissue and

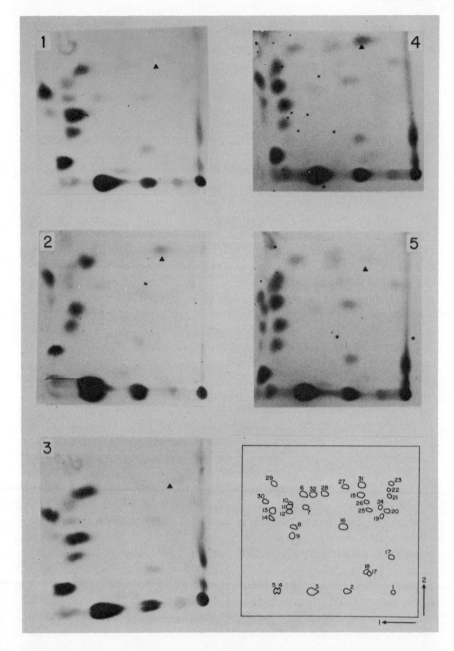

FIGURE 19. Autoradiographic demonstration of the influence of denervation on the content of [³H]-dansyl derivatives of low molecular weight compounds from olfactory tissues of mice. Ethanolic extracts were reacted with [³H]-dansyl chloride and aliquots spotted in the lower right-

cerebrospinal fluid (Abraham *et al.*, 1962; Perry *et al.*, 1968; Yockey and Marshall, 1969) and carnosine to be present primarily in muscle (Waley, 1966) with only in traces in nervous tissue, it seemed probable that we were dealing with homocarnosine. To test this, extracts were subjected to paper electrophoresis at pH 10.0 (Figure 20); since imidazoles were indicated, diazotized sulfanilic acid was used as a detection system. It was surprising and rapidly apparent that the compound present in the olfactory bulb and epithelium, which decreased on denervation, coelectrophoresed with authentic carnosine but not with homocarnosine nor with gly-L-his, L-his-L-ala or L-ala-L-his (Margolis, 1974). Furthermore, this compound was absent from lung, a source of respiratory epithelium, a fact indicating its probable location in the receptor cells of the olfactory epithelium. In addition, the compound comigrated with the major diazotized sulfanilic acid reactive compound from muscle, a known source of carnosine. The reactivity of the compound with diazotized sulfanilic acid indicated it to be an imidazole derivative without ring substituents, thus eliminating anserine (β-ala-*N*-methyl-L-his) from consideration. Evaluation of tissue extracts by ion exchange chromatography demonstrated the coelution of the unknown compound with authentic carnosine and its disappearance from the bulb on deafferentation (Table 12). Finally, acid hydrolysis of the imidazole fraction from mouse olfactory epithelium extracts generated β-ala and L-his in equimolar amounts.

These various data taken together proved the presence of carnosine in the primary olfactory pathway of the mouse and demonstrated it to be present at a higher concentration than that previously reported for any histidine peptide in any region of the mammalian nervous system (Abraham

---

hand corner of polyamide TLC plates (7.5 × 7.5 cm). Development in the first dimension was with 3% formic acid followed by heptane: *n*-butanol: glacial acetic acid (3:3:1) in the second dimension. The plates were exposed to X-ray film for 2 months. On each autoradiograph the location of carnosine and homocarnosine is indicated (▲). Brain without olfactory bulbs, 18 μg (1); olfactory bulbs, 14 μg (2); olfactory bulbs 1 wk after intranasal irrigation with $ZnSO_4$, 18 μg (3); olfactory epithelium, sham operated, 10 μg (4); olfactory epithelium 10 days after bulbectomy, 8 μg (5). The final panel indicates the relative positions of the dansyl derivatives of a variety of compounds: origin 1; taurine 2; dansic acid 3; GABA 6; glutamate 8; aspartate 9; alanine and β-alanine 10; glycine and dansylamide 11; glutamine 13; serine 14; carnosine and homocarnosine 15; bisdansyl lysine 16; 5-hydroxytryptophan 17; tryptophan 18; serotonin 19; tyrosine 20; norepinephrine 21; dopamine 22; tyramine 23; dopa 24; tryptamine 25; octopamine 26; histamine 27; proline 28; epinephrine 29; histidine 30; anserine 31; α-amino *N*-acetyl histidine 32. In addition, the dansyl derivatives of hydroxylysine, ornithine, 1-methyl-histidine, 3-methylhistidine, arginine, *i*-leucine, phenylalanine, methionine, threonine, cysteine, valine, leucine, 2-thienyl alanine, 2-thienyl serine, norleucine, norvaline, and α-amino-β-guanidopropionic acid were distinguishable in mobility from carnosine and homocarnosine at spot 15.

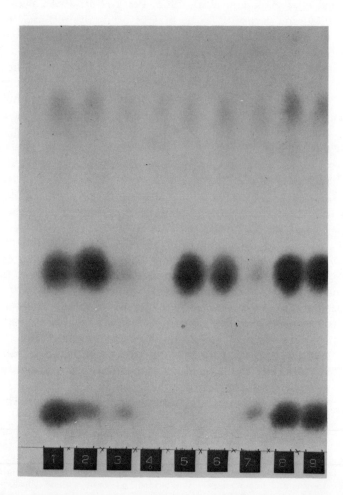

FIGURE 20. Paper electrophoresis of tissue extracts. Ethanol extracts equivalent to 50 mg of fresh tissue were placed at the origin and were subjected to electrophoresis at pH 10 in 0.1 *M* sodium borate buffer at 25 V/cm for 4 hr. The positive electrode was at the top of the figure. Alkaline-diazotized sulfanilic acid was used to visualize the imidazole compounds. Carnosine and homocarnosine (50 nmole each) lanes 1 and 9; olfactory bulb, lane 2; cerebral hemispheres, lane 3; lung, lane 4; olfactory epithelium, lane 5; skeletal muscle, lane 6; olfactory bulbs 15 days after peripheral deafferentation, lane 7; olfactory bulb plus 50 nmole each of carnosine and homocarnosine, lane 8. The origin is at the bottom and the order of increasing mobility toward the positive electrode at the top of the figure is: homocarnosine, carnosine, histidine. (From Margolis, 1974.)

TABLE 12. Amino Compounds[a] in Olfactory Tissues of Mice

Compound	Olfactory			Whole brain[c]
	Epithelium	Bulbs	Bulbs after $ZnSO_4$[b]	
Phosphoserine	0.3	0.1	0.1	0.1
Phosphoethanolamine	1.1	1.1	1.1	1.4
Taurine	22.1	16.3	13.0	10.2
Aspartic acid	1.4	3.5	3.2	3.6
Threonine	<0.2	0.3	0.4	0.3
Serine	0.5	0.7	0.8	0.8
Asparagine and glutamine	2.3	4.7	4.9	4.8
Glutamic acid	3.0	9.7	8.5	11.9
Glycine	1.6	0.5	0.7	1.0
Alanine	<0.2	0.5	0.5	0.4
γ-Aminobutyric acid	<0.2	6.1	5.5	2.7
Carnosine	2.5	2.2	ND	ND

[a] Ethanol extracts of tissues were analyzed on an amino acid analyzer using a physiological fluid elution program. Results are in nanomoles per milligram of tissue. The following amino compounds were present (in all samples) at less than 0.2 nmole per milligram of tissue: valine, isoleucine, leucine, tyrosine, phenylalanine, β-alanine, lysine, histidine, arginine, and ethanolamine. ND, not detected.
[b] Twenty-four days after deafferentation with zinc sulfate.
[c] Whole brain excluding olfactory bulbs. (From Margolis, 1974.)

et al., 1962; Enwonu and Worthington, 1974; Himwich and Agrawal, 1969; Kanazawa and Sano, 1967; Marshall and Yockey, 1968; Perry et al., 1968, 1971; Yockey and Marshall, 1969). The occurrence of carnosine at high contents in mouse olfactory bulbs was simultaneously and independently reported at the 1974 meeting of the American Society for Neurochemistry by our laboratory (Margolis and Armona, 1974) and that of Neidle and Kandera (1974). The presence of this compound in high content in a specific region of the nervous system and its susceptibility to manipulation by denervation suggests it is important to the function of the olfactory chemoreceptor neurons, conceivably functioning as a neurotransmitter or involved in modulating transmitter function.

3.4. Studies of Carnosine, a Micromolecular Marker of the Primary Olfactory Pathway

It seems pertinent at this point to gain some information about the biological distribution of carnosine in the olfactory pathway, and the time-course of decrease following denervation, as well as about the enzymes

TABLE 13. Effect of Central and Peripheral Denervation on Carnosine Content of
the Primary Olfactory Pathway of Female Mice

Tissue	Treatment	Carnosine[a] (nmoles)/tissue (mg)
Olfactory bulb	Control	0.87
	2 days after intranasal zinc sulfate	0.73
	5 days after intranasal zinc sulfate	0.13
	8 days after intranasal zinc sulfate	0.10
	90 days after intranasal zinc sulfate	0.09
Olfactory epithelium	Control	0.95
	4 days after bulbectomy	0.32
	10 days after bulbectomy	0.09
	90 days after bulbectomy	1.0

[a] Tissue was extracted with ethanol and reacted with [^{3}H]-dansyl-Cl and subjected to two-dimensional chromatography on polyamide thin-layer plates and the orange fluorescent dansyl-carnosine spot cut off the plate, eluted, and counted in a scintillation counter.

involved in its metabolism. Nearly 90% of the carnosine content of olfactory bulb disappears in about 1 week following intranasal irrigation with zinc sulfate solution and remains low for at least 3 months (Table 13). In the olfactory epithelium a similar rapid loss of carnosine is seen following bulbectomy. However, the olfactory epithelium contrasts with the olfactory bulb in that this loss appears to be reversible in the epithelium at long time intervals after surgery (Table 13). This observation was quite unexpected since the olfactory marker protein does not reappear at long-time intervals following bulbectomy (Margolis et al., 1974). The possibility that this apparent recovery of carnosine is related to the reported postbulbectomy regeneration of olfactory chemoreceptor neurons (Graziadei and DeHan, 1973; Metcalf, 1973) is the subject of current studies.

The synthetic enzyme carnosine synthetase has been studied extensively in muscle (Kalyankar and Meister, 1959; Stenesh and Winnick, 1960), but only recently has it been reported to occur in cerebral tissues (Skaper et al., 1973). Utilizing a modification of the published assay for cerebral tissues, we were able to demonstrate carnosine synthetase activity in the olfactory pathway of mice (Table 14). Our ability to demonstrate the occurrence of this synthetase activity in muscle is in agreement with earlier reports and with the known high levels of carnosine in that tissue. On the other hand, lung, a very poor source of carnosine, has no demonstrable activity by this assay, a result indicating that it is not respiratory epithelial cells which are the source of this activity in the nasal olfactory epithelium. Extracts of cerebellum showed virtually no carnosine synthetase activity under these assay conditions, an indication of the much higher concentration

TABLE 14. Carnosine Synthetase Activity[a] in Mouse Tissues

Tissue	Treatment	cpm/mg tissue/hr
Olfactory bulbs	—	170
Olfactory bulbs	11 days after intranasal zinc sulfate.	< 10
Olfactory epithelium	—	140
Olfactory epithelium	6 days after bulbectomy	< 10
Cerebellum	—	< 10
Lung	—	< 10
Skeletal muscle	—	80

[a] Tissue extracts were prepared as described by Skaper et al. (1973), with the addition of 2 mM dithiothreitol throughout. Enzyme activity was measured as the conversion of $[^{14}C]$-β-ala to $[^{14}C]$-carnosine separated by ion exchange chromatography.

of this enzyme in the olfactory pathway as compared to the cerebellum. The effect of denervation is clear, in that carnosine synthetase activity decreases dramatically (Table 14) as does the level of carnosine (Table 13) and that of the marker protein (Tables 6, 8), although other enzymes (Table 9) and low-molecular-weight compounds are unaltered (Table 12). Very preliminary results indicate that the activity of the degradative enzyme, carnosinase, is present in both olfactory bulb and cerebellum and is not grossly altered following intranasal zinc sulfate treatment (unpublished observations). Carnosine is present in olfactory tissue of both male and female rat, mouse, and hamster. It is present as well in olfactory bulbs of rabbit, guinea pig, and dog (unpublished observations).

The occurrence of carnosine and the enzyme responsible for its synthesis in high concentrations in the primary olfactory pathway of several species prompts a variety of questions as to the possible function of this compound.

3.5. Possible Approaches to Function and Utility of Carnosine and the Enzymes Involved in Its Metabolism

The dipeptide carnosine (β-ala-L-his) is present in higher content in the primary olfactory pathway than in any other brain region tested by us or reported by others. The localization of both carnosine and the enzyme responsible for its synthesis in the primary olfactory pathway, and their response to denervation is similar to the results obtained with the olfactory marker protein. There are, however, several differences. Unlike the marker protein, carnosine is also present in muscle, a nonneural tissue, and is present in low contents in other brain areas. In addition, carnosine, but not the marker protein, reappears in the olfactory epithelium after the initial, rapid, postbulbectomy decrease. Nevertheless, it is difficult to avoid the feeling that these marker components are somehow related to each other and to the function of the chemoreceptor neurons.

What is the function of carnosine in the olfactory pathway and how could it be related to the marker protein? While attempts to postulate function for the marker protein suffer at this time from total lack of any known biological activity which can be ascribed to the protein, carnosine suffers from perhaps a surfeit of biological activities which have been ascribed to it, and to related compounds. The very existence of any biological activity is of course encouraging, but sorting out the probable from the improbable is difficult. About 35 years ago it was reported that only L-carnosine but not homocarnosine nor other histidine dipeptides has hypotensive activity in the cat (Hunt and du Vigneaud, 1939). The high content of carnosine in muscle has generated data suggesting that it functions as a buffer and regulates glycogen metabolism (Davey, 1960; Quereshi and Wood, 1960) and is involved in regulating the function of the neuromuscular junction (Severin, 1964). Whether any of these reports relate to its function in the primary olfactory pathway is presently unknown.

Carnosine is an excellent metal chelator and has been reported to form copper chelate complexes which are polymeric (Vallee and Wacker, 1970). Copper, zinc, and manganese are present in high levels in the olfactory bulb (Donaldson et al., 1973) and are required cofactors for carnosinase (Rosenberg, 1960), and both copper and zinc have been implicated in chemoreception (Schechter et al., 1972). The juxtaposition of these observations suggests possible functional interactions between these divalent metals, carnosine, and olfactory chemoreception. The possibility that carnosine may be a novel dipeptide neurotransmitter or transmitter precursor has not escaped our notice, especially since many amino compounds are being considered as transmitter candidates in vertebrates (Aprison and Werman, 1968; Krnjevic, 1974; Iversen et al., 1973). Rat brain slices are reported to have a much greater avidity for carnosine than for homocarnosine (Abraham et al., 1964).

Carnosinase activity is present in olfactory bulb tissue (unpublished observations) but is reportedly absent from muscle (Hanson and Smith, 1964) suggesting that the role of carnosine may be different in muscle and olfactory tissue. The occurrence of carnosinase further suggests that carnosine may function as a storage form of β-alanine or L-histidine. The possible involvement of β-alanine in sensory systems has been noted in some recent publications (Bruun et al., 1974; McBride et al., 1974). An approach to some of these questions of function may be available through genetics, since hereditary disorders of β-alanine and carnosine metabolism are known to exist in man (Schriver and Perry, 1972) and may occur in animals as well.

In addition to the considerations of possible functions of carnosine in the primary olfactory pathway are questions of its utility as a tool in studying this particular neural pathway. Many of the considerations discussed in regard to the utility of the acidic marker protein apply here as well and will not be considered again. However, unlike the marker protein, which never recovers following bulbectomy, carnosine levels in the olfactory epithelium do return to normal. The olfactory receptor neurons have been reported to degenerate following bulbectomy (Clark, 1957; SenGupta, 1967; Takagi, 1971) and then to be replaced from staminal cells in the olfactory muscosa (Clark, 1957; SenGupta, 1967; Takagi, 1971; Graziadei and Dehan, 1973; Metcalf, 1973; Andres, 1966). Indeed, the olfactory receptor neurons are thought to undergo continual replacement and turnover in normal animals (Moulton and Fink, 1972; Moulton, 1974; Graziadei and Metcalf, 1971; Metcalf, 1973). Perhaps the reappearance of carnosine levels following the postbulbectomy decrease represents an early biochemical index of receptor cell replacement, while the level of the marker protein cannot recover until functional synapses are reformed. If this postulate is true, it offers an elegant two-pronged approach to the study of the neuroembryology of this pathway as discussed earlier, as well as to the questions of chemoreceptor cell turnover and function.

4. FINAL SUMMARY AND COMMENTS

At the beginning of this chapter I presented a case indicating the general need for cell-specific markers as useful probes of function within the nervous system. The general thrust of this argument was the desirability, indeed the necessity, of being able to monitor selectively the biochemical behavior of a single cell type in the midst of a variety of dissimilar cell types interacting with it. The approach taken was to search for examples of cell-specific genetic expression. The feasibility of this approach has been illustrated by the studies from my own laboratory which have demonstrated the existence of a macromolecule uniquely localized in the olfactory chemoreceptor neurons. The macromolecule, an acidic marker protein of low molecular weight, appears to be unaffected by changes in endocrine status of the animal, increases postnatally, is present in the olfactory chemoreceptor neurons of virtually all vertebrates, and is subject to selective alteration following denervation procedures. In addition we have been able to present preliminary evidence for the existence of a low-molecular-weight compound in rodent nervous tissue which, along with the enzyme responsible for its synthesis, is highly localized to the primary olfactory chemoreceptor neurons. The compound, the dipeptide carnosine (β-ala-L-his), is present in the olfactory pathway of mouse, rat, hamster, guinea pig, rabbit, and dog, and at least in the mouse is subject to alteration in quantity following either central or peripheral denervation. Possible functions of these two markers have been considered as well as experimental approaches to elucidate said functions. In addition, potential uses of these materials as probes to learn something of the neurons that they mark have been considered, as well as the potential interrelationships of these two markers to each other.

Imidazole derivatives are very reactive components of biological systems and by way of concluding I should like to comment briefly on what seems to be the ubiquitous occurrence of histidine derivatives in excitable tissues, i.e., nerve and muscle. The specific derivative observed varies from species to species, but some representative seems always to be present. Thus we find the dipeptides carnosine, homocarnosine, anserine, homoanserine, cetasine, and ophidine (Waley, 1966) as well as histamine (Green, 1970), N-acetylhistidine (Baslow et al., 1969), and TRF (pyroglutamylhistidyl-prolinamide (Brownstein et al., 1974). But even more intriguing is the frequent appearance of an α-N-acylated histidine derivative in association with a "marker protein." From the olfactory placode (Sinclair, 1971) a tissue derives which possesses carnosine and the olfactory marker protein. From the visual placode the lens of the eye derives (Sinclair, 1971), possessing N-acetylhistidine (Baslow et al., 1969) and the α, β, and γ-crystallins (Kuck, 1970). The auditory placode (Sinclair, 1971) appears to give rise to unique marker proteins (Davies, 1970) although no evidence for a histidine peptide is yet forthcoming. Muscle contains carnosine and anserine (Davey, 1960) and a characteristic marker protein, actomyosin. Whether these observations are merely a series of coincidences or an indication of some functional relatedness is totally unknown.

ACKNOWLEDGMENTS

At various times during the course of these studies I had the talented assistance of Brian Copeland, Janet Feldman, Donna Ferriero, Angelica Keller, Nelson Roberts, and Ivana Santic. Alina Dugan has given dedicated secretarial assistance for many years.

I appreciate permission to use previously unpublished material taken from a thesis to be submitted by Angelica Keller to the Graduate Department of Biochemistry of CUNY. For permission to reproduce previously published materials I thank: Academic Press, Elsevier Scientific Publishing Co., *Journal of Biological Chemistry*, Pergamon Press, Raven Press, *Science*, and *Scientific American.*

5. REFERENCES*

Abraham, D., Pisano, J. J., and Udenfriend, S., 1962, The distribution of homocarnosine in mammals, *Arch. Biochem. Biophys.* **99**:210–213.

Abraham, D., Pisano, J. J., and Udenfriend, S., 1964, Uptake of carnosine and homocarnosine by rat brain slices, *Arch. Biochem. Biophys.* **104**:160–165.

Adler, J., 1972, Chemoreception in bacteria, *in Olfaction and Taste IV* (D. Schneider, ed.), pp. 70–80, Wissenschaftiche Verlag, MBH, Stuttgart.

Airhart, J., Sibiga, S., Sanders, H., and Khairallah, E. A., 1973, An ultramicromethod for quantitation of amino acids in biological fluids, *Anal. Biochem.* **53**:132–140.

Alberts, J., 1974, Producing and interpreting experimental olfactory deficits, *Physiology and Behavior* **12**:657–670.

Altman, J., 1969, Autoradiographic and histological studies of postnatal neurogenesis. IV. Cell proliferation and migration in the anterior forebrain with special reference to persisting neurogenesis in the olfactory bulb, *J. Comp. Neurol.* **137**:433–457.

Andres, K. H., 1966, Der feinbau der regio olfactoria von makrosmatikern, *Zeitschr. f. Zellforsch.* **69**:140–154.

Aprison, M. H., and Werman, R., 1968, A combined neurochemical and neurophysiological approach to identification of central nervous system transmitters, *Neurosci. Res.* **1**:143–174.

Ash, K. O., Bransford, J. E., and Koch, R. B., 1966, Studies on dispersions of rabbit olfactory cells, *J. Cell Biol.* **29**:554–561.

Balcar, V. J., and Johnston, G. A. R., 1973, High affinity uptake of transmitters: Studies on the uptake of L-asparate, GABA, ʳ-glutamate and glycine in cat spinal cord, *J. Neurochem.* **20**:529–539.

Baslow, M. H., Turplaty, P., and Lenney, J. F., 1969, *N*-acetylhistidine metabolism in the brain, heart and lens of the goldfish, *Carassius Auratus in vivo*: Evidence of rapid turnover and a possible intermediate, *Life Sciences* **8**:535–541.

Baradi, A. F., and Bourne, G. H., 1959, Histochemical localization of cholinesterase in gustatory and olfactory epithelia, *J. Histochem. & Cytochem.* **7**:2–7.

Beidler, L. M. (ed.), 1971, Chemical senses, in: *Handbook of Sensory Physiology*, part 1, Olfaction, Vol. 4, Springer–Verlag, Berlin.

Berger, B., 1971*a*, Etude ultrastructurale de la degenerescence wallerienne experimentale d'un nerf entierement amyelinique: le nerf olfactif. I. Modifications axonales, *J. Ultrastructure Res.* **37**:105–118.

Berger, B., 1971*b*, Etude ultrastructurale de la degenerescence wallerienne experimentale d'un nerf entierement amyelinique: le nerf olfactif. II. Reactions cellulaires, *J. Ultrastructure Res.* **37**:479–494.

Berger, B., 1973, Degenerescence transsynaptique dans le bulbe olfactif du lapin, apres desafferentation peripherique, *Acta Neuropath. (Berlin)* **24**:128–152.

Bignami, A., Eng, L., Dahl, D., and Uyeda, C., 1972, Localization of the glial fibrillary acidic protein in astrocytes by immunofluorescence, *Brain Res.* **43**:429–435.

* In order to maintain a bibliography of reasonable proportions, it was frequently necessary to choose references which seemed to offer the interested reader facilitated access to related literature. I apologize to those whose work has not been cited directly as a result of these decisions.

Bondy, S. C., and Margolis, F. L., 1971, Sensory deprivation and brain development, *in Brain and Behavior Research* (J. Bures, E. R. John, P. G. Kostuk, and L. Pickenhain, eds.), Vol. 4, pp. 3–54, Fisher Verlag, Jena.

Bovet, D., Bovet-Nitti, F., and Oliverio, A., 1969, Genetic aspects of learning and memory in mice, *Science* **163**:139–149.

Bradford, H. F., 1972, Cerebral cortex slices and synaptosomes: *In vitro* approaches to brain metabolism, *in Methods of Neurochemistry* (R. Fried, ed.), Vol. 3, pp. 155–202, Dekker, New York.

Brownstein, M. J., Palkovits, M., Saavedra, J., Bassiri, R., and Utiger, R., 1974, Thyrotropin releasing hormone in specific nuclei of the brain, *Science* **185**:267–269.

Bruun, A., Ehinger, B., and Forsberg, A., 1974, *In vitro* uptake of β-alanine into rabbit retinal neurons, *Exptl. Brain Res.* **19**:239–247.

Calissano, P., Moore, B., and Friesen, A., 1969, Effect of calcium ion on S-100, a protein of the nervous system, *Biochemistry* **8**:4318–4326.

Cheal, M. L., and Sprott, R. L., 1971, Social olfaction: A review of the role of olfaction in a variety of animal behaviors, *Psychol. Reports* **29**:195–243.

Clark, W. L. G., 1957, Inquiries into the anatomical basis of olfactory discrimination, *Proc. Roy. Soc. (London)* **B146**:299–319.

Cuenod, M., Marko, P., and Niederer, E., 1973, Disappearance of particulate tectal protein during optic nerve degeneration in the pigeon, *Brain Res.* **49**:422–426.

Dahlstrom, A., Fuxe, K., Olson, L., and Ungerstedt, U., 1965, On the distribution and possible function of monoamine nerve terminals in the olfactory bulb of the rabbit, *Life Sciences* **4**:2071–2074.

Dannies, P., and Levine, L., 1971, Structural properties of bovine brain S-100 protein, *J. Biol. Chem.* **246**:6276–6283.

Davey, C. L., 1960*a*, Effects of carnosine and anserine on glycolytic reactions in skeletal muscle, *Arch. Biochem. Biophys.* **89**:296–302.

Davey, C. L., 1960*b*, The significance of carnosine and anserine in striated skeletal muscle, *Arch. Biochem. Biophys.* **89**:303–308.

Davidoff, R. A., Graham, L. T., Shank, R. P., Werman, R., and Aprison, M. H., 1967, Changes in amino acid concentrations associated with loss of spinal interneurons, *J. Neurochem.* **14**:1025–1031.

Davies, W. E., 1970, The disc electrophoretic separation of proteins from various parts of the guinea pig brain, *J. Neurochem.* **17**:297–303.

Donaldson, J., St. Pierre, T., Minnich, J. L., and Barbeau, A., 1973, Determination of Na^+, K^+, Mg^{2+}, Cu^{2+}, Zn^{2+} and Mn^{2+} in rat brain regions, *Can. J. Biochem.* **51**:87–92.

Dusenbery, D. B., 1973, Countercurrent separation, a new method for studying behavior of small aquatic organisms, *Proc. Nat. Acad. Sci. (U.S.A.)* **70**:1349–1352.

Easton, D., 1965, Impulses at the artifactual nerve end, *Cold Spring Harbor Symp. on Quant. Biol.* **30**:15–28.

Enwonwu, C. O., and Worthington, B. S., 1974, Regional distribution of homocarnosine and other ninhydrin-positive substances in brains of malnourished monkeys, *J. Neurochem.* **22**:1045–1052.

Estable-Puig, J. F., and De Estable, R. F., 1969, Acute ultrastructural changes in the rat olfactory glomeruli after peripheral deafferentation, *Exptl. Neurol.* **24**:592–602.

Filogamo, G., and Marchisio, P. C., 1971, Acetylcholine system and neural development, *Neurosci. Res.* **4**:29–64.

Fish, W., Mann, K., and Tanford, C., 1969, The estimation of polypeptide chain molecular weights by gel filtration in 6 *M* guanidine hydrochloride, *J. Biol. Chem.* **244**:4989–4994.

Fonnum, F., 1972, Application of microchemical analysis and subcellular fractionation techniques to the study of neurotransmitters in discrete areas of mammalian brain, *Adv. in Biochem. Psychopharmocol.* **6**:75–88.

Gainer, H., 1972a, Electrophysiological behavior of an endogeneously active neurosecretory cell, *Brain Res.* **39**:403–418.

Gainer, H., 1972b, Patterns of protein synthesis in individual identified molluscan neurons, *Brain Res.* **39**:369–385.

Gainer, H., 1972c, Effects of experimentally induced diapause on the electrophysiology and protein synthesis patterns of identified molluscan neurons, *Brain Res.* **39**:387–402.

Gainer, H., and Wollberg, Z., 1974, Specific protein metabolism in identifiable neurons of *Aplysia californica, J. Neurobiol.* **5**:243–261.

Getchell, M., and Gesteland, R., 1972, The chemistry of olfactory reception: Stimulus specific protection from sulphydryl reagent inhibition, *Proc. Nat. Acad. Sci. (U.S.A.)* **69**:1494–1498.

Giacobini, E., 1968, Chemical studies on individual neurons, *Neurosci. Res.* **1**:1–71.

Graham, L. T., Jr., 1973, Distribution of glutamic acid decarboxylase activity and GABA content in the olfaction bulb, *Life Sciences* **12**:443–447.

Graziadei, P. P. C., 1971, The olfactory mucosa of vertebrates, *in Handbook of Sensory Physiology* (L. Beidler, ed.), Vol. 4, pp. 29–58, Springer–Verlag, Berlin.

Graziadei, P. P. C., and Metcalf, J. F., 1971a, Autoradiographic and ultrastructural observations on the frogs olfactory mucosa, *Zeitschr. f. Zellforschung* **16**:305–318.

Graziadei, P. P. C., and Metcalf, J. F., 1971b, Neuronal dynamics in the olfactory mucosa of the adult vertebrates, *Amer. Anat.* **10**:11.

Graziadei, P. P. C., and Dehan, R. S., 1973, Neuronal regeneration in frog olfactory system, *J. Cell Biol.* **59**:525–530.

Green, E. (ed.), 1967, *Biology of the Laboratory Mouse*, McGraw-Hill Book Co., New York.

Green, J. P., 1970, Histamine, *in Handbook of Neurochemistry* (A. Lajtha, ed.), Vol. IV, pp. 221–250, Plenum Press, New York.

Griffith, A. L., LaVelle, A., and Catsimpoolas, N., 1970, Isoelectric focussing of soluble brain proteins and changes associated with development, *Brain Res.* **24**:537–546.

Gross, G., 1973, The effect of temperature on the rapid axoplasmic transport in C-fibers, *Brain Res.* **56**:359–363.

Hamilton, C., Henkin, R., Weir, G., and Kliman, B., 1973, Olfactory status and response to clomiphene in male gonadotrophin deficiency, *Ann. Int. Med.* **78**:47–55.

Hanson, H., and Smith, E., 1949, Carnosinase: An enzyme of swine kidney, *J. Biol. Chem.* **179**:789–801.

Heimer, L., 1968, Synaptic distribution of centripetal and centrifugal nerve fibers in the olfactory system of the rat. An experimental anatomical study, *J. Anat.* **103**:413–432.

Heimer, L., 1971, Pathways in the brain, *Sci. Amer.* **225** (July):48–60.

Heimer, L., 1972, The olfactory connections of the diencephalon in the rat, *Brain Behav. Evol.* **6**:484–523.

Henkin, R., Keiser, H., and Bronzert, D., 1972, Histidine dependent zinc loss, hypogensia, anorexia and hypogensia, *J. Clin. Invest.* **51**:44a.

Henry, K., Buckholz, N., and Bowman, R., 1969, Genetics of memory, *Science* **165**:1148.

Herrold, K., 1964, Induction of olfactory neuroepithelial tumors in syrian hamsters by diethylnitrosamine, *Cancer* **17**:114–121.

Herschman, H. R., 1971, Synthesis and degradation of a brain-specific protein (S-100 protein) by clonal cultured human glial cells, *J. Biol. Chem.* **246**:7569–7571.

Himwich, W., and Agrawal, H., 1969, Amino acids, *in Handbook of Neurochemistry* (A. Lajtha, ed.), Vol. I, pp. 33–52, Plenum Press, New York.

Hinds, J., 1972a, Early neuron differentiation in the mouse olfactory bulb. I. Light microscopy, *J. Comp. Neurol.* **146**:233–252.

Hinds, J., 1972b, Early neuron differentiation in the mouse olfactory bulb. II. Electron microscopy, *J. Comp. Neurol.* **146**:253–276.

Hunt, M., and duVigneaud, V., 1939, A further contribution on the relationship of the structure of L-carnosine to its depressor activity, *J. Biol. Chem.* **127**:727–735.

Iversen, L. L., Kelly, J. S., Minchin, M., Schon, F., and Snodgrass, S. R., 1973, Role of amino acids and peptides in synaptic transmission, *Brain Res.* **62**:567–576.

Iversen, L. L., and Neal, M. J., 1968, The uptake of ^{3}H-GABA by slices of rat cerebral cortex, *J. Neurochem.* **15**:1141–1149.

Jakumeit, H. D., 1971, Neuroblastoma of the olfactory nerve, *Acta Neurochirurg.* **25**:99–108.

Jankovic, B. D., Rakic, L., Veskov, R., and Horvat, J., 1968, Effect of intraventricular injection of anti-brain antibodies on defensive conditioned reflexes, *Nature* **218**:270–271.

Kalyankar, G., and Meister, A., 1959, Enzymatic synthesis of carnosine and related β-alanyl and γ-aminobutyryl peptides, *J. Biol. Chem.* **234**:3210–3218.

Kanazawa, A., and Sano, I., 1967, A method of determination of homocarnosine and its distribution in mammalian tissues, *J. Neurochem.* **14**:211–214.

Keller, A., and Margolis, F., 1975, Immunological studies with the rat olfactory protein, in *J. Neurochem.* (in press).

Kim, S. U., 1972, Light and electron microscopic study of neurons and synapses in neonatal olfactory bulb cultured *in vitro, Exptl. Neurol.* **36**:336–349.

Kristensson, K., and Olsson, Y., 1971, Uptake of exogenous proteins in mouse olfactory cells, *Acta Neuropathol. (Berlin)* **19**:145–154.

Krnjević, K., 1974, Chemical nature of synaptic transmission in vertebrates, *Physiol. Rev.* **54**:419–540.

Kuck, J., 1970, Chemical constituents of the lens, *in Biochemistry of the Eye* (C. Graymore, ed.), pp. 183–260, Academic Press, New York.

Kuhar, M. J., 1973, Neurotransmitter uptake: A tool in identifying neurotransmitter-specific pathways, *Life Sciences* **13**:1623–1634.

Kuhar, M. J., Sethy, V. H., Roth, R. H., and Aghajanian, G. K., 1973, Choline: Selective accumulation by central cholinergic neurons, *J. Neurochem.* **20**:581–593.

Kurihara, K., and Koyama, N., 1972, High activity of adenylcyclase in olfactory and gustatory organs, *Biochem. Biophys. Res. Comm.* **48**:30–34.

Labhart, A., 1974, Clinical Endocrinology, p. 470, Springer–Verlag, New York.

Levine, J. D., and Wyman, R. J., 1973, Neurophysiology of flight in wild-type and a mutant *Drosophila, Proc. Nat. Acad. Sci. (U.S.A.)* **70**:1050–1054.

Loyber, I., Perassi, N., Palma, J., and Lecuona, F., 1972, Effects on serum proteins of stimulation of olfactory bulbs in spinal rats, *Exptl. Neurol.* **34**:535–542.

MacPherson, C., and Chinerman, J., 1971, Effects of intraventricular injections of brain iso-antibodies on learning, *Exptl. Neurol.* **31**:45–52.

Margolis, F. L., 1971, Search for S-100 protein variants in inbred strains and neurological mutants of the mouse, Third International Meeting of the International Society for Neurochemistry, Budapest, Hungary, Abstract 25.

Margolis, F. L., 1972a, Solid phase radioimmune assay using ^{3}H-labeled antigen for the mouse olfactory bulb specific protein, *Anal. Biochem.* **50**:602–607.

Margolis, F. L., 1972b, A brain protein unique to the olfactory bulb, *Proc. Nat. Acad. Sci.(U.S.)* **69**:1221–1224.

Margolis, F. L., 1974, Carnosine in the primary olfactory pathway, *Science* **184**:909–911.

Margolis, F. L., and Armona, D., 1974, Carnosine: Is it a neurotransmitter in the primary olfactory pathway? *Trans. Amer. Soc. Neurochem.* **5**:118.

Margolis, F. L., and Tarnoff, J. F., 1973, Site of biosynthesis of the mouse brain olfactory bulb protein, *J. Biol. Chem.* **248**: 451–455.

Margolis, F. L., Roberts, N., Ferriero, D., Feldman, J., 1974, Denervation in the primary olfactory pathway of mice: Biochemical and morphological effects, *Brain Res.* **81**:469–483.

Marshall, F. D., and Yockey, W. C., 1968, The effects of various agents on the levels of homocarnosine in rat brain, *Biochem. Pharmacol.* **17**:640–642.

Marshall, J., and Henkin, R., 1971, Olfactory activity, menstrual abnormalities and oocyte status, *Ann. Int. Med.* **75**:207–211.

McBride, W. J., Shank, R. P., Freeman, A. R., and Aprison, M. H., 1974, Levels of free amino acids in excitatory, inhibitory and sensory axons of the walking limbs of the lobster, *Life Sciences* **14**:1109–1120.

McMorris, F. A., Nelson, P., and Ruddle, F., 1973, Contributions of clonal systems to neurobiology, *Neurosci. Res. Prog. Bull.* **11**:414–536.

Meisami, E., and Manoochehri, S., 1974, Effect of destruction of olfactory mucosa on the activity of the Mg and Na–K–ATPase in the olfactory bulbs and cerebellum of developing rats, *Fed. Proc.* **33**:418.

Metcalf, J. F., 1973, Renewal and regeneration of olfactory neurons in adult mice, Society for Neuroscience, Third Annual Meeting, p. 158.

Moore, B. W., and McGregor, D., 1965, Chromatographic and electrophoretic fractionation of soluble proteins of brain and liver, *J. Biol. Chem.* **240**:1647–1653.

Moscona, A. A., 1971, Control mechanisms in hormonal induction of glutamine synthretase in the embryonic neural retina, *in Hormones in Development* (M. Hamburgh, and E. Barrington, eds.), pp. 169–189, Appleton-Century-Crofts, New York.

Moulton, D. G., 1974, Cell renewal in the olfactory epithelium of the mouse, *in* Conference on odors: Evaluation, utilization and control, *in Ann. New York Acad. Sci.* (W. S. Cain, ed.), **237**:52–61.

Moulton, D. G., and Beidler, L. M., 1967, Structure and function in the peripheral olfactory system, *Physiol. Rev.* **47**:1–52.

Moulton, D. G., and Fink, R. P., 1972, Cell proliferation in the olfactory epithelium, *in Olfaction and Taste IV* (D. Schneider, ed.), pp. 20–26, Wissenschaftliche Verlag, Stuttgart.

Nandy, K., and Bourne, G. H., 1966, Histochemical study of the oxidative enzymes in the olfactory bulb of the rat, *Acta Histochem.* **23**:86–93.

Neidle, A., Kandera, J., and Lajtha, A., 1973, The uptake of amino acids by the intact olfactory bulb of the mouse: A comparison with tissue slice preparations, *J. Neurochem.* **20**:1181–1193.

Neidle, A., and Kandera, J., 1974, A histidine derivative isolated from mouse olfactory bulb, *Trans. Amer. Soc. Neurochem.* **5**:169.

Neuhoff, V., Briel, G., and Maelicke, A., 1971, Characterization and micro-determination of histidine as its dansyl compounds, *Arzneim. Forschr.* **21**:104–107.

Nieuwenhuys, R., 1967, Comparative anatomy of olfactory tracts and centers, *Prog. Brain Research* **23**:1–64.

Nir, Y., Beemer, A., and Goldwasser, R. A., 1965, West Nile virus infection in mice following exposure to a viral aerosol, *Brit. J. Exptl. Pathol.* **46**:443–449.

Ortman, R., 1957, Uber succinodehydrogenase in olfactrischen system, *Acta Anat.* **30**:542–565.

Ostroy, S. E., and Pak, W. L., 1973, Protein differences associated with a phototransduction mutant of Drosophila, *Nature New Biology* **243**:120–121.

Ottoson, D., 1963, Some aspects of the function of the olfactory system, *Pharm. Revs.* **15**:1–42.

Perry, T. L., Berry, K., Hansen, S., Diamond, S., and Mok, C., 1971, Regional distribution of amino acids in human brain obtained at autopsy, *J. Neurochem.* **18**:513–519.

Perry, T. L., Hansen, S., Stedman, D., and Love, D., 1968, Homocarnosine in human cerebrospinal fluid: An age dependent phenomenon, *J. Neurochem.* **15**:1203–1206.

Phillips, D., and Martin, G., 1972, Heart rate conditioning of anosmic rats, *Physiol. and Behav.* **8**:33–36.

Pinching, A. J., and Powell, T. P. S., 1971, Ultrastructural features of transneuronal cell degeneration in the olfactory system, *J. Cell Sci.* **8**:253–287.

Pinching, A. J., and Powell, T. P. S., 1972*a*, A study of terminal degeneration in the olfactory bulb of the rat, *J. Cell Sci.* **10**:585–619.

Pinching, A. J., and Powell, T. P. S., 1972*b*, Experimental studies on the axons intrinsic to the glomerular layer of the olfactory bulb, *J. Cell Sci.* **10**:637–655.

Pohorecky, L., Larin, F., and Wurtman, R., 1969, Mechanism of changes in brain norepinephrine levels following olfactory bulb lesions, *Life Sciences* **8**:1309–1317.

Quereshi, Y., and Wood, T., 1960, The effect of carnosine on glycolysis, *Biochim. Biophys. Acta* **60**:190–192.

Ralph, P., Nakoinz, I., and Cohen, M., 1973, Antibody dependent cellular immunity in newborn mice, *Nature New Biology* **245**:157–158.

Rappoport, D., and Daginwala, H., 1968, Changes in nuclear RNA of brain induced by olfaction in catfish, *J. Neurochem.* **15**:991–1006.

Reiss, M., 1970, The hypothalamo-hypophyseal complex, *in Handbook of Neurochemistry* (A. Lajtha, ed.), pp. 463–505, Plenum Press, New York.

Roberts, P. J., Keen, P., and Mitchell, J. F., 1973, The distribution and axonal transport of free amino acids and related compounds in the dorsal sensory neuron of the rat, as determined by the dansyl reaction, *J. Neurochem.* **21**:199–209.

Rosenberg, A., 1960, The activation of carnosinase by divalent metal ions, *Biochim. Biophys. Acta* **45**:297–316.

Rush, R., Kindler, S., and Udenfriend, S., 1975, Solid phase radioimmunoassay on polystyrene beads and its application to dopamine-β-hydroxylase, *Clin. Chem.* **21**:148–150.

Sabin, A. B., and Olitsky, P. K., 1937, Influence of host factors on neuroninvasivness of vesicular stomatitis virus instilled in the nose. I. Effect of age on the invasion of the brain by virus instilled in the nose, *J. Exp. Med.* **66**:15–34.

Sachs, H., Pearson, D., Shainberg, A., Shin, S., Bryce, G., Malamed, S., and Mowles, T., 1974, Studies on the hypothalamo-neurohypophysial complex in organ culture, *in International Symposium on Recent Studies of Hypothalamic Function* (K. Lederis, ed.), S. Karger Press, Basel, pp. 50–66.

Schechter, P., Friedwald, W., Bronzert, D., Raff, M., and Henkin, R., 1972, Idiopathic hypogeusia: A description of the syndrome and a single blind study with zinc sulfate, *in Neurobiology of the Trace Metals Zinc and Copper* (C. C. Pfeiffer, ed.), pp. 125–140, Academic Press, New York.

Schneider, D. J., 1973, Proteins of the nervous system, Raven Press, New York.

Schrier, B. K., and Thompson, E. J., 1974, On the role of glial cells in the mammalian nervous system. Uptake, excretion and metabolism of putative neurotransmitters by cultured glial tumor cells, *J. Biol. Chem.* **249**:1769–1780.

Schriver, C. R., and Perry, T. L., 1972, Disorders of β-alanine and carnosine metabolism, *in Metabolic Basis of Inherited Disease* (J. Stanbury, J. Wyngaarden, and D. Fredrickson, eds.), pp. 476–490, McGraw-Hill, New York.

Scott, J., and Pfaffman, C., 1972, Characteristics of responses of lateral hypothalamic neurons to stimulation of the olfactory system, *Brain Research* **48**:251–264.

SenGupta, P., 1967, Olfactory receptor reaction to the lesion of the olfactory bulb, *in Olfaction and Taste II* (Hayashi, T., ed.), pp. 193–201, Pergamon Press, New York.

Severin, S. E., 1964, Problems concerned with the biological activity of naturally occurring imidazole compounds, in *Proceedings of the Sixth International Congress of Biochemistry*, pp. 45–61, New York.

Shaskan, E. G., and Snyder, S. H., 1970, Kinetics of serotonin accumulation into slices from rat brain: Relationship to catecholamine uptake, *J. Pharm. Exptl. Therap.* 175:404–418.

Shepherd, G. M., 1970, The olfactory bulb as a simple cortical system: Experimental analysis and functional implications, in *The Neurosciences* (F. O. Schmitt, ed.), Second Study Program, pp. 539–551, Rockefeller Press, New York.

Shepherd, G. M., 1972, Synaptic organization of the mammalian olfactory bulb, *Physiol. Revs.* 52:864–917.

Shooter, E. M., and Einstein, E. R., 1971, Proteins of the nervous system, *Ann. Rev. Biochem.* 40:635–652.

Siefert, K., and Ule, G., 1967, Die ultrastructure der riechschleimaut der neugeborenen und jugendlichen weissen maus, *Zeitschr. f. Zellforsch.* 76:147–169.

Sinclair, J. G., 1971, Reflections on the role of receptor systems for taste and smell, *Int. Rev. Neurobiol.* 14:159–171.

Singh, N., Grewal, M., and Austin, J., 1970, Familial anosmia, *Arch. Neurol.* 22:40–44.

Skaper, S. D., Das, S., Marshall, F. D., 1973, Some properties of a homocarnosine–carnosine synthetase isolated from rat brain, *J. Neurochem.* 21:1429–1445.

Snyder, S., Logan, W., Bennett, J. P., and Arregui, A., 1973, Amino acids as central nervous transmitters: Biochemical studies, *Neurosci. Res.* 5:131–157.

Snyder, S. H., Yamamura, H. I., Pert, C. B., Logan, W. J., and Bennett, J. P., 1973, Neuronal uptake of neurotransmitters and their precursors. Studies with "transmitter" amino acids and choline, in *New Concepts of Neurotransmitter Regulation* (A. Mandell, ed.), pp. 195–222, Plenum Press, New York.

Steiner, G., and Schonbaum, E., 1972, *Immunosympathectomy*, Elsevier Publishing Co., New York.

Stenesh, J. J., and Winnick, T., 1960, Carnosine–anserine synthetase from muscle, 4. Partial purification of the enzyme and further studies of β-alanyl peptide synthesis, *Biochim. Biophys. Acta* 77:575–581.

Steward, O., Lynch, G., and Cotman, C., 1973, Histochemical detection of orthograde degeneration in the central nervous system of the rat, *Brain Res.* 54:65–73.

Takagi, S. F., 1971, Degeneration and regeneration of the olfactory epithelium, in *Handbook of Sensory Physiology* (L. M. Beidler, ed.) IV–1, pp. 76–94, Springer–Verlag, Berlin.

Taylor, A., 1968, Autosomal trisomy syndromes: A detailed study of 27 cases of Edward's Syndrome and 27 cases of Patau's Syndrome, *J. Med. Genetics* 5:227–252.

Vallee, B. L., and Wacker, W. E. C., 1970, Metalloproteins, in *The Proteins* (H. Neurath, ed.), Vol. 5, p. 86, Academic Press, New York.

Van den Bergh, J. G., 1973, Effects of central and peripheral anosmia on reproduction of female mice, *Physiol. and Behavior.* 10:257–261.

Villet, R. H., 1974, Involvement of amino and sulphydryl groups in olfactory transduction in silk moths, *Nature* 248:707–708.

Wahlsten, D., 1972, Genetic experiments with animal learning: A critical review, *Behav. Biol.* 7:143–182.

Waley, S. G., 1966, Naturally occurring peptides, *Adv. Protein Chem.* 21:2–112.

Ward, S., 1973, Chemotaxis by the nematode *Caenorhabditis elegans*: Identification of attractants and analysis of the response by use of mutants. *Proc. Nat. Acad. Sci. (U.S.A.)* 70:817–821.

Waterman, R. E., and Meller, S. M., 1973, Nasal pit formation in the hamster: A transmission and scanning electron microscope study, *Devel. Biol.* 34:255–266.

Weiss, P., and Holland, Y., 1967, Neuronal dynamics and axonal flow. II. The olfactory nerve as a model test object, *Proc. Nat. Acad. Sci. (Washington)* **57**:258–264.

Whitten, W. K., 1956, The effect of removal of the olfactory bulb on the gonads of mice, *J. Endocrinol.* **14**:160–163.

Wilson, D., 1974, Protein synthesis and nerve cell specificity, *J. Neurochem.* **22**:465–467.

Winans, S., and Powers, J., 1974, Neonatal and two-stage olfactory bulbectomy: Effects on male hamster sexual behavior, *Behav. Biol.* **10**:461–471.

Woolf, C. M., 1972, Genetic analysis of geotactic and phototactic behavior in selected strains of *Drosophila pseudoobscura*, *Behav. Genet.* **2**:93–106.

Wurtman, R., 1970, Pineal hormones, *in Handbook of Neurochemistry* (A. Lajtha, ed.), pp. 451–461, Plenum Press, New York.

Yockey, W. C., and Marshall, F. D., 1969, Incorporation of [^{14}C] histidine into homocarnosine and carnosine of frog brain *in vivo* and *in vitro*, *Biochem. J.* **114**:585–588.

CHAPTER 7

APOMORPHINE AND ITS RELATION TO DOPAMINE IN THE NERVOUS SYSTEM

THEODORE L. SOURKES

Department of Psychiatry
McGill University
Montreal, Quebec, Canada

AND
SAMARTHJI LAL

Department of Psychiatry
McGill University
Montreal General Hospital and Queen Mary Veterans' Hospital
Montreal, Quebec, Canada

1. APOMORPHINE IN THE CONTEXT OF DOPAMINE FUNCTIONS

1.1. Introduction

Apomorphine was synthesized from morphine over one hundred years ago and was soon recognized as a powerful emetic agent. Its ability to induce

stereotypic behavior in experimental animals—a repetitious pattern involving chewing, licking, and gnawing movements—was noted in the earliest
pharmacotoxicological research with the alkaloid (Harnack, 1874). Whereas
its emetic activity brought apomorphine into therapeutics as one of the
earliest synthetic medicinal agents, until recently little attention was paid to
its stereotypic properties with the exception of the work of Morita (1915) and
Amsler (1923). However, a number of developments have brought it into
focus. In 1948, Dordoni in Italy found that apomorphine decreased decerebrate rigidity in dogs. Similar observations led Schwab *et al.* (1951) to use
subemetic doses of apomorphine in patients with Parkinson's disease, a
condition in which rigidity is one of the cardinal symptoms. Improvement in
rigidity and tremor was definite but transient. Further investigators confirmed these findings (Struppler and von Uexküll, 1953; von Uexküll, 1953).
However, the requirements for parenteral administration, the short duration
of action of apomorphine, and the problem of its stability limited therapeutic application; thus interest quickly waned. Schwab and his associates
(1951) did describe an oral mixture containing apomorphine which was
stable and which produced improvement, but it was less effective than
injected apomorphine. In 1970, the anti-Parkinsonian effect was restudied by
Cotzias and his colleagues.

The similarity of the stereotyped behavior induced by apomorphine to
that seen with amphetamine was another impressive factor, playing a role at
a time when the latter drug was attaining considerable prominence through
its nonmedical and socially widespread use. A further development that has
brought renewed interest in apomorphine as a research tool is the work on
dopamine that led to the introduction of the L-dopa treatment for Parkinson's
disease. The structures of apomorphine, amphetamine, and dopamine are
shown in Figure 1.

Dopamine had been synthesized early in this century at the time that
epinephrine and norepinephrine were first prepared, and dopa (3,4-di-
hydroxyphenylalanine) was synthesized a few years later. This amino acid
was also isolated from *Vicia faba* by Markus Guggenheim, who, many years
later, recalled that after consuming a large sample of the compound he had
experienced violent vomiting (Sourkes, 1972c). In Borison and Wang's
review of mechanisms of emesis (Borison and Wang, 1953), dopa is not listed
among the drugs capable of stimulating the trigger zone of the emetic center
in the medulla oblongata. This is now considered a significant action of dopa,
the precursor of dopamine. Dopamine is formed from dopa by enzymic
decarboxylation; if this step is prevented by giving animals a suitable
decarboxylase inhibitor, dopa does not evoke vomiting.

Since apomorphine is believed to act by mimicking a physiological
action of dopamine at certain receptor sites in the CNS, it is useful to ex-

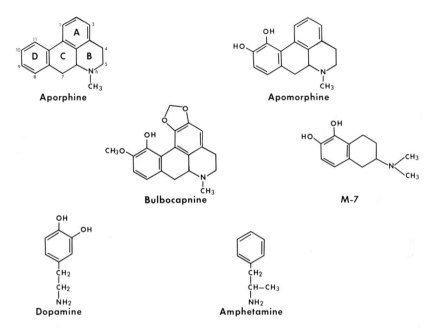

FIGURE 1. Structure of aporphine, apomorphine, and some other compounds referred to in the text.

amine its chemical, biochemical, and pharmacological properties from the perspective of its newly appreciated significance as a prototypic dopamine-receptor agonist. There are dopamine-receptor sites in the body elsewhere than near the emetic center, and these are being carefully evaluated for their responsiveness to apomorphine. Because of this intimate association, it is necessary to characterize the dopamine-containing neural systems and to describe briefly what is known of their specific characteristics.

1.2. Dopamine-Containing Neural Systems

1.2.1. Neurochemical Roles of Dopamine

Dopamine (3-hydroxytryamine; 3,4-dihydroxyphenylethylamine) was identified in the early 1950s as a normal constituent of urine and some tissues; this finding justified the earlier claims that the body makes use of the compound as an intermediary in the biosynthesis of epinephrine and norepinephrine. However, after 1957, when it was discovered that most of the dopamine in the brain is localized in a specific region—the striatum—that contains very little norepinephrine or dopamine-β-hydroxylase, it became clear that dopamine must have some other role than merely serving as a metabolic precursor. Its function was then assumed to be related to those of the striatum. The striatum consists of the caudate nucleus and putamen, two of the major structures among the so-called basal ganglia of the brain. These large, anatomically distinct masses of gray matter lying at the base of the brain have many connections between one another, as well as to and from other regions of the brain (Poirier and Sourkes, 1972; Sourkes *et al.*, 1975). Among the bodily functions that they regulate are the tone and the posture of the limbs. These are achieved in conjunction with the extrapyramidal, or striopallidal, system (Poirier and Sourkes, 1972; Sourkes *et al.*, 1975), that is to say, structures apart from the cerebral cortex that project to the spinal cord.

Diseases of the basal ganglia include Parkinson's disease, Huntington's chorea, Wilson's disease (hepatolenticular degeneration), kernicterus, and some others (Sourkes, 1972*a*; Sourkes *et al.*, 1975). We now know that dopamine-containing fibers that course from the substantia nigra, a structure possessing a distinctive melanin pigment, to the striatum are degenerate in Parkinson's disease. In drug-induced Parkinsonism, occurring as a side effect of treatment with certain major tranquilizers, the fibers are intact but the dopamine they release is blocked from acting by the neuroleptic drug. In the natural disease, the striatum is deficient in dopamine, although ordinarily it is exceedingly rich in this substance. Because of this fact, Parkinson's disease has been listed as one of several types of "dopamine-deficiency" diseases (Hornykiewicz, 1972).

One can easily reproduce certain features of Parkinson's disease in experimental animals by surgical intervention, i.e., by interrupting the nigrostriatal fibers with a stereotaxically placed brain lesion. In the monkey, it is feasible to interfere with these fibers and little else. In the rat, one cuts the medial forebrain bundle, a major trunk line in which the dopamine-containing fibers run for a distance. In the first 12–24 hr after axotomy, there is an increase in their dopamine content because of physiological inactivity and failure to release the material that is continuing to be synthesized. Thereafter, degenerative processes set in and the neuronal contents disappear.

Normally, dopamine is released at synapses in the striatum and certain other brain centers. This release is regulated and at least two mechanisms have been postulated for it. The first would act through a postsynaptic receptor site and would involve another neuronal pathway and at least one other transmitter. This system would "report back" to the substantia nigra at the level of the cell bodies of the nigrostriatal fibers. The other mechanism would operate locally through the nerve endings, or varicosities (swellings along the length of the fine nonmyelinated terminations that lend them a "beaded" appearance), from which the dopamine is released. In the second instance, it is postulated that dopamine, once in the synaptic space, exerts a back-up "transsynaptic" action on a receptor site on the external membrane of the presynaptic termination; this action is transmitted in some manner all the way through the nerve ending, with the net result of slowing down synthesis of the transmitter in the fiber (Andén et al., 1969). At the present time, the second mechanism is more favored than is the neuronal feedback hypothesis. The problem has important practical consequences, for if function is to be influenced in these regions by drugs or other means, one must know how regulation is maintained there.

There are other dopamine-containing tracts in the brain (Dresse, 1972; Ungerstedt, 1973). One of these, in the lowest part of the brain, seems to receive impulses from the body which funnel into the *area postrema* (Borison and Wang, 1953). This area is exquisitely sensitive to emetic agents like apomorphine, which act in the chemoreceptor ("trigger") zone that projects short fibers to the emetic center in the medulla oblongata. The chemoreceptor zone is notably one of the few areas of the brain that is relatively unprotected by a blood–brain barrier.

Barnett has observed a hypotensive effect of apomorphine in anesthetized cats which is antagonized by haloperidol, and he postulates that the lowering of blood pressure by this alkaloid mimics a midbrain dopaminergic system normally functioning through the vasomotor centers (Barnett and Fiore, 1971). The vasodilatory effect is probably responsible for the hypothermia caused by apomorphine (Schelkunov and Stabrovskii, 1971; Barnett et al., 1972).

Dopamine fibers have been identified in the olfactory tract (Dahlström and Fuxe, 1964b; Ungerstedt, 1971a, 1973). This fact suggests that dopamine may ultimately be concerned with the defensive and food-gathering activities of lower animals and therefore would be of interest in ethological studies. There is some clinical evidence that dopamine is involved in olfaction in humans also (Constantinidis and De Ajuriaguerra, 1970), but this sensory modality has been little explored.

Dopamine is found in the retina, from which it is released by the action of light on that tissue (Kramer, 1971; Kramer et al., 1971). Thus, the compound may play some role in the mediation of at least two of the special senses (cf. Crow and Arbuthnott, 1972).

There are dopamine-containing neurons in the hypothalamus—in the median eminence and the infundibulum—and they innervate neuroendocrine cells that secrete releasing factors (Dahlström and Fuxe, 1964a; Dresse, 1972; Ungerstedt, 1971a). Dopamine-containing neurons of this kind would transmit signals received from the preoptic region of the brain to the RF (releasing factor)-secreting fibers.

Recently dopamine has been tentatively recognized as a mediator in the superior cervical sympathetic ganglion, where it is said to stimulate adenyl cyclase. In fact, apomorphine is a very potent inhibitor of cerebral phospho-diesterase, much more effective than theophylline (Nahorski *et al.*, 1973). This inhibition may be responsible for increasing the formation of adenosine 3′,5′-monophosphate during synaptic activity (Kebabian and Greengard, 1971; Clement-Cormier *et al.*, 1974).

Finally, dopamine-containing fibers have been identified in the cerebral cortex by means of the histofluorescence technique (Thierry *et al.*, 1973*a,b*; Hökfelt *et al.*, 1974*a,b*). Naturally, great interest is attached to this finding, for it may well associate an action of dopamine with synaptic function at the highest levels of integration in the CNS. Furthermore, because of the development of major tranquilizing drugs whose action is more prominent on biological actions of dopamine than those of other monoamines, there is the real possibility that cortical dopamine plays a role in those mental processes that go awry in the major psychoses.

1.2.2. *Model of the Dopaminergic Terminal and Its Synaptic Connections*

It is always useful in dealing with a complex subject to have some kind of model from which to work. Knowledge of synaptic structure, biochemistry, and mechanisms is growing (Van Heyningen, 1959; DeRobertis, 1967; Cotman and Taylor, 1972), especially in regard to cholinergic synapses (DeRobertis, 1971), but a clearer picture is emerging also about events at adrenergic and dopaminergic synapses (Sourkes, 1973). For synaptic transmission involving dopamine, the model must include a cell body that is protected by a membrane with some predilection for uptake and transport of tyrosine, the precursor of the catecholamines. In addition, it must contain the enzymes tyrosine hydroxylase (EC 1.14.3a) and dopa decarboxylase (EC 4.1.1.26), along with components responsible for axonal transport of the enzymes, the products of their action, and the vesicular bodies in which the amine is stored at the peripheral endings of the fiber. The varicosities that stud these very fine, nonmyelinated terminations along their length contain the mass of monoamine storage vesicles. Release of the amine through exocytosis (Douglas, 1968) into the space external to the terminal makes the amine available for diffusion, or transport by some other means, through a short distance to the dendrites or other portions of an adjacent neuron. This process occurs when a physiological stimulus fires the dopamine fiber so that the postsynaptic site, sometimes visualized in electron micrography as a thickening or "plate" on the dendrite, is affected in a manner that leads to a change in excitability of that postsynaptic fiber. Some of the features of dopaminergic systems are presented in an idealized version in Figure 2.

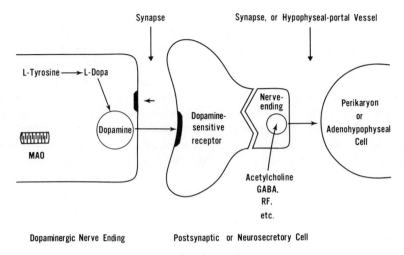

FIGURE 2. Schematic model of dopaminergic systems in the CNS.

Once dopamine has been released into the synaptic cleft it may suffer different fates. Some may be carried away in the capillaries and will undergo metabolism peripherally, primarily in the liver. Another portion may be metabolized locally through O-methylation, deamination, and further oxidation. The terminal metabolite in this process is HVA (homovanillic acid). HVA accumulates locally to a certain extent, the amount apparently depending upon the species, but is normally removed by a probenecid-sensitive transport mechanism. If dopamine is released within the nerve ending, as through leakage from vesicular stores or through the action of a drug like reserpine, it is attacked by monoamine oxidase (MAO; EC 1.4.3.4), an enzyme in the external membrane of the mitochondria; the product is then further oxidized through the action of aldehyde dehydrogenase (EC 1.2.1.3) so that DOPAC (3,4-dihydroxyphenylacetic acid) is formed. Since catechol O-methyl transferase (COMT; EC 2.1.1.6) is not found in these monoamine-containing neurons, DOPAC is converted to HVA only after it crosses the membrane of the neuronal termination.

The enzymes of biosynthesis are located intraneuronally, for they soon disappear (4–10 days) from the striatum when the nerve fibers are interrupted by a lesion that initiates anterograde degeneration. The more fibers damaged by the imposed lesion, the greater will be the cell loss in the substantia nigra.

The sketch of the central dopaminergic synapse in Figure 2 takes into account the onward connections of the system governed by dopamine release. If the central structure depicted releases ACh, GABA, or another transmitter substance, the last cell in the scheme is to be regarded as a neuron; it may be distant from the first one or may even synapse with it to provide a regulatory feedback. On the other hand, if dopamine causes the secretion of a RF (releasing factor) in the hypothalamus, the structure in the center of Figure 2 is to be looked upon as a neuroendocrine cell whose product, the RF, will be carried in the specialized and highly localized hypothalamo–hypophyseal portal system to the anterior pituitary gland, where the corresponding hormone will be secreted. Some neuroendocrine cells secrete factors that ultimately inhibit the release of an adenohypophyseal hormone, and the RIF (release-inhibiting factor) will also be carried in the localized portal circulatory system from the hypothalamus where it is produced.

1.2.3. Behavioral Effects of Dopamine

Dopamine has certain behavioral effects of interest to the experimenter and the clinician. First of all, in Parkinson's disease the deficiency of cerebral dopamine results in tremor and rigidity of the limbs, as well as akinesia (lack of volitional movement). These effects are overcome by use of L-dopa, to one extent or another. An akinetic state can be produced in monkeys if they are given very large doses of α-methyltyrosine, of the order of 1.5–2.0 g over a period of many hours. This drug effectively, but gradually, causes the cessation of catecholamine synthesis through its inhibitory action on tyrosine hydroxylase. Of course, other actions may be involved. The animals fall into a retarded, though waking, state which resembles catatonia (Bédard et al., 1970; Larochelle et al., 1971). This state can be temporarily but repeatedly reversed by giving the animal L-dopa, which is converted to dopamine and probably some norepinephrine in the brain. Catecholamine formation bypasses the inhibited enzyme in this way, but the effect of the amino acid is brief, and that of α-methyltyrosine long-lasting. The cataleptic state probably results from overwhelming loss of striatal stores of dopamine bilaterally, stemming from massive blockade of its synthesis by α-methyltyrosine. A reduction in dopaminergic activity might relieve inhibition of cholinergic fibers that pass from striatum to cerebral cortex (Zetler and Thörner, 1973). Experimental catatonia and catalepsy are general reaction patterns of the CNS (De Jong, 1945) brought about by many different drugs and treatments; they are related to certain psychiatric phenomena and may even serve as a model of Parkinsonian akinesia, which also responds to L-dopa. The production of catalepsy with α-methyltyrosine in a higher mammal is the first example of (a) its induction by a substance whose biochemical mode of action is clearly defined, and (b) its reversal by another substance that specifically overcomes the induced biochemical deficiency.

There are a number of drugs that produce tremor of the limbs in experimental animals, but only a few reproduce the typical Parkinsonian rhythm; these drugs mainly are neuroleptics, or major tranquilizers, and cholinergic agents. Among the former, reserpine achieves the effect by causing a depletion of cerebral dopamine (among other monoamines). The phenothiazines, haloperidol and pimozide, apparently block the action of dopamine at important postsynaptic receptor sites so that there is effective interference with the action of fibers governed by dopamine even though the amount of dopamine present in the terminals is more or less normal.

Experimental tremor has been produced in monkeys following the introduction of certain types of lesions in the ventromedial tegmentum. Analysis of the histopathological changes produced has demonstrated that at least two systems are involved (Sourkes *et al.*, 1975): the nigrostriatal dopaminergic pathway and the rubro(small-celled)-olivo-cerebellorubral loop. Interruption of either alone does not result in the appearance of postural tremor, but if both are interrupted tremor results. Two drugs are of considerable experimental significance here. α-Methyltyrosine, in a dose of 150–250 mg/kg (less than required for the production of catalepsy), administered to a monkey with a lesion of the loop through the red nucleus and other structures, causes postural tremor of the limbs; the tremor comes on gradually, apparently as catecholamine contents decline and the nigrostriatal tract becomes inoperative. On the other hand, if only the nigrostriatal tract is interrupted, tremor can be induced by giving the animals harmaline or harmine (2–3 mg/kg); these β-carbolines seem to interfere with the function of the rubro-olivo-cerebellorubral loop, perhaps at the level of the olivary nucleus (Lamarre and Puil, 1974).

In addition to specific surgical lesions as a means of interfering with the action of nigrostriatal tract, some investigators have produced electrolytic lesions in the caudate nucleus or have used a suction device to remove parts of that structure. In either case, the lesion is nonspecific in that both pre- and postsynaptic organization may be damaged, and usually there is no histological control. Nevertheless, these techniques have provided some useful behavioral models for testing drug action, such as the "head-turning" test.

The compound 2,4,5-trihydroxyphenethylamine ("6-hydroxydopamine") has been widely studied for its ability to damage dopaminergic fibers (Malmfors and Thoenen, 1971). It seems to be taken up into the nerve endings where it undergoes oxidation, with the production of hydrogen peroxide, the deleterious agent. Destruction of the nigrostriatal fibers by any means is thought to result eventually in a supersensitivity of the intact postsynaptic receptors to dopamine (Schoenfeld and Uretsky, 1972; Ungerstedt, 1973).

A century ago the pharmacologist Harnack (1874) tested apomorphine in rabbits, a species that does not respond to the drug by vomiting. Soon after the first injection, the animals began to chew, lick, and bite on the cage wire in a repetitive, stereotyped manner. More recently it has been claimed that this behavioral stereotypy is evoked by intracerebral injection of apomorphine or dopamine into the region of the striatum (Smelik and Ernst, 1966; Ernst and Smelik, 1966). The behavioral pattern, or a very similar one, can also be evoked with amphetamine. The action of amphetamine, however, appears to be presynaptic. The "neurological substrate" for this behavior has been regarded first of all as the striatum (or nigrostriatal tract) (Amsler, 1923; Ernst, 1965; Smelik and Ernst, 1966). However, this interpretation has been challenged by the work of Costall *et al.* (1972) and McKenzie (1972); the latter author (McKenzie, 1972; McKenzie *et al.*, 1973) regards the tuberculum olfactorium and perhaps other structures as also being important.

Other behavioral effects of dopamine have been conjectured. For example, the excited state produced in cats by morphine ("mania") has been attributed to the release of dopamine on receptors of neurons involved in the manic response (Dhasmana *et al.*, 1972). However, the role of dopamine in these other phenomena, if any, must still be clarified by additional experiments. Apomorphine-induced aggression in rats has been attributed to enhanced stimulation of dopamine-sensitive receptors (McKenzie, 1971). Pigeons given apomorphine exhibit stereotyped pecking activity (Burkman, 1960).

1.2.4. *Dopamine Receptors: Agonists and Antagonists*

This subject has been reviewed from the neuropharmacological aspect by several authors (Hornykiewicz, 1971; Woodruff, 1971; Sourkes, 1973). Apomorphine is of special interest in this connection because of its dopamine-like action at a number of receptor sites; it may be regarded as the model agonist in such cases, at least for striatal receptors (Ernst, 1965; Smelik and Ernst, 1966; Andén *et al.*, 1967; Roos, 1969; Ungerstedt *et al.*, 1969; Etevenon *et al.*, 1970; Boissier *et al.*, 1971; Costall and Naylor, 1973), although McKenzie (1974) dissents from this view. The drug as prepared from morphine is levorotatory; its enantiomer is essentially devoid of biological activity (Neumeyer *et al.*, 1973a; Saari *et al.*, 1973). Other substances besides apomorphine are known to stimulate one or more types of dopamine receptor (Borison and Wang, 1953). Among the aporphines, apocodeine (10-*O*-methylapomorphine; 11-hydroxy-10-methoxyaporphine) is less active than apomorphine on the nigrostriatal system (Lal *et al.*, 1972a). The nigrostriatal receptor action has been assessed in several ways: by induction of stereotyped behavior, by antagonism of reserpine sedation, by reduction of the content of HVA in the striatum, and head- and body-turning in animals with striatal lesions. In some of these tests, 10,11-methylenedioxyaporphine is also less active than apomorphine (Lal et al., 1972a); this compound and apocodeine probably act only after they have been dealkylated to apomorphine. Isoapocodeine (10-hydroxy-11-methoxyaporphine) (Cannon et al., 1972), 10,11-dimethoxyaporphine (Lal et al., 1972a; Neumeyer et al., 1973a; Saari et al., 1973), (−)morphothebaine (2,11-dihydroxy-10-methoxyaporphine), 2,10,11-trihydroxyaporphine, 1,2,10,11-tetrahydroxyaporphine, 8,9-dibromo-10,11-dihydroxyaporphine, and the 10,11-quinone of Δ_{6a}-apomorphine (Lal et al., 1972a) are all pharmacologically inactive. The auto-oxidation products of apomorphine are also inert (Kaul and Brochmann-Hanssen, 1961; Burkman, 1963a).

Aporphine itself is inactive in inducing stereotyped behavior in rats and is only one-tenth as active as apomorphine in exerting a vasodepressor effect in the urethanized rabbit (Pinder et al., 1971).

Granchelli and his colleagues (Granchelli et al., 1971) have tested some new aporphines in rats bearing a unilateral lesion of the caudate nucleus. Apomorphine causes the animals to turn toward the intact side. 7-Hydroxy- and 11-hydroxyaporphine act similarly but more weakly. Ginos et al. (1972) claim that 10,11-diacetoxyaporphine, a derivative with an emetic effect (Tiffeneau and Porcher, 1915), is active in this test in mice. Isoapomorphine (9,10-dihydroxyaporphine), 1,2-dihydroxyaporphine, and 1,2,9,10-tetra-hydroxyaporphine all have weak biological activity (Neumeyer et al., 1973b).

TABLE 1. Effect of N-Substitution on Stereotyped Behavior (SB), Emesis and Straub Tail Response[a]

N-Substituent	Compound	SB (mouse)	SB (pigeon)	Emesis (pigeon)	Emesis (dog)	Straub tail (mouse)
CH$_3$	Apomorphine	1.0	1.0	±	1.0	+[b]
H	Norapomorphine	0.04	−	+ +	0.01	+
C$_2$H$_5$	N-Ethylnorapomorphine	3.25	2.95	±	3.0	+
nC$_3$H$_7$	N-n-propylnorapomorphine	1.14	1.28	±	1.20	+
CH$_2$CH=CH$_2$	N-Allylnorapomorphine	0.27	0.48	±	0.75	+
C≡CH	N-Propargylnorapomorphine	−	−	±	−	−
CH$_2$—◁	N-Cyclopropylmethyl norapomorphine	0.02	0.06	±	−	+
CH$_2$C$_6$H$_5$	N-Benzylnorapomorphine	−	−	±	−	−
CH$_2$CH$_2$C$_6$H$_5$	N-Phenethylnorapomorphine	−	−	±	−	−

[a] Based on data of Koch et al. (1968); Hensiak et al. (1965). Results expressed as potency relative to apomorphine: − effect absent, + effect present, ± mild effect, + + marked effect.
[b] Shemano and Wendel (1964).

By extending the length of the nitrogen substituent from methyl group in apomorphine to a *n*-propyl group, Neumeyer *et al.* (1973*a*) were able to obtain an aporphine with increased biological activity. The activities of this and other *N*-substituted noraporphines are shown in Table 1. Norapomorphine has approximately the same convulsive and lethal activity as apomorphine in mice, but it has extremely low potency in evoking the gnawing syndrome in that species or emesis in the dog (Koch *et al.*, 1968).

Dopa and *m*-tyrosine are agonists after their decarboxylation to dopamine and *m*-tyramine (3-hydroxyphenethylamine), respectively. α-Methyl-*m*-tyrosine may be in the same category (Dorris and Shore, 1971; 1974).

Certain ergot alkaloids, such as ergocornine, 2-bromo-α-ergocryptine, and agroclavine, stimulate dopamine receptors.

Emetine and cephaeline (desmethylemetine), ipecac alkaloids that are emetic by central action, are devoid of action on the nigrostriatal tract (Lal *et al.*, 1972*a*).

Some novel synthetic compounds are now available as dopamine receptor stimulants. Among them are Trivastal (Corrodi *et al.*, 1971; 1972) and NBTI (Menon *et al.*, 1972). The former, also known as Pirebedil and ET-495, is 1-(2″-pyrimidyl)-4-piperonyl piperazine. NBTI is 2-(*p*-nitrobenzylthio)-imidazoline (3H)·HCl.

The *N*-methyl derivative of dopamine, epinine, has been tested in several biological systems. It is active on dopamine receptors in the renal vascular bed (Goldberg *et al.*, 1968; Bell and Lang, 1973), a locus where apomorphine has weaker activity, and in the nervous system of *Helix* (Woodruff and Walker, 1969), where apomorphine is inactive (Pinder *et al.*, 1972). Dextrorotatory apomorphine has no effect on renal hemodynamics (Saari *et al.*, 1972).

Dopamine activates the adenyl cyclase of rat erythrocytes (Sheppard and Burghardt, 1971), caudate nucleus (Garelis and Neff, 1974), nucleus accumbens, and tuberculum olfactorium (Horn *et al.*, 1974). The action on the red cell enzyme, matched by epinine, has led Sheppard and Burghardt (1971) to postulate the presence of a dopamine receptor on the erythrocyte membrane. Although apomorphine is inactive in this test system, it acts like dopamine in the caudate nucleus (Kebabian *et al.*, 1972).

In regard to dopamine-receptor antagonism, the neuroleptics (other than reserpine and its congeners) generally possess this activity (van Rossum, 1966; York, 1972). Various phenothiazines, haloperidol, and other compounds have been used effectively. Some of these substances block other types of receptor as well, but perphenazine, haloperidol, pimozide, and spiroperidol among the synthetic compounds seem to be relatively specific in antagonizing dopaminergic actions, including those of apomorphine (Nielsen and Lyon, 1973; Cools, 1971; Rotrosen *et al.*, 1972*a*).

Bulbocapnine, a naturally occurring alkaloid, and the phenethylamine derivatives O-methyltyrosine and dimethyldopamine are also antagonists (Ernst, 1965; Tseng et al., 1973). The structure of bulbocapnine is shown in Figure 1; the orientation of its 6a-carbon atom places it in the S-series.

Apomorphine is not an agonist in all dopamine-mediated systems. It opposes the action of dopamine in causing contraction of rat vas deferens and rabbit spleen preparations (Ferrini and Miragoli, 1972) and at high doses prevents the action of dopamine on the renal vascular bed (Goldberg et al., 1968). Moreover, in the spinal cord, which lacks dopaminergic fibers, the action of apomorphine, a direct one, is not identical with that of dopamine (Schlosser et al., 1972).

2. CHEMISTRY OF APOMORPHINE

2.1. Synthesis

(−)-Apomorphine is prepared from morphine by hydrolysis with strong mineral acids; this method has been used for over 100 years. The absolute stereochemistry of this isomer is designated as 6aR. The dextrorotatory isomer (6aS) has been synthesized (Saari et al., 1973) by resolution of (±)-10, 11-dimethoxyaporphine, a compound that was made almost 50 years ago by Späth and Hromatka (1929).

Racemic apomorphine has now been obtained by total synthesis (Neumeyer et al., 1970; 1973a).

2.2. Phenolic Oxidative Coupling

Recently there has been much interest in whether the suggestion of Barton and Cohen (1957), regarding the possible role of a dienone–phenol type of rearrangement in the conversion of benzyl–tetrahydroisoquinolines to aporphines in plants, might also be applicable to the animal organism (Sourkes, 1971). The first model substrate considered for such a reaction has been tetrahydropapaveroline (norlaudanosoline), an alkaloid that can be formed from dopamine, as shown in Figure 3, through the action of mono-amine oxidase of animal tissues and nonenzymic coupling (Holtz et al., 1964). This compound would give rise to the positional isomers 1,2,9,10- and 1,2,10,11-tetrahydroxynoraporphine (Figure 3).

The search for additional substrates of the tetrahydropapaveroline type was suggested by Sourkes (1970; 1971) in connection with the use of large

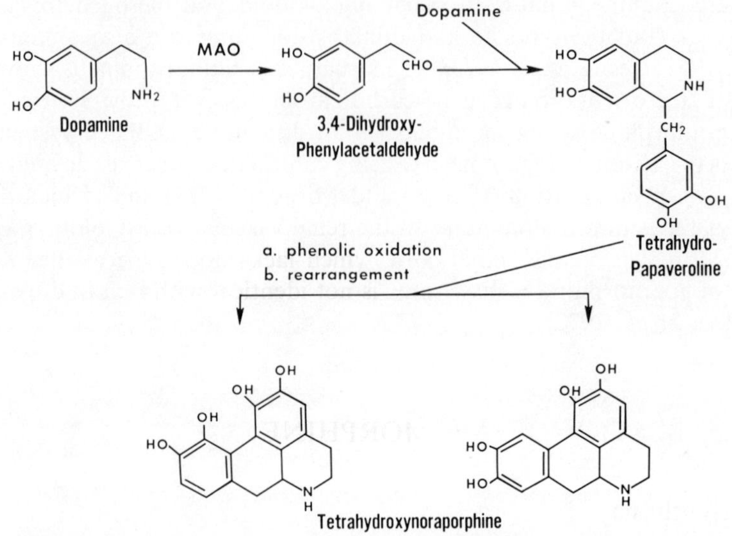

FIGURE 3. Hypothetical formation of noraporphines from dopamine and tetrahydropapaveroline.

doses of L-dopa in the treatment of Parkinson's disease. The argument runs that there is the possibility of the conversion of L-dopa not only to dopamine but also to significant amounts of other metabolites which would ordinarily not be encountered. Amine, aldehyde, and keto derivatives could enter into the formation of Schiff's bases with appropriate compounds, and these might then be converted to pharmacologically active products (Sourkes, 1970). There have been several developments since this suggestion was made. Sandler and his colleagues (1973) have reported the identification, in significant concentrations, of tetrahydropapaveroline and salsolinol (the tetrahydroisoquinoline, or THIQ, formed by condensation of dopamine with acetaldehyde), in the urine of patients with Parkinson's disease during oral treatment with L-dopa. Thus, the postulated condensations occur under physiological conditions and yield at least one substrate for noraporphine formation.

The condensation of catecholamines with acetaldehyde, the first product of metabolism of ethanol, to yield THIQs or further products, has been proposed by several groups as a factor in the genesis of the alcohol-dependent state (Davis and Walsh, 1970; Cohen and Collins, 1970; Sprince et al., 1972). In fact, tetrahydropapaveroline has been identified in brain of rats given dopa combined with ethanol (Turner et al., 1974).

The possibility that aporphines might be formed through enzymic action from benzyl–THIQs requires systematic study of the structural requirements in substrates, and identification of products. Such work is now under way in the laboratories of Brossi, Teitel, and others. For example, the THIQ (1 *R*)-(−)-laudanosoline methiodide can be made to undergo oxidative coupling under the influence of peroxidase, with formation of an aporphine methiodide having the same absolute configuration as the reactant (Brossi *et al.*, 1973). The procedure is an efficient one for preparation of certain types of alkaloids and is being investigated now on a broad scale (Teitel *et al.*, 1974).

   The earlier chemistry of apomorphine and related compounds has been reviewed in several monographs (Manske, 1954; Shamma and Slusarchyk, 1964; Shamma, 1967; Shamma and Hillman, 1969). Over 70 naturally occurring aporphine alkaloids have now been isolated and many of them have been structurally characterized.

2.3. Conformational Relation to Dopamine

   Investigators have sought to identify that portion of the apomorphine molecule responsible for its dopaminelike action on mammalian receptors. The proposal that different receptors are affected by dopamine and apomorphine, respectively, has been rejected recently (Rekker *et al.*, 1972). Moreover, the view of Kier and Truitt (1970), derived from calculations based on molecular orbital theory that the nonhydroxylated ring of apomorphine provides the proper fit, is not now accepted. Pinder has theorized that it is the dihydroxytetrahydroaminonaphthalene moiety of the molecule that accounts for its activity (Pinder *et al.*, 1971; 1972), and evidence for this has been brought forward by Cannon (1974). Cannon has synthesized the proposed pharmacophore and has shown it to be a potent centrally acting emetic, which also stimulates gnawing behavior in the mouse. The substance, M-7, is racemic 5,6-dihydroxy-2-dimethylaminotetralin (Figure 1). In both M-7 and apomorphine, interatomic distances are similar to those in dopamine. Cannon states that "the ring structure of apomorphine cannot be disrupted without destroying dopaminelike effects. ... The precise arrangement of oxygen atoms in apomorphine represents not just the optimum, but about the only arrangement which will permit proper *in vivo* interaction with one type of dopamine receptors."

2.4. Properties of Apomorphine

   Apomorphine hydrochloride is a pharmacopoeial drug in Great Britain, U.S.S.R., and other countries. In the United States it falls within the regulations concerned with narcotics. The National Formulary contains a monograph on the drug. Apomorphine hydrochloride forms minute, glistening, colorless crystals which readily undergo autooxidation, especially under alkaline conditions, to yield greenish material. However, even a deeply pigmented solution may still contain as much as 98% of the original apomorphine (Burkman, 1963b). The oxidation product in more concentrated solutions is insoluble in the alkaline aqueous medium, but it can be dissolved with difficulty in diethyl ether to yield a purple solution; chloroform solutions are blue and those in 95% ethanol are green. Solutions of apomorphine that are oxidized by iodine give an emerald-green product; on extraction with ether a deep ruby-red solution results. Kaul and Brochmann-Hanssen (1961) think that during autooxidation the piperidine ring is opened, with loss of the nitrogen.

Sensitive fluorometric methods have been developed for measuring apomorphine (Van Tyle and Burkman, 1971; Smith *et al.*, 1973).

3. BIOCHEMISTRY OF APOMORPHINE

3.1. Metabolism

Apomorphine is rapidly absorbed from the subcutaneous tissues and mucous membranes. This leads quickly to nausea, salivation, and vomiting in susceptible species. Recent recognition of the more versatile actions of apomorphine in the CNS has generated studies of its pharmacokinetics and metabolism. Thus, it has been estimated that within 8 min of injecting apomorphine intraperitoneally in mice, only one-half the administered dose can be detected in the body and excreta as unchanged apomorphine (Kaul and Conway, 1971). The half-life of apomorphine in the brain is of the same order, 7.6 min (Van Tyle and Burkman, 1971). The rate of degradation of apomorphine is not accelerated in mice by prior administration of substances such as phenobarbital or SKF-525A that stimulate the activity of drug-metabolizing microsomal enzymes, but it is diminished by estradiol. Mice that have already received apomorphine metabolize a further dose of the alkaloid at a greater rate (Kaul and Conway, 1971). Thus, apomorphine favors its own metabolism, but neither the mode of induction of metabolizing enzymes nor which enzymes are increased under the influence of apomorphine is known.

In mice receiving apomorphine, the peak level of the drug in the brain is reached in less than 1 min. At that time, 3% of the dose is present in that organ. Since the effective content of apomorphine in the brain for causing the gnawing syndrome in 50% of a group of mice is about 0.3 μg/g of brain

(Van Tyle and Burkman, 1972), it may be calculated that this level would be obtained in 55 to 60 min with a dose of 2 mg/kg, and in 70–75 min with a dose five times as great. These times correspond fairly well to the duration of stereotyped behavior.

Two major pathways of metabolism have been noted for apomorphine, viz., conjugation with glucuronic acid and O-methylation. Conjugates of apomorphine, at first called "bound" apomorphine (Kaul et al., 1961a), have been separated from the urine of mice, rats, rabbits, and horses, and they have been characterized as a mixture of the 10- and 11-O-monoglucuronides. The former predominates in a ratio of 7:3 (Kaul et al., 1961b; Kaul and Conway, 1971), indicating the less hindered character of the 10-position. It is not known if the conjugates are biologically active but, if they are at all, the activity must be considerably less than that of apomorphine. This fact is deduced from experiments with rats given acetoaminophen (N-acetyl-p-aminophenol) along with apomorphine; such animals exhibit stereotyped behavior for much longer periods than other animals receiving apomorphine alone (Missala et al., 1973). Acetoaminophen is readily glucuronidated in vivo and presumably competes successfully with apomorphine for available glucuronidyl groups. The results also indicate that glucuronidation is a quantitatively significant pathway in the metabolism of apomorphine.

Evidence that apomorphine is a substrate for COMT has come from studies in vivo (Belenky et al., 1966) and others in vitro (White and McKenzie, 1971; Cannon et al., 1972; McKenzie and White, 1973; Missala et al., 1973). The major product is apocodeine, but some isoapocodeine is also formed (Cannon et al., 1972). For example, with the supernatant fraction of rat liver as enzyme source, suitably supplemented with $MgCl_2$ and S-adenosyl-methionine, the rate of production of O-methylapomorphine was 270–300 nmol/g original liver/hr, the limits being observed at pH 7.8 and pH 9.1, respectively. The ratios of apocodeine to isoapocodeine at the two pHs were 81 and 67 (Cannon et al., 1972). Dopamine is methylated predominantly in the meta-position, and the meta:para ratio varies from 6.9 at pH 8.1 to 3.5 at pH 9.1 (Creveling et al., 1972). The apparent K_m for apomorphine was 1.4 mM with both liver and brain enzymes; corresponding values for dopamine were 0.26 and 0.23 mM (McKenzie and White, 1973).

The ability of apomorphine to act as a substrate for COMT and therefore as an inhibitor of the enzyme's action on dopamine has led McKenzie (1974) to propose protection of synaptic dopamine as a mode of action of apomorphine.

Conversion of apomorphine to apocodeine entails, as already mentioned, a reduction of pharmacological activity. This can be circumvented experimentally by administering to animals a COMT inhibitor, such as pyrogallol, 3,4-dimethoxy-5-hydroxybenzoic acid, tropolone, or 8-hydroxyquinoline

(Missala *et al.*, 1973; McKenzie and White, 1973). The result is a prolongation of the apomorphine-induced stereotyped behavior. Costall and Naylor (1973) have observed a reduction in the intensity of this behavior with pyrogallol. However, these authors used smaller doses of the compound than did others and did not administer it before the apomorphine.

Apocodeine can be demethylated to apomorphine. A second product found with apomorphine in the urine of apocodeine-treated animals is norapomorphine (Smith and Cook, 1973; Smith *et al.*, 1973). Whether the *N*-demethylation occurs with apomorphine itself or only when one of its hydroxyls is methylated is not known. Only small quantities of free apomorphine are excreted in the urine. In the rat, which excretes a slightly acidic urine, this comprises 3–4% of a dose; none is detectable in the normally alkaline urine of horse and rabbit (Kaul *et al.*, 1961*a*).

3.2. Neurochemical Actions of Apomorphine

3.2.1. *Catecholamine-Containing Structures*

Blocking agents of the dopamine-receptor induce an increased release of the amine into the synaptic cleft where a portion of the dopamine is then metabolized to HVA. Since transport of HVA across the cerebral–blood barrier is slow, some accumulation of the terminal metabolite is detectable in dopamine-rich regions of the brain (e.g., striatum) under the influence of neuroleptics (Sourkes, 1972*b*). Conversely, receptor stimulants ought to deactivate feedback regulation and cause a decreased formation and accumulation of HVA. This is actually the case with apomorphine (Roos, 1969; Lahti *et al.*, 1972; Lal *et al.*, 1972*a*), as well as with apocodeine and 10,11-methylenedioxyaporphine, but not with 10,11-dimethoxyaporphine (Lal *et al.*, 1972*a*). Within certain limits of dosage, the biochemical actions of thiothixene and chlorpromazine, as detected by the content of striatal HVA, are prevented by administration of apomorphine (Lahti *et al.*, 1972).

The content of dopamine remains essentially unaltered (Andén *et al.*, 1967; Nybäck *et al.*, 1970) after apomorphine, but the drug reduces the level of norepinephrine in brains of the cat, mouse, and rat (Vogt, 1954; Nybäck *et al.*, 1970; Benesova and Benes, 1970; Balakleevsky, 1971), apparently by accelerating its utilization (Persson and Waldeck, 1970) or by inhibiting tyrosine hydroxylase and the rate of renewed synthesis of catecholamines (Goldstein *et al.*, 1970; Kehr *et al.*, 1972). However, with very large doses of apomorphine, the cerebral dopamine content can be made to decrease as well (Andén *et al.*, 1973).

The diminished activity of dopaminergic fibers under the influence of apomorphine has been demonstrated in another manner. Animals injected with labeled tyrosine acquire labeled catecholamines in the brain through normal processes of biosynthesis and lose this material at a measurable rate. The administration of apomorphine retards the loss of labeled dopamine from the brain but may accelerate the turnover and even the loss of [^{14}C]-norepinephrine (Waldeck, 1970; Andén and Bédard, 1971). The inhibition of biosynthesis of dopamine from [^{14}C]-tyrosine in the rat striatum has also been demonstrated *in vitro* with two dopamine-receptor agonist agents— apomorphine and Trivastal (Goldstein *et al.*, 1970; 1973).

The inhibition of tyrosine hydroxylase by apomorphine has proved to be more complex than that by catecholamines. Kinetic studies indicate that the inhibition may be of a cooperative nature, the cooperativity being eliminated by mild heating of the enzyme, among other treatments. Moreover, borate, which binds to vicinal hydroxyl groups, affects the inhibition by apomorphine differently than that with catecholamines, so that there may be separate binding sites or mechanisms for these substances. Thus, cooperative effects may play a role in the regulation of adrenal medullary tyrosine hydroxylase (Quik and Sourkes, 1974).

Farnebo and Hamberger (1971) have shown that apomorphine decreases dopamine release following electrical field stimulation of neostriatal slices preincubated with tritiated dopamine. These authors consider that the drug acts by a transsynaptic negative feedback mechanism. Symchowicz *et al.* (1971) state that apomorphine does not affect uptake of dopamine into synaptosomes of the caudate nucleus.

3.2.2. *Cholinergic Mechanisms*

Apomorphine causes the content of ACh in the basal ganglia of the rat to decrease (Kunz *et al.*, 1971), and it abolishes the increased release of ACh from the caudate nucleus of the cat also given chlorpromazine (Stadtler *et al.*, 1973). By contrast, Sethy and Van Woert (1974) record opposite results, viz., an increased level of ACh in the rat given apomorphine.

Whereas apomorphine decelerates the turnover of brain dopamine (see above), anticholinergics do so to but a small extent (Andén and Bédard, 1971). However, the effects of the latter drugs are seen only in animals that have previously received a neuroleptic (haloperidol); such treatment inhibits the action of apomorphine.

These results indicate that dopamine exerts an inhibitory influence on certain cholinergic fibers and that these probably favor turnover of dopamine. Stadtler and his colleagues (1973) therefore propose the existence of an interdependent network, consisting of both types of fiber, in the striatum.

3.2.3. Serotonin-Mediated Functions

The behavioral stereotypy induced by apomorphine is potentiated by reserpine, but not by α-methyl-p-tyrosine (Rotrosen *et al.*, 1972*b*). Since reserpine decreases 5-HT and catecholamine levels, and α-methyl-p-tyrosine only the catecholamines, there is the possibility that diminished contents of cerebral 5-HT are crucial for appearance of the stereotypy. However, drugs that cause increases or decreases in 5-HT levels or that antagonize its action do not influence the effect of apomorphine stereotypy (Rotrosen *et al.*, 1972*b*). The results are said to be different if apomorphine-induced locomotor stimulation is measured (Grabowska *et al.*, 1973*a*). In this case, 5-hydroxytryptophan, the precursor of 5-HT *in vivo*, antagonizes apomorphine, and p-chlorophenylalanine, which inhibits the synthesis of 5-HT, potentiates apomorphine-induced locomotor activity. Although the interpretation of these interactions is not clear, Grabowska *et al.* (1973*a*) point out that at the time that the short-lived locomotor stimulation is diminishing, 5-HT and 5-hydroxyindoleacetic acid in brain are beginning to increase under the influence of apomorphine. The increases are evident in the cortex, striatum, hippocampus, and especially the mesencephalic area including the raphe nuclei. These authors postulate a dopaminergic–serotoninergic sequence of fibers to account for the monoamine changes.

Balakleevsky (1971) and Grabowska and her colleagues (1973*a*) think that apomorphine may accelerate the turnover of 5-HT in the brain stem, for example, by an indirect mechanism involving dopamine receptors (Grabowska *et al.*, 1973*b*). However, Tagliamonte *et al.* (1971) and Lal *et al.* (1972*a*) did not observe any changes in the content of 5-HT or 5-hydroxyindoleacetic acid in the brain of the rat after apomorphine.

Despite suggestions of an involvement of 5-HT, the gnawing syndrome in the rat brought about by apomorphine (Ernst, 1972) and bulbocapnine-induced catatonia (Tseng and Walaszek, 1970*b*) are considered to be basically mediated by dopaminergic mechanisms.

4. NEUROPHARMACOLOGY OF APOMORPHINE

4.1. Stereotyped Behavior

Apomorphine causes a repetitive pattern of behavior in a variety of animal species (Harnack, 1874; Amsler, 1923) in a sufficiently characteristic way to be designated as stereotyped behavior (SB). During this SB, normal activities are inhibited. Elicitation of SB in the mouse, rat, and pigeon has been used as an index of central dopaminergic activity.

4.1.1. *Rat*

Within minutes of administration of apomorphine (10 mg/kg intra-peritoneally) the rats develop continuous sniffing, licking, or biting (i.e., SB). Initially, some rearing on the hind legs and sniffing directed upward occurs and a slight increase in forward locomotion accompanies the SB, but within 10 min the SB is directed toward the floor. The animals develop ptosis (which never occurs after amphetamine), and normal activities such as grooming, social interaction, forward locomotion, and feeding are inhibited. Thus, the rubric of "eating automatism" applied by Ungerstedt (1971*d*) is misleading. Retropulsion, which may accompany amphetamine-induced SB is never seen. During the terminal 10 min there is a gradual return to normal activities which interrupt the SB and a diminution of ptosis until at last the animals group together and fall asleep (Lal and Sourkes, 1973). The duration (Lal and Sourkes, 1973) and intensity (McKenzie, 1972) of SB are proportional to the logarithm of the dose. At low doses (0.5 mg/kg), the SB is delayed in onset and intermittent, and ptosis is variable; at higher doses (30 mg/kg) exophthalmos may occur and convulsions (50 mg/kg) may interrupt the SB (Lal and Sourkes, 1973). A certain percentage of rats (10.8 %) fail to develop SB even with the relatively large dose of 10 mg/kg. There is no effect of sex. Cage size has no effect on SB; however, if the wire grid size is too fine, biting does not occur but sniffing and licking persist (Lal and Sourkes, 1973). Dresse and Niemegeers (1961), who gave seven injections at 90-min intervals, and Lal and Sourkes (1973), who gave daily injections of apomorphine for 7 days, found no effect of repeated injection on the duration of SB. On the other hand, Divac (1972) reported, though without details, that the duration and distinctiveness of SB decrease with repeated treatment. The latency of onset of SB decreases with repeated administration (Dresse and Niemegeers, 1961).

Rudimentary SB consisting of intermittent tongue protrusion can be elicited by both amphetamine and apomorphine at least as early as 2 days of age (Lal and Sourkes, 1973). Following apomorphine injection (10 mg/kg i.p.) the 2-day-old animals exhibit some initial head rearing, crawling, and dispersion in the cage; within 10 min the animals remain motionless with limbs extended. Only after a delay of 60 min from the time of injection does the rat assume a partial hunched posture and then commence intermittent tongue protrusion. This behavior terminates 2–3 hr after injection in con-trast to 70 min in the adult. With advancing age, the latent period and termin-ation time decrease, the sedative effect is attenuated, and the SB becomes a continuous phenomenon. Ptosis becomes manifest as soon as eye opening occurs (14–16 days of age) and at 20 days the pattern of response is indistin-guishable from the adult (Lal and Sourkes, 1973). The failure of Kellogg and

Lundborg (1972) to detect SB until 21 days of age may be related to the smaller dose used (1 mg/kg) and the shorter duration of observation (1–2 hr). The SB described by Kellogg and Lundborg in their 21-day-old rats was actually an intense grooming and digging response rather than the recognized SB, consisting of sniffing, licking, and biting.

Randrup and Munkvad (1970) have accumulated much evidence implicating striatal dopaminergic mechanisms in the development of drug-induced SB. Amsler (1923) was able to abolish the response by ablating the striatum bilaterally. Ernst and Smelik (1966) elicited SB after a delay of 30–40 min by stereotaxic placement of crystalline apomorphine in the globus pallidus and also the dorsal, but not ventral, part of the caudate nucleus. Recently, the role of the striatum in apomorphine SB has been called into question. Thus, McKenzie (1972) found that 24–48 hr, and Divac (1972) 30–40 days, after bilateral lesions of the neostriatum SB was similar to that in intact animals even though 50–80 % of the neostriatum was destroyed (Divac, 1972). Wolfarth *et al.* (1973) noted an enhancement of SB 2 days after bilateral striatal lesions, but SB returned to normal by day 8. Of course, it is possible that the residual neostriatal tissue was sufficient to mediate the apomorphine response. Further observations by McKenzie (1972) have shown that lesions of the nucleus accumbens, and olfactory bulbs have no effect on SB but bilateral lesions of the tuberculum olfactorium either abolished the response (in 45 % of rats) or markedly diminished it.

Following acute lesions of the substantia nigra, spontaneous SB develops and persists for 4–6 days (Costall *et al.*, 1972). During this stage, amphetamine increases the intensity of SB but the intensity of apomorphine-induced SB is diminished, possibly owing to a raised dopaminergic threshold occasioned by persistent release of dopamine. However, 14 days after the lesion, apomorphine SB was absent or markedly reduced whereas amphetamine SB was unaffected. These findings have led Costall *et al.* (1972) to postulate that apomorphine SB does not stem from a direct action of the drug on dopamine receptors but does require an effective dopaminergic nigrostriatal pathway, and, further, that this system is nonessential for amphetamine SB. In contrast, Schoenfeld and Uretsky (1972) noted an enhancement of apomorphine SB after intraventricular injection of 6-hydroxydopamine and Ungerstedt (1971d) described a similar effect after selective bilateral destruction of the nigrostriatal pathway with intracerebral 6-hydroxydopamine. The enhancement was attributed to denervation supersensitivity of the striatal dopamine receptors, a phenomenon that could also explain the enhancement of rotational behavior after unilateral lesion of the nigrostriatal pathway with 6-hydroxydopamine (Ungerstedt, 1971c).

Administration of α-methyltyrosine or α-methyldopa, which depletes brain dopamine, abolishes amphetamine SB but not apomorphine SB. MAO inhibitors enhance amphetamine SB but have no effect on that caused by apomorphine. This result suggests that apomorphine SB is not dependent on endogenous catecholamines in contrast to the action of amphetamine (Ernst, 1967).

p-Chlorophenylalanine (Ernst, 1972; Rotrosen et al., 1972b), an inhibitor of serotonin synthesis; methysergide, a serotonin antagonist; and tryptophan (Rotrosen et al., 1972b) have all been administered with apomorphine but do not affect SB. Thus, there is no evidence from these experiments that a serotonergic mechanism modulates apomorphine SB.

The duration of SB is unaffected by reserpine when apomorphine is given 3 hr after reserpine (Lal et al., 1972a), but when given 20 hr after, both the duration and intensity are increased (Rotrosen et al., 1972b). The latter effects may be related to increased sensitivity of dopamine receptors (Ungerstedt, 1971c). However, there is no information on the effect of reserpine on the biodisposition of apomorphine. In fact, drug interaction studies often have been interpreted without information on the possible effects of the second drug on apomorphine metabolism.

Neuroleptics characteristically inhibit apomorphine SB; this inhibition provides an accurate prediction of clinical antipsychotic potency (Janssen et al., 1960; 1967). The more potent inhibitors of apomorphine SB are the most effective in inducing Parkinsonism and in exerting antiemetic activity, whereas the weak neuroleptics are less effective in inducing Parkinsonism, antagonizing apomorphine SB and, in the dog, apomorphine emesis (Janssen et al., 1960). Recently, the mean effective content of neuroleptic in brain required to inhibit apomorphine SB has been determined (Lewi et al., 1970; Heykants et al., 1970). Many drugs which inhibit apomorphine emesis in dogs also antagonize apomorphine SB. However, a dissociation in these effects does occur. Thus, metoclopramide (Laville and Margarit, 1964) and dextromoramide (Janssen et al., 1960) inhibit apomorphine emesis in dogs but are ineffective as antagonists of SB. As yet, no compound is known which inhibits apomorphine SB but does not inhibit emesis in dogs (Janssen et al., 1960).

Increasing the dose of apomorphine overcomes the blockade of neuroleptics. The antagonistic effect of neuroleptics toward apomorphine decreases with repeated injection of the tranquilizer. Thus, Asper et al. (1973) found that the ED_{50} of apomorphine to overcome neuroleptic blockade decreased by 75% after 7–14 daily doses of neuroleptic.

In addition to neuroleptic agents (Janssen et al., 1960), morphine (Kuschinsky and Hornykiewicz, 1972), methadone (Sasame et al., 1972), bulbocapnine, p-methoxyphenylethylamine, and 3,4-dimethoxyphenylethylamine (but not 3,5-dimethoxyphenylethylamine) also induce catalepsy in rats and inhibit apomorphine SB (Ernst, 1965). Conversely, catalepsy induced by various means—e.g., with morphine (Kuschinsky and Horny-kiewicz, 1972), methadone (Sasame *et al.*, 1972), reserpine (Lal *et al.*, 1972*a*), or by bilateral lesions of the medial forebrain bundle at the diencephalic level of the subthalamus (Boissier *et al.*, 1971; Etevenon *et al.*, 1970)—is antagon-ized by apomorphine. Rats treated in this way develop SB.

Vedernikov (1970) observed that morphine prolonged apomorphine SB in nontolerant but not in tolerant rats. This potentiation, rather than inhibition as noted by Janssen *et al.* (1960), may be related to the differences in relative doses of the two drugs used.

α- and β-blockers (Simon *et al.*, 1972), antihistamines, muscle relaxants, barbiturates, and CNS stimulants are ineffective in blocking SB (Janssen *et al.*, 1960). Boissier *et al.* (1968), however, did note antagonism with large doses of yohimbine, dihydroergotamine, and bretylium; the significance of these findings is unclear. Costall *et al.* (1972) found that the cholinergic agent arecoline inhibits apomorphine SB; this result fits in with the concept of a counterbalancing dopaminergic–cholinergic system in the striatum (Scheel-Krüger, 1970; see also Section 3.2.2).

4.1.2. *Mouse*

In contrast to its effects in the rat, apomorphine induces only weak SB behavior in the mouse consisting of sniffing, licking, and biting (Scheel-Krüger, 1970; Pedersen, 1967; Frommel, 1965). Nevertheless, this species is frequently used in the assessment of central dopamine agonists. The SB is markedly potentiated by anticholinergic (Scheel-Krüger, 1970; Ther and Schramm, 1962) and thymoleptic drugs (Pedersen, 1967). Whereas physostig-mine inhibits the anticholinergic potentiation of apomorphine SB (Scheel-Krüger, 1970), that due to thymoleptics is not affected (Pedersen, 1967). Only large doses of the neuroleptic spiramide, a potent inhibitor of apomorphine SB in the rat, antagonize the anticholinergic potentiation of apomorphine SB (Scheel-Krüger, 1970). The thymoleptic potentiation of apomorphine SB is inhibited to a greater degree by the neuroleptic flupenthixol than is the anti-cholinergic potentiation (Pedersen, 1967).

Fekete *et al.* (1970) have claimed that reserpine antagonizes and iproni-azid enhances apomorphine SB. Their finding is in contrast to that of Ther and Schramm (1962), who found no inhibition with reserpine, but inhibition with high doses of iproniazid. Ernst (1967), however, found no effect of either of these two drugs in the rat. Also, Fekete *et al.* (1970) noted that pretreatment with either L-dopa or 5-hydroxytryptophan, each with a MAO inhibitor, potentiated apomorphine SB, and they concluded that apomorphine induces SB by an indirect effect on catecholamines. However, their results were based on the number of holes gnawed; Rotrosen *et al.* (1972*b*) have pointed out that, if reserpine potentiated apomorphine SB, as in their own findings in the rat, then as a result of retardation of locomotor activity the concentrated gnawing would be confined to one area and the number of holes would be expected to be decreased. A further criticism is that the authors failed to use appropriate controls, i.e., to study the independent effects, if any, of dopa or 5-hydroxytryptophan combined with an MAO inhibitor.

4.1.3. *Guinea Pig*

Apomorphine induces stereotyped chewing in the guinea pig which is not modified by anticholinergic drugs (Frommel *et al.*, 1965) but, as in the rat, is inhibited by morphine and neuroleptics (Srimal and Dhawan, 1970). Also, as in the rat, α-methyldopa blocks SB owing to amphetamine but not apomorphine. On the other hand, α-methyltyrosine, in contrast to its complete inhibition of apomorphine SB in the rat, is only partially effective in the guinea pig (Srimal and Dhawan, 1970). Both in the hyperthyroid guinea pig (Klawans *et al.*, 1973) and the guinea pig recently treated chronically with chlorpromazine (Klawans and Rubovits, 1972), the threshold dose of apomorphine required to induce SB is decreased. These findings have been attributed to an enhancement of striatal dopamine-receptor sensitivity, and it has been proposed that these treatment states may be considered as models of hyperthyroid chorea and tardive dyskinesia in man, respectively (Klawans *et al.*, 1973; Klawans and Rubovits, 1972).

4.1.4. *Pigeon*

In pigeons, SB after apomorphine takes the form of repetitive pecking. This result was referred to by Amsler (1923) as "Zwangspicken." The behavioral pattern was rediscovered by Koster (1957) and Burkman *et al.* (1957), who described it as a "feeding hallucination" and as a "pecking response," respectively. Though most extensively studied in the pigeon, this SB can also be elicited in other avian species such as sparrows, to a lesser extent in parrots and hens, and also in quails if they are grouped in a wire cage (Deshpande *et al.*, 1961). Chaney and Kare (1966), however, were able to elicit pecking in the herring gull and cowbird, but not in chickens, even when they were injected intravenously with 20 mg/kg body weight.

Though the type of movements are similar to those observed in pecking for grain, the birds ignore any grain placed in the cage. The syndrome is unrelated to starvation and insulin is without effect on it (Deshpande *et al.*, 1961). SB occurs even if the bird is made blind (Dhawan and Saxena, 1960). Some of the parameters of this behavior have been investigated by Burkman (1960) and Dhawan and Saxena (1960), and recently Van Tyle and Burkman

(1970) have described an electronic monitoring system to estimate the intensity of apomorphine SB. The latent period decreases with dose; the rate of pecking increases with dose to a maximum and then plateaus; and the duration of SB is proportional to the logarithm of the dose. Some pigeons are remarkably refractory, even to doses 30 times larger than the ED_{50} (Dhawan and Saxena, 1960).

Chronic administration decreases the latent period of onset, which returns to basal levels within a week of stopping the drug (Dhawan and Saxena, 1960). No tolerance or increased sensitivity occurs over a 5-wk period of drug administration (Burkman, 1961; Dhawan and Saxena, 1960). However, weak conditioning effects may develop following repeated injections of apomorphine in some birds (Burkman, 1961). Distracting stimuli such as vigorous thumping, exposure to a bright light, induction of fear by moving a dog close to the cage, or emesis may temporarily reduce the pecking, and, if the bird is placed in a dark room, the SB may even be completely abolished (Dhawan and Saxena, 1960). Preconditioning of the pigeon to peck a Skinner-type key could qualitatively affect the SB, but this effect occurred in only one of the five trained birds (Weissman, 1966).

Neuroleptics (Deshpande *et al.*, 1961; Burkman, 1961, 1962; Gupta and Dhawan, 1965; Dhawan *et al.*, 1961), except reserpine (Dhawan *et al.*, 1961), as well as tricyclic antidepressants (Gupta *et al.*, 1969) and morphine (Dhawan *et al.*, 1961; Weissman, 1966), antagonize apomorphine SB in the pigeon. The structure–activity relationships have been studied in detail by Gupta and Dhawan (1965). Although chlorpromazine antagonizes apomorphine-induced SB in the pigeon, its sulfoxide metabolite does not. Interestingly, the sulfoxide of chlorpromazine does not inhibit amphetamine SB in the rat (Lal and Sourkes, 1972). Anticholinergics, antihistamines, and anticonvulsants are without effect.

Additional drugs exert an antagonistic effect against apomorphine SB: orphenadrine (Gupta *et al.*, 1969), barbiturates, cortisone, nicotine (4 mg/kg) (Deshpande *et al.*, 1961), caffeine, LSD, yohimbine (Dhawan *et al.*, 1961), and hydroxyzine (Burkman, 1961). Others, such as histamine, lobeline, testosterone, progesterone, sodium taurocholate, and nicotine in small doses (0.2–0.4 mg/kg) intensify the response (Deshpande *et al.*, 1961). The mechanisms underlying the inhibition and potentiation have not been studied. How far the execution of SB is antagonized, rather than inhibition of central processes necessary to induce SB, requires consideration. Also, how far the enhancing effect on SB is due to interference with the metabolism of apomorphine remains to be explored.

The failure of Burkman (1961) to observe morphine-induced antagonism of apomorphine SB may be related to the smaller dose used compared to that employed by Dhawan *et al.* (1961). Interestingly, *d*-amphetamine

(Deshpande *et al.*, 1961) and methamphetamine (Dhawan and Saxena, 1960) do not induce SB in pigeons.

Antipecking activity of drugs parallels their blockade of conditioned avoidance response in rats; to a lesser degree there is a correlation between antipecking activity and antiemetic effects in the dog (Gupta and Dhawan, 1965; Burkman, 1962). However disparities exist; thus, thioproperazine is an extremely potent antiemetic in dogs but is relatively weak in antagonizing apomorphine SB in the pigeon (Gupta and Dhawan, 1965). It is possible to dissociate emetic and pecking effects in the pigeon, as observations with promethazine and nicotine show. In emetic doses, these have antipecking activity (Deshpande *et al.*, 1961).

4.1.5. Dog

Doses of apomorphine in excess of the emetic dose induce in the dog incessant running behavior which may be interrupted with emesis. The duration of running increases with dose. This behavior was first described by Feser (1873) and recently rediscovered by Nymark (1972). Dopamine antagonists inhibit this behavior (Nymark, 1972).

4.2. Aggressive Behavior

Apomorphine may induce aggression (AB) in rats (Senault, 1968; 1970; 1971; 1972; 1973; 1974; McKenzie, 1971) consisting of defensive stances and actual fighting. In septal-lesioned rats as well as rats known to kill, aggression is directed toward inanimate objects and mice, respectively, whereas after apomorphine the behavior is directed toward members of the same species (McKenzie, 1971). The induction of aggressive behavior by apomorphine is not correlated with shock-induced aggression or muricidal behavior (Senault, 1970). In fact, apomorphine actually suppresses the increase in foot shock aggression induced by intracisternal injection of 6-hydroxydopamine (Thoa *et al.*, 1972), though this may be in part related to competition of SB over AB. These data suggest that the latter three forms of AB mentioned are dependent on different mechanisms.

Apomorphine-induced AB is influenced by strain; thus Wistar rats are more prone to AB than the Long-Evans or Holtzman strains (Senault, 1970). Among Wistar rats, Senault (1970) distinguished three categories of animals regarding apomorphine response when combined with auditory stimuli: (a) those that showed no aggression (61.9 %); (b) those that showed a moderate short-lasting AB (21.7 %); and (c) those that showed marked AB (16.4 %). Only in the latter group was this behavior reproducible and extensively studied.

Within a certain dose range, apomorphine-induced AB increases with dose as does the number of pairs of rats that develop AB. When not fighting, the rats display SB. Pairs of rats quickly develop a dominant or subordinate role which is never reversed. When two subordinate rats are placed together they usually engage only in defensive maneuvers (McKenzie, 1971). Placement of a treated rat with an untreated animal results in AB, but this is more pronounced if both rats are treated (Senault, 1970).

Environmental factors modify the apomorphine response. Sound enhances the duration and frequency of combat. This fact has led Senault (1970) to incorporate the use of auditory stimuli at regular intervals into his experimental design of apomorphine-induced AB. Pinching of the tail also increases the number of pairs of rats which engage in AB and decreases the dose of apomorphine needed to induce fighting (McKenzie, 1971). Increasing the dimension of the cage decreases the duration of combat (Senault, 1970). Prior isolation of adults enhances AB, especially if they have been isolated in opacified Makrolon boxes. The enhancement of aggressive response can be attenuated by keeping the animals in groups following their isolation. Isolation of young rats at weaning for 2 months results in enhancement of AB if they are kept in wire cages, but not if isolated in Makrolon boxes. One month after grouping, the enhanced AB is attenuated (Senault, 1971).

More male Wistar rats show apomorphine-induced AB than do females (Senault, 1970). McKenzie (1971) was unable to induce AB in female Long-Evans rats. Hypophysectomy reduces the duration of apomorphine-induced AB. Prepubertal castration (especially if performed at 5 days of age), but not postpubertal castration, reduces the proportion of rats that become aggressive but does not abolish AB. Prolonged treatment of male, female, and castrated rats with high doses of testosterone from the time of weaning increases the proportion of aggressive animals; treatment of adult rats is ineffective (Senault, 1972).

The aggressive response is age-dependent. Thus, young rats show much less AB both in terms of numbers developing the aggressive response and the duration of AB than do adults (Senault, 1970; McKenzie, 1971). McKenzie (1971) found that AB did not develop until the 49th day of age, and then only if very large doses of apomorphine were given.

Bulbectomy, destruction of the anterior part of the striatum, or septal lesions enhance apomorphine-induced AB without facilitating its appearance in nonaggressive rats. Lesions of the amygdala and substantia nigra (especially the pars compacta) exert an inhibitory effect (Senault, 1973).

Neuroleptics (except reserpine) and morphine antagonize AB, as in the case of SB. However, in contrast to SB, minor tranquilizers, anticholinergic agents, and antidepressants also exert an antagonistic effect (Senault, 1970; Dlabač, 1973). Reserpine administered 2 hr before apomorphine lowers the threshold for AB (McKenzie, 1971). In rats sensitive to apomorphine phenoxybenzamine (a central α-adrenergic blocking agent) almost completely inhibits AB; partial inhibition follows administration of diethyldithiocarbamate, FLA 63, and 5-hydroxytryptophan (Senault, 1974). Parachlorophenylalanine, which induces mouse-killing behavior (Sheard, 1969), α-methyltyrosine, α-methyldopa, and MAO inhibitors have little effect on AB. In rats not sensitive to the actions of apomorphine, however, pretreatment with reserpine or MAO inhibitors (and to a lesser extent with α-methyldopa) sensitizes the rats to the action of apomorphine. This sensitizing effect of reserpine and MAO inhibitors is abolished by diethyldithiocarbamate. In nonaggressive rats, a combination of clonidine (a noradrenergic receptor agonist) plus apomorphine is effective in inducing AB (Senault, 1974). A lesser degree of AB was also observed with Trivastal and clonidine. These data have led Senault (1974) to conclude that dopamine-receptor stimulation, together with participation of the noradrenergic system, is necessary for apomorphine-induced AB.

The AB associated with morphine abstinence in morphine-dependent rats is enhanced by administration of apomorphine, and this enhanced AB is not blocked by α-methyltyrosine but is blocked by methadone (Puri and Lal, 1973).

4.3. Rotational Behavior

Unilateral injection of dopamine and apomorphine, or placement of crystals of these substances into the caudate nucleus of the rat, induces turning toward the opposite side (Ungerstedt *et al.*, 1969). This turning or rotational behavior has been further studied in rodents with (a) unilateral destruction of the caudate nucleus or (b) unilateral destruction of the nigrostriatal pathway (electrothermically or by 6-hydroxydopamine). Such behavior can be quantified by use of a rotometer (Ungerstedt, 1971*b*). Rotational behavior, spontaneous or drug-induced, is believed to be an expression of an imbalance of dopamine transmission in the CNS (Ungerstedt, 1971*b*). Following unilateral removal of the caudate nucleus, both the nigrostriatal pathway and the caudatal dopamine receptors are destroyed, but in the animals with a lesion of the nigrostriatal pathway the receptors remain intact, though denervated.

In the unilaterally caudate-lesioned animal, drugs that act by releasing endogenous dopamine, such as amphetamine, and drugs acting directly on dopamine receptors, such as apomorphine, cause rotational behavior toward the lesioned side. After administration of α-methyltyrosine, only the action of directly acting compounds elicits this response (Andén *et al.*, 1967;

Lotti, 1971). In rodents with selective unilateral destruction of the nigro-striatal pathway the indirectly acting compounds cause rotation toward the side of the lesion whereas apomorphine or Trivastal (Corrodi *et al.*, 1972) induces turning behavior toward the intact side. The denervated receptors on the lesioned side are believed to be supersensitive to apomorphine; hence, an enhanced apomorphine effect occurs at the site of the denervated receptors (Ungerstedt, 1971c; Von Voigtlander and Moore, 1973). L-Dopa induces a similar effect to that of apomorphine, but its action is inhibited if the animals receive pretreatment with a dopa–decarboxylase inhibitor. Apparently, the caudate nucleus still contains enough decarboxylase, despite lesioning of the nigrostriatal tract, to permit the biosynthesis of an effective amount of dopamine (Ungerstedt, 1971c).

Neuroleptics, except reserpine, block turning behavior. After reserpine, the behavior is enhanced, especially on the third day after the administration of this drug. Large doses of apomorphine induce the stereotypy, which then interferes with the rotational behavior (Ungerstedt, 1971c).

4.4. Miscellaneous Behavioral Effects

4.4.1. *Rat*

In addition to SB, apomorphine may increase motility (Maj *et al.*, 1972), produce agitation (Janssen *et al.*, 1967) and induce heightened and prolonged exploration (Carlsson, 1972). The motility can be blocked not only by neuroleptics (other than reserpine), but also by phenoxybenzamine. The effect of the neuroleptics can be overcome with larger doses of apomorphine. These data and the fact that inhibitors of tyrosine hydroxylase and dopamine-β-hydroxylase produce partial antagonism of motility has led Maj and his colleagues (1972) to consider the importance not only of dopamine-receptor stimulation but also of noradrenergic transmission in locomotor behavior. Maj *et al.* (1972) and Persson and Waldeck (1970) postulate that apomorphine stimulates dopamine receptors which in turn causes an increased flow of impulses to noradrenergic neurons. The latter cells then release their transmitter norepinephrine.

Weissman (1971) has described "cliff-jumping" behavior after intravenous apomorphine. This drug is much more active in inducing the effect than is morphine or tetrabenazine and desmethylimipramine given together. L-Dopa and amphetamine are ineffective.

4.4.2. *Mouse*

In the mouse, 1 mg/kg apomorphine given subcutaneously induces psychomotor excitement (agitation) but no SB (Frommel, 1965). This excitement is neutralized by anticholinergic agents. However, the agitation described by Frommel was measured by an electronic recording device which amplified vibrations. In view of the fact that anticholinergics facilitate the development of SB (Scheel-Krüger, 1970), it is possible that the observed neutralization of agitation by such drugs simply represents conversion of agitation to SB.

Apomorphine increases locomotion in mice (Andén *et al.*, 1973). Scheel-Krüger (1970) noted that administration of 10 mg/kg apomorphine induces rearing in addition to increased locomotion; at 15 mg/kg, the rearing behavior extends to climbing activity; and at doses of 30–40 mg/kg, rearing and climbing behavior lead to characteristic attempts to escape from the cage (jumping behavior also occurs). Various authors have focused on one or other of these behavioral manifestations. Thus, Gouret (1973) concentrated on rearing behavior induced by apomorphine (10 mg/kg given s.c.) and noted that not only neuroleptics, but also bulbocapnine and fentanyl (catatonia-inducing cholinomimetics) inhibit this behavior. Similar inhibition was noted with yohimbine and propranolol. Gouret (1973) also suggested that inhibition of mouse rearing might be a useful screening procedure for cataleptic agents. Hester *et al.* (1970) have used antagonism of apomorphine-induced cage climbing to assess CNS effects of a new series of butyrophenones. Combination of apomorphine with clonidine or α-methyldopa markedly increases motor activity and induces pronounced jumping behavior. The effect with clonidine is not mediated through a drug interaction influencing brain apomorphine levels (Andén *et al.*, 1973). These data point to the importance of noradrenergic mechanisms in modifying motor activity.

Cotzias and coworkers (Cotzias, 1971; Cotzias *et al.*, 1971*a*) have investigated the phenomenon of "mouse-falling" in the Swiss albino Hale–Stoner strain which is induced by both apomorphine and dopa. Cotzias' group uses "mouse falling" as a model for L-dopa-induced involuntary movements in man. The strain of mouse appears to be a critical factor in eliciting this behavior. Whereas L-dopa-induced falling is antagonized by DOPAC or dopamine, these agents have no effect on the apomorphine-induced falling. There is a further difference; both L-dopa and apomorphine cause turning toward the side of the lesion in mice with a unilateral lesion of the caudate nucleus. In this behavior the action of dopa is blocked by melatonin, but not that of apomorphine (Cotzias *et al.*, 1971*b*).

4.5. Emetic Action

Apomorphine induces emesis in a wide variety of animal species including man, but the sensitivity of species varies widely. Thus, the effective dose of intravenous apomorphine in the cat is about 1000 times the dose in the dog (Bhargava *et al.*, 1961). The monkey (*Macacus cyclopis*) is resistant (Peng and Wang, 1962). Emesis may occur in certain avian species such as the pigeon (Burkman, 1960), herring gull, and cowbird but not in the chicken (Chaney and Kare, 1966).

Both apomorphine and emetine act directly on the chemoreceptor trigger zone of the area postrema of the medulla oblongata which lies on the floor of the fourth ventricle in the dog (Borison and Wang, 1953; Bhargava *et al.*, 1961; Share *et al.*, 1965) and cat (Borison *et al.*, 1960). Takaori *et al.* (1968; 1970) have studied the behavior of single neurons of the Nucleus tractus solitarii in the encéphale isolé preparation of the cat. Apomorphine increased the frequency of spontaneous discharge, whereas metoclopramide and chlorpromazine blocked it. Local application of apomorphine to the area postrema increases the firing rate from the Nucleus tractus solitarii; chlorpromazine reduces the number of units responding to the drug.

Over 300 papers have appeared in the last 25 years on apomorphine emesis in the dog, the model species in which to assess antiemetic agents. Niemegeers (1971), in an extensive review of this literature, pointed out that many of the discrepant findings are due to different doses, routes of administration, and criteria for assessment of antiemetic activity, as well as to differences in the time interval between administration of the antiemetic agent and apomorphine.

Repeated administration of apomorphine decreased the number of emeses per episode of vomiting (Dresse and Niemegeers, 1961), but emesis always occurred even in animals tested frequently over a period of years (Niemegeers, 1971). Large doses of apomorphine (in contrast to small doses) may actually induce an antiemetic effect (Borison and Wang, 1953). In dogs, in which an experimental neurosis has been induced, the threshold for induction of emesis is increased (Toldy, 1962).

The emetic response is present in the puppy by 2–5 days of age; it increases in sensitivity until the ED_{50} for apomorphine approaches the adult value by 30 days of age (Pi and Peng, 1971). This result suggested that the function of the chemoreceptor trigger zone and its neural connections with the vomiting center are present soon after birth and the system reaches maturity at approximately 4 weeks.

Neuroleptics antagonize apomorphine emesis (Niemegeers and Janssen, 1965). Bhargava and Chandra (1963) have studied the structure–activity relationships of phenothiazines in relation to their antagonism toward apomorphine-induced emesis. Kazdova *et al.* (1972) have found a good correlation between duration of antiemetic effect of long-acting neuroleptics in dogs and the duration of inhibition of the conditioned avoidance response in rats. Glycine has also been reported to antagonize apomorphine emesis (Koster, 1964); the mechanism of its action is unknown.

4.6. Hemodynamic and Temperature Effects

The cardiovascular and renal effects of dopamine result from actions on α- and β-adrenergic receptors and on specific dopamine receptors in the renal and mesenteric vascular beds (Goldberg, 1972). In the dog, dopamine dilates the renal vascular bed by a noradrenergic mechanism. N-Methyldopamine is equally effective, whereas apomorphine is much weaker, and amphetamine is ineffective (Goldberg et al., 1968). In addition to the agonistic effects on renal blood flow of dog kidney, apomorphine attenuates dopamine-induced renal vasodilation; bulbocapnine acts similarly (Goldberg and Musgrave, 1971). In the phenoxybenzamine-treated cat, apomorphine does not antagonize vasodepressor effects of dopamine (Dhasmana et al., 1969), whereas bulbocapnine does so not only in the cat but also in the rabbit and guinea pig (Tseng and Walaszek, 1970a).

Attenuation of dopamine effects by apomorphine has also been observed in the isolated rat vas deferens (Simon and van Maanen, 1971).

Apomorphine lowers the blood pressure in a dose-related manner in the anesthetized cat; this hypotensive effect is antagonized by haloperidol and abolished by spinal transsection (Barnett and Fiore, 1971). It is often implied that all apomorphine effects are the result of its action on dopamine receptors. Recently, Finch and Haeusler (1972) have produced evidence that the centrally mediated hypotensive action of apomorphine (in the urethanized rat) does not involve a central dopaminergic action, but is due to an increase in efferent vagal activity.

Apomorphine abolishes halothane-induced shivering (Nikki, 1969), increases peripheral blood flow (Richter, 1964), and induces a dose-dependent fall in body temperature in the mouse which is blocked by dopamine antagonists (Barnett et al., 1972; Fuxe and Sjöqvist, 1972). The hypothermic effect may be related to the centrally mediated hypotensive action of apomorphine (Barnett et al., 1972). In the rabbit, however, apomorphine induces a hyperthermia which is also blocked by dopamine antagonists (Hill and Horita, 1972). In both of these species, amphetamine induces hyperthermia.

4.7. Aversive Conditioning

Apomorphine can be used to induce a conditioned taste aversion in rats by administering the drug 30 min after presenting a particular solution (Rozin, 1969). The aversion is mediated subcortically (Best and Zuckerman, 1971). It does not occur if metrazol is given as an amnesic agent during the conditioning period (Ahlers and Best, 1972). Rats with lesions in the ventromedial nucleus of the hypothalamus learn less rapidly than controls to avoid a solution that was associated with apomorphine; during extinction they lose the aversion more rapidly. Rats lesioned after learning to avoid water containing saccharin continue to avoid; they lose this avoidance behavior during extinction at the same rate as controls (Gold and Proulx, 1972). In rats given a distinctive fluid during recovery from an injection of apomorphine, there is an increase in the intake of the fluid conditionally paired with recovery from the effects of the drug (Green and Garcia, 1971).

4.8.   Learned Behavior

Apomorphine decreases electrical self-stimulation in the rat; however, if it is given after injection of α-methyltyrosine, it restores this behavior within 2 hr. L-Dopa is ineffective in such an experiment (St. Laurent et al., 1973). The reduction in self-stimulation by apomorphine (1.5 mg/kg) stems from interference by the SB that is induced. However, with only half that dose, the tendency to stereotypic movements is overcome by doubling the current, i.e., the reward stimulus, and self-stimulation increases above normal levels (Liebman and Butcher, 1973). L-Dopa also decreases the rate of self-stimulation, but doubling the current restores the normal rate.

Apomorphine decreases the rate of lever pressing in rats maintained on a variable interval schedule of food reinforcement. In tetrabenazine-injected animals, apomorphine and amphetamine partially restore the rate— amphetamine is the more effective drug (Butcher and Andén, 1969). In a free operant avoidance situation, apomorphine may increase the rate of bar pressing (Butcher, 1968).

4.9.   Linguomandibular Reflex

Apomorphine has been investigated for its effects on the linguomandibular reflex in cats, which has been studied as a model for detecting potential anti-Parkinsonian agents (Barnett and Fiore, 1973). The effect of the drug on the spontaneous twitching of the branchiomeric muscles of the rat, which has been proposed as a model for the assessment of drugs acting on dopaminergic mechanisms (Bieger et al., 1972), has also been studied. Apomorphine and dopa both inhibit the linguomandibular reflex in a dose-dependent manner. Whereas the effect of apomorphine is blocked by haloperidol, that of L-dopa is not (Barnett and Fiore, 1973). Intracarotid injections of apomorphine increase the spontaneous twitching of the branchiomeric muscles; chronic lesions in the striatum diminish the effect (Bieger et al., 1972).

4.10.   Analgesia and Addiction

Apomorphine increases the pain threshold during SB and, on disappearance of the behavioral syndrome, the pain threshold returns to normal. If morphine is then given, the increase in pain threshold is less than in control rats administered morphine (Vedernikov, 1969). This postapomorphine SB-antagonism to morphine analgesia can itself be antagonized by the administration of amphetamine prior to morphine (Vedernikov, 1969). Apomorphine antagonism to morphine analgesia has also been described in the mouse (VanderWende and Spoerlein, 1973).

Lorenzetti and Sancilio (1970) have shown that apomorphine suppresses the writhing-wet shake syndrome in morphine-dependent rats and is a more potent agent in this respect than is codeine. These authors have pointed out that the dose of various antagonists of this syndrome correlates well with their human addiction liability and infer that apomorphine may have such addictive potential. Similar speculations based on the high Straub index of apomorphine in the mouse, compared with that of known addicting drugs, have been made by Shemano and Wendel (1964). However, in contrast to the analgesic effects of addiction agents, apomorphine is devoid of this property (Shemano and Wendel, 1964). Despite the long history of clinical use of apomorphine, addiction to this compound has never been described. Further, nonaddicting drugs such as haloperidol also block withdrawal symptoms in morphine-dependent rats, and apomorphine actually aggravates the withdrawal aggression in this species (Puri and Lal, 1973) so that it is difficult to accept the speculations of Lorenzetti and Sancilio (1970).

5.   CLINICAL USES

Soon after apomorphine was synthesized, it was quickly established as a powerful emetic for use in clinical practice and continues to be of use in the emergency treatment of accidental poisoning (Tattersall, 1971). The ready ability of this agent to induce nausea and vomiting has led to its use in aversion therapy for such conditions as alcoholism (Dent, 1934; Quinn and Kerr, 1963) and homosexuality (McConaghy, 1969; 1970). Quinn and Kerr (1963) have pointed to the difficulties in establishing a conditioned aversion to alcohol with the apomorphine procedure and, in fact, results have been disappointing. Antagonism of apomorphine-induced emesis in volunteers serves as a means to evaluate antiemetic agents (Shields et al., 1971).

Patients with the dumping syndrome after gastrectomy can have similar dumping symptoms induced with apomorphine. This result has led to its use as a preoperative dumping test prior to gastric resection and as a diagnostic aid for the evaluation of gastric-operated patients with dumpinglike symptoms (Fenger et al., 1972).

Since 1899, when apomorphine was found to be a remarkably effective sedative in the treatment of delirium tremens (Tompkins, 1899; Douglas, 1899), a large body of literature has appeared on the treatment of alcoholism with this agent. Emphasis has been placed on a specific anticraving property of apomorphine on alcoholism (see Schlatter and Lal, 1972, for literature citations) and addiction to other drugs (Dent, 1953); however, Schlatter and Lal (1972) were unable to substantiate the therapeutic claims in terms of abstinence from alcohol. One of the problems in assessing anticraving effects lies in the absence of an objective measure of craving. In a double-blind study, apomorphine in subnauseating doses and distilled water were equally effective in eliminating subjectively rated craving (Lal and de la Vega, unpublished data).

The limitations of L-dopa therapy in Parkinson's disease, namely the development of involuntary movements (McDowell et al., 1971), diurnal intermittency of therapeutic effects (Cotzias et al., 1972b), mental symptoms (Murphy, 1973), and unresponsiveness (Lieberman et al., 1972) in a significant number of cases has led to an awakening interest in apomorphine as a therapeutic agent. Apomorphine was first shown to be effective in the treatment of Parkinson's disease by Schwab et al. (1951). Since then this effect has been confirmed by several studies (Struppler and von Uexküll, 1953; Von Uexküll, 1953; Braham et al., 1970; Castaigne et al., 1971; Cotzias et al., 1970). Improvement with this drug also occurs in subjects unresponsive to L-dopa (Cotzias et al., 1972a). In addition, apomorphine enhances the therapeutic results of L-dopa (Düby et al., 1972; Cotzias et al., 1972a), especially tremor (Strian et al., 1972), and diminishes or prevents L-dopa-induced dyskenesias (Düby et al., 1972). On the other hand, apomorphine itself may induce mild buccolingual and head movements as well as choreo-athetoid movements in patients (Cotzias et al., 1970; 1972a; Düby et al., 1972) or monkeys (Sassin et al., 1972) that have experienced similar movements with L-dopa. Unfortunately, the duration of therapeutic effects of apomorphine is short. Schwab et al. (1951) obtained a more prolonged improvement with oral apomorphine, but this was less effective than the injected drug. Recently, Strian et al. (1972) and Cotzias et al. (1972a) have experimented with large oral doses of the drug either alone or in combination with L-dopa or L-dopa plus a dopa–decarboxylase inhibitor. Results have been encouraging, but unfortunately some patients have developed a reversible uremia (Cotzias et al., 1972a). In addition to improving tremor in

Parkinsonism, apomorphine also antagonizes oxotremorine-induced tremor in mice (Everett et al., 1971).

Apomorphine has been shown to suppress acute neuroleptic-induced dyskinesias (Gessa et al., 1972); its effect on tardive dyskinesias is unknown. Reports have shown beneficial effects of apomorphine in some cases of dystonia musculorum deformans (Braham et al., 1973) but not in others (Cotzias et al., 1970), as well as improvement in Sydenham's chorea (Feldman et al., 1945). It should be borne in mind that apomorphine also has a sedative effect, and hence has found widespread application in the past in the treatment of agitation and excitement accompanying a wide variety of psychiatric and neuropsychiatric disorders (Feldman et al., 1945). It has also been used to treat the excitement associated with the usage of scopolamine in the management of labor (White, 1952). It is well known that anxiety increases involuntary movements, and that sedation and sleep diminish such movements, so that some of the beneficial effects of apomorphine may not be related to dopamine-receptor agonistic action but to a nonspecific sedative effect. Unfortunately, studies with apomorphine have all compared this agent with an inactive placebo, namely physiological saline.

The rapid effect of apomorphine on neurological symptoms could lend itself to use as an investigational tool to predict response to L-dopa in conditions such as Huntington's chorea and dystonia musculorum deformans. In general, these conditions are not improved or are actually worsened by this amino acid. However, in certain cases, dopa gives rise to dramatic therapeutic amelioration (Tan et al., 1972; Rajput, 1973). Also, observations on the response to apomorphine might serve to delineate the role of dopaminergic mechanisms in a variety of extrapyramidal disorders. In this regard, apomorphine does not aggravate the abnormal movements of Huntington's chorea (Lal et al., 1973c), a result that does not support the view that hypersensitivity of dopaminergic receptors underlies the disturbance of movements in this condition (Klawans, 1970).

There is evidence that dopamine plays a role at the hypothalamic level in the modulation of anterior pituitary secretion in the rat (Fuxe and Hökfelt, 1969; Hökfelt and Fuxe, 1972; Kamberi et al., 1971a; 1971b; Schneider and McCann, 1970; Müller et al., 1970) possibly by affecting the release of releasing factors. Following administration of L-dopa in man, serum growth hormone (HGH) increases (Boyd et al., 1970) and prolactin falls (Kleinberg, 1971). The ability of L-dopa to release HGH has led to its use as a preliminary screening agent to assess growth hormone reserve. However, some normal subjects do not respond to L-dopa or the rise in HGH is delayed. L-Dopa is a precursor of dopamine and norepinephrine; it may alter the turnover of serotonin (Goodwin et al., 1971) so that the mechanism by which L-dopa affects anterior pituitary secretion is unclear.

This has led to the introduction of apomorphine as a pharmacological agent to investigate hypothalamic–adenohypophyseal function (Lal et al., 1972b).

Apomorphine (0.75 mg s.c.) causes a prompt increase in HGH levels in normal subjects with a peak at 30–60 min (Lal et al., 1972b; 1973a; Brown et al., 1973). This increase is unrelated to changes in serum glucose or cortisol (Lal et al., 1973b). Men have a significantly higher peak response than do women (Ettigi et al., 1974). Growth hormone response to apomorphine is increased in women on oral contraceptive medication (Ettigi et al., 1974). Chlorpromazine (Lal et al., 1973a) and glucose loading antagonize (Ettigi et al., 1974) the HGH response; glucose loading also antagonizes L-dopa–induced HGH release (Mims et al., 1973). The anticholinergic agent benztropine, which potentiates apomorphine effects on the striatum of the mouse (Scheel-Krüger, 1970), has no potentiating effect on apomorphine-induced HGH release in man (Lal et al., 1973b). In acromegalic subjects both L-dopa and apomorphine cause a decrease in HGH (Chiodini et al., 1974). Parkinsonian patients show a diminished HGH response to apomorphine, possibly because of a degeneration of hypothalamic dopaminergic neurones (Brown et al., 1973).

In normal subjects, apomorphine also decreases prolactin but larger doses are required than to increase HGH (Lal et al., 1973a). A much more pronounced decrease occurs in patients with hyperprolactinemia, either secondary to pituitary prolactin-secreting tumors or in patients with amenorrhea and galactorrhea following a course of oral contraceptive medication or following a normal delivery (Martin et al., 1974). The decrease in prolactin coincides with an elevation of HGH. The magnitude of decrease in these patients is similar following apomorphine (0.75 mg s.c.), L-dopa (0.5 g p.o.), or 2-bromo-α-ergocryptine (2.5 mg p.o.) administered as a single dose (Martin et al., 1974). Apomorphine has no effect on chlorpromazine-induced elevation of prolactin in normal subjects (Lal et al., 1973a). Recently Shaar et al. (1973) have shown that apomorphine decreases prolactin secretion by incubated rat anterior pituitaries.

Apomorphine has no effect on serum follicle-stimulating hormone or luteinizing hormone (Lal et al., 1973a).

In a comparative study of apomorphine (0.75 mg s.c.) and L-dopa (0.5 g p.o.), apomorphine was more effective in releasing HGH, both in terms of promptness of response and number of patients responding. The mean peak was also much sharper than that after L-dopa (Lal et al., 1975). This fact points to the potential advantage of apomorphine over L-dopa as a screening agent to assess HGH secretory reserve.

Tesarova and Molcan (1966) and Tesarova (1968; 1972) have reported (in uncontrolled studies) that administration of 0.5–1.0 mg of apomorphine subcutaneously three times daily for 12–14 days to neurotic and to mentally healthy subjects induces a clinical picture of psychotic depression. In a double-blind study, Lal and de la Vega (Lal, 1974) were unable to confirm these findings, since both experimental and control subjects showed improvement in depression as evaluated clinically and by depression rating scales. Also, none of the subjects developed schizophrenic pathology. This fact is of interest in view of the fact that not only depressive symptoms but also schizophrenic symptoms may occur following use of L-dopa (Murphy, 1973), and overactivity of dopaminergic mechanisms have been implicated in the pathophysiology of schizophrenia (Klawans *et al.*, 1972). However, Strian *et al.* (1972) did notice paranoid symptoms with sexual coloring in some patients receiving apomorphine in addition to L-dopa and a dopa decarboxylase inhibitor. Since disorientation accompanied these symptoms it suggests a picture of an organic confusional state more than a schizophrenic state. In view of the postulated deficiency of dopamine in retarded depressions (van Praag and Korf, 1970), apomorphine has also been administered to patients with psychomotor retardation occurring as part of the symptomatology of manic-depressive psychosis, depressed unipolar type. No change in psychomotor retardation or mood was noted in the two patients investigated (Lal, 1974).

L-Dopa causes spontaneous penile erections (Yaryura-Tobias *et al.*, 1970). Similar findings have been noted following oral apomorphine (Schlatter and Lal, 1972) and subcutaneous injection of subemetic doses of apomorphine (Lal and de la Vega, unpublished data). Dopamine-containing fibers have been described in the retina, but administration of apomorphine (0.75 mg s.c.) to blindfolded subjects fails to elicit photic stimulation (Lal and Sourkes, unpublished data).

6. REFERENCES

Ahlers, R. H., and Best, P. J., 1972, Retrograde amnesia for discriminated taste aversions—a memory deficit, *J. Comp. Physiol. Psychol.* **79**:371–376.

Amsler, C., 1923, Beiträge zur Pharmakologie des Gehirns, *Naunyn-Schmiedebergs Arch. Exptl. Path. Pharmakol.* **97**:1–14.

Andén, N. E., and Bédard, P., 1971, Influence of cholinergic mechanisms on the function and turnover of brain dopamine, *J. Pharm. Pharmacol.* **23**:460–462.

Andén, N. E., Rubenson, A., Fuxe, K., and Hökfelt, T., 1967, Evidence for dopamine receptor stimulation by apomorphine, *J. Pharm. Pharmacol.* **19**:627–629.

Andén, N. E., Carlsson, A., and Häggendahl, J., Adrenergic mechanisms, 1969, *Annu. Rev. Pharmacol.* **9**:119–134.

Andén, N. E., Strömbom, U., and Svensson, T. H., 1973, Dopamine and noradrenaline receptor stimulation: Reversal of reserpine-induced suppression of motor activity, *Psychopharmacologia (Berlin)* **29**:289–298.

Asper, H., Baggiolini, M., Burki, H. R., Lauener, H., Ruch, W., and Stille, G., 1973, Tolerance phenomena with neuroleptics, catalepsy, apomorphine stereotypies, and striatal dopamine metabolism in the rat after single and repeated administration of loxapine and haloperidol, *Eur. J. Pharmacol.* **22**:287–294.

Balakleevsky, A. I., 1971, Neurohormonal mechanism of apomorphine and γ-hydroxybutyrate activity in the brain, *Proceedings of the Third International Meeting of the International Neurochemical Society*, Budapest.

Barnett, A., and Fiore, J. W., 1971, Hypotensive effects of apomorphine in anesthetized cats, *Eur. J. Pharmacol.* **14**:206–208.

Barnett, A., and Fiore, J. W., 1973, The effect of antiparkinson drugs on the linguomandibular reflex in cats, *Eur. J. Pharmacol.* **21**:178–182.

Barnett, A., Goldstein, J., and Taber, R. I., 1972, Apomorphine-induced hypothermia in mice: A possible dopaminergic effect, *Arch. Int. Pharmacodyn.* **198**:242–247.

Barton, D. H. R., and Cohen, T., 1957, Some biogenic aspects of phenol oxidation, *in Festschrift Professor Dr. Arthur Stoll*, pp. 117–141, Birkhäuser, Basel.

Bédard, P., Larochelle, L., Poirier, L. J., and Sourkes, T. L., 1970, Reversible effect of L-dopa on tremor and catatonia induced by α-methyl-*p*-tyrosine, *Canad. J. Physiol. Pharmacol.* **48**:82–84.

Belenky, M. L., Vitolinya, M. A., and Baumanis, E. A., 1966, The influence of apomorphine on adrenaline inactivation in cats, *Bull. Eksper. Biol. Med.* **61**:54–55.

Bell, C., and Lang, W. J., 1973, Neural dopaminergic vasodilator control in the kidney, *Nature New Biol.* **246**:27–29.

Benesova, O., and Benes, V., 1970, Apomorphine and monoamines in the brain of rats, *Activ. Nerv. Sup. (Prague)* **12**:238–239.

Best, P. J., and Zuckerman, K., 1971, Subcortical mediation of learned taste aversion, *Physiol. and Behavior* **7**:317–320.

Bhargava, K. P., and Chandra, O., 1963, Antiemetic activity of phenothiazines in relation to their chemical structure, *Brit. J. Pharmacol.* **21**:436–440.

Bhargava, K. P., Gupta, P. C., and Chandra, O., 1961, Effect of ablation of the chemoreceptor trigger zone (CT zone) on the emetic response to intraventricular injection of apomorphine and emetine in the dog, *J. Pharmacol. Exptl. Ther.* **134**:329–331.

Bieger, D., Larochelle, L., and Hornykiewicz, O., 1972, A model for the quantitative study of central dopaminergic and serotoninergic activity, *Eur. J. Pharmacol.* **18**:128–136.

Boissier, J. R., Simon, P., and Guidicelli, J. F., 1968, Effets centraux de quelques substances adréno- et/ou sympatholytiques. III. Ptosis, catalepsie, antagonisme vis-à-vis de l'apomorphine et de l'amphétamine, *Arch. Int. Pharmacodyn.* **171**:68–80.

Boissier, J. R., Etevenon, P., Piarroux, M. C., and Simon, P., 1971, Effects of apomorphine and amphetamine in rats with a permanent catalepsy induced by diencephalic lesion, *Res. Commun. Chem. Pathol. Pharmacol.* **2**:829–836.

Borison, H. L., and Wang, S. C., 1953, Physiology and pharmacology of vomiting, *Pharmacol. Rev.* **5**:193–230.

Borison, H. L., Rosenstein, R., and Clark, W. G., 1960, Emetic effect of intraventricular apomorphine after ultrasonic decerebration in the cat, *J. Pharmacol. Exptl. Ther.* **130**:427–430.

Boyd, A. E., Lebovitz, H. E., and Pfeiffer, J. B., 1970, Stimulation of growth hormone secretion by L-dopa, *New Engl. J. Med* **283**:1425–1429.

Braham, J., and Sarova-Pinhas, I., 1973, Apomorphine in dystonia musculorum deformans, *Lancet* **1**:432–433.

Braham, J., Sarova-Pinhas, I., and Goldhammer, Y., 1970, Apomorphine in Parkinsonian tremor, *Brit. Med. J.* **3**:768.

Brossi, A., Ramel, A., O'Brien, J., and Teitel, S., 1973, Enzymatic oxidative coupling of optically active laudanosoline and its methiodide, *Chem. Pharm. Bull.* **21**:1839–1840.

Brown, W. A., van Woert, M. H., and Ambani, L. M., 1973, Effect of apomorphine on growth hormone release in humans, *J. Clin. Endocrinol. Metabol.* **37**:463–465.

Burkman, A. M., 1960, The characteristics of an apomorphine response, *J. Amer. Pharm. Assoc. Sci. Ed.* **49**:558–559.

Burkman, A. M., 1961, Antagonism of apomorphine by chlorinated phenothiazines, *J. Pharm. Sci.* **50**:156–160.

Burkman, A. M., 1962, Potent anti-apomorphine action of fluphenazine in pigeons, *Arch. Int. Pharmacodyn.* **137**:396–403.

Burkman, A. M., 1963a, Loss of biological activity of apomorphine from auto-oxidation, *J. Pharm. Pharmacol.* **15**:461–465.

Burkman, A. M., 1963b, Some kinetic and thermodynamic characteristics of apomorphine degradation, *J. Pharm. Sci.* **54**:325–326.

Burkman, A. M., Tye, A., and Nelson, J. W., 1957, Antiemetics in the pigeon, *J. Amer. Pharm. Assoc.* **46**:140–144.

Butcher, L. L., 1968, Effects of apomorphine on free operant–avoidance behavior in the rat, *Eur. J. Pharmacol.* **3**:163–166.

Butcher, L. L., and Andén, N. E., 1969, Effects of apomorphine and amphetamine on schedule-controlled behavior reversal of tetrabenazine suppression and dopaminergic correlates, *Eur. J. Pharmacol.* **6**:255–264.

Cannon, J. G., 1974, Chemistry of apomorphine and closely related systems, *Proc. Am. Chem. Soc.*, 167th National Meeting, Los Angeles, California, April, 1974.

Cannon, J. G., Smith, R. V., Modiri, A., Sood, S. P., Borgman, R. J., Aleem, M. A., and Long, J. P., 1972, Centrally acting emetics. 5. Preparation and pharmacology of 10-hydroxy-11-methoxyaporphine (isoapocodeine). *In vitro* enzymatic methylation of apomorphine, *J. Med. Chem.* **15**:273–276.

Carlsson, S. G., 1972, Effects of apomorphine on exploration, *Physiol. and Behavior* **9**:127–129.

Castaigne, P., Laplane, D., and Dordain, G., 1971, Clinical experimentation with apomorphine in Parkinson's disease, *Res. Commun. Chem. Pathol. Pharmacol.* **2**:154–158.

Chaney, S. G., and Kare, M. R., 1966, Emesis in birds, *J. Amer. Vet. Med. Assoc.* **149**:938–943.

Chiodini, P. G., Liuzzi, A., Botalla, L., Cremascoli, G., and Silvestrini, F., 1974, Inhibitory effect of dopaminergic stimulation on growth hormone release in acromegaly, *J. Clin. Endocrinol. Metab.* **38**:200–206.

Clement-Cormier, Y. C., Kebabian, J. W., Petzold, G. L., and Greengard, P., 1974, Dopamine-sensitive adenylate cyclase in mammalian brain: A possible site of action of antipsychotic drugs, *Proc. Nat. Acad. Sci. (U.S.A.)* **71**:1113–1117.

Cohen, G., and Collins, M., 1970, Alkaloids from catecholamines in adrenal tissue: Possible role in alcoholism, *Science* **167**:1749–1751.

Constantinidis, J., and De Ajuriaguerra, J., 1970, Syndrome familial avec tremblement parkinsonien et anosmie et sa thérapeutique par la L-dopa associée à un inhibiteur de la décarboxylase, *Thérapeutique (Semaine des Hôpitaux)* **46**:263–269.

Cools, A. R., 1971, The function of dopamine and its antagonism in the caudate nucleus of cats in relation to the stereotyped behavior, *Arch. Int. Pharmacodyn.* **194**:259–269.

Corrodi, H., Fuxe, K., and Ungerstedt, U., 1971, Evidence for a new type of dopamine receptor stimulating agent, *J. Pharm. Pharmacol.* **23**:989–991.

Corrodi, H., Farnebo, L. O., Fuxe, K., Hamberger, B., Ungerstedt, U., 1972, ET495 and brain catecholamine mechanisms: Evidence for stimulation of dopamine receptors, *Eur. J. Pharmacol.* **20**:195–204.

Costall, B., and Naylor, R. J., 1973, On the mode of action of apomorphine, *Eur. J. Pharmacol.* **21**:350–361.

Costall, B., Naylor, R. J., and Olley, J. E., 1972, The substantia nigra and stereotyped behavior, *Eur. J. Pharmacol.* **18**:95–106.

Cotman, C. W., and Taylor, D., 1972, Isolation and structural studies on synaptic complex from rat brain, *J. Cell Biol.* **55**:696–711.

Cotzias, G. C., 1971, Levodopa in the treatment of Parkinsonism, *J. Amer. Med. Assoc.* **218**: 1903–1908.

Cotzias, G. C., Papavasiliou, P. S., Fehling, C., Kaufman, B., and Mena, I., 1970, Similarities between neurologic effects of L-dopa and of apomorphine, *New Engl. J. Med.* **282**:31–33.

Cotzias, G. C., Tang, L., Ginos, J. Z., Nicholson, A. R., Jr., Papavasiliou, P. S., 1971*a*, Block of cerebral actions of L-dopa with methyl receptor substances, *Nature* **231**:533–535.

Cotzias, G. C., Tang, L. C., Miller, S. T., and Ginos, J. Z., 1971*b*, Melatonin and abnormal movements induced by L-dopa in mice, *Science* **173**:450–452.

Cotzias, G. C., Lawrence, W. H., Papavasiliou, P. S., Düby, S. E., Ginos, J. Z., and Mena, I., 1972*a*, Apomorphine and Parkinsonism, *Trans. Amer. Neurol. Assoc.* **97**:156–159.

Cotzias, G. C., Papavasiliou, P. S., Düby, S. E., Steck, A. J., and Ginos, J. Z., 1972*b*, Some newer metabolic concepts in the treatment of Parkinsonism, *Neurology* **22**(5): Part 2, 82–85.

Creveling, C. R., Morris, N., Shimizu, H., Ong, H. H., and Daly, J., 1972, Catechol *O*-methyltransferase. IV. Factors affecting the *m*- and *p*-methylation of substituted catechols, *Mol. Pharmacol.* **8**:398–409.

Crow, T. J., and Arbuthnott, G. W., 1972, Function of catecholamine-containing neurones in mammalian central nervous system, *Nature New Biol.* **238**:245–246.

Dahlström, A., and Fuxe, K., 1964*a*, Evidence for the existence of monoamine-containing neurons in the central nervous system. I. Demonstration of monoamines in the cell bodies of brain stem neurons, *Acta Physiol. Scand.* **62**: Suppl. 232, 55 pp.

Dahlström, A., and Fuxe, K., 1964*b*, The adrenergic innervation of the nasal mucosa of certain mammalians, *Acta Otolaryngologica* **59**:65–72.

Davis, V. E., and Walsh, M. J., 1970, Alcohol, amines and alkaloids: A possible biochemical basis for alcohol addiction, *Science* **167**:1005–1007.

Dent, J. Y., 1934, Apomorphine in the treatment of anxiety states, with especial reference to alcoholism, *Brit. J. Inebriety* **32**:65–88.

Dent, J. Y., 1953, Apomorphine in the treatment of addiction to "other drugs," *Brit. J. Addiction* **50**:43–46.

DeJong, H. H., 1945, *Experimental catatonia*, Williams and Wilkins, Baltimore.

DeRobertis, E., 1967, Ultrastructure and cytochemistry of the synaptic region, *Science* **156**:907–914.

DeRobertis, E., 1971, Molecular biology of synaptic receptors, *Science* **171**:963–971.

Deshpande, V. R., Sharma, M. L., Kherdikar, P. R., and Grewal, R. S., 1961, Some observations on pecking in pigeons, *Brit. J. Pharmacol.* **17**:7–11.

Dhasmana, K. M., Dixit, K. S., Dhawan, K. N., and Gupta, G. P., 1969, Blockade of depressor response of dopamine, *Japan J. Pharmacol.* **19**:168–169.

Dhasmana, K. M., Dixit, K. S., Jaju, B. P., and Gupta, M. L., 1972, Role of central dopaminergic receptors in manic response of cats to morphine, *Psychopharmacologia (Berlin)* **24**:380–383.

Dhawan, B. N., and Saxena, P. N., 1960, Apomorphine-induced pecking in pigeons, *Brit. J. Pharmacol.* **15**:285–289.

Dhawan, B. N., Saxena, P. N., and Gupta, G. P., 1961, Antagonism of apomorphine-induced pecking in pigeons, *Brit. J. Pharmacol.* **16**:137–145.

Divac, I., 1972, Drug-induced syndromes in rats with large, chronic lesions in the corpus striatum, *Psychopharmacologia (Berlin)* **27**:171–178.

Dlabać, A., 1973, Apomorphine-induced aggressivity in rats and its alterations, *Activ. Nerv. Suppl. (Prague)* **15**:2.

Dordoni, F., 1948, Sugli effeti dell'associazione morfina-apomorfina nel cane. I. Vomito, depressione del sistema nervoso e ipotonia muscolare, *Boll. Soc. Ital. Biol. Sper.* **24**:228–231.

Dorris, R. L., and Shore, P. A., 1971, Localization and persistence of metaraminol and α-methyl-*m*-tyramine in rat and rabbit brain, *J. Pharmacol. Exptl. Ther.* **179**:10–14.

Dorris, R. L., and Shore, P. A., 1974, Interaction of apomorphine, neuroleptics and stimulants with α-methyl-*m*-tyramine, a false dopaminergic transmitter, *Biochem. Pharmacol.* **23**:867–872.

Douglas, C. J., 1899, Alcoholism, *N.Y. Med. J.* **70**:626–628.

Douglas, W. W., 1968, Stimulus-secretion coupling: The concept and clues from chromaffin and other cells, *Brit. J. Pharmacol.* **134**:451–474.

Dresse, A., 1972, Topographie des systèmes catécholaminergiques et tryptaminergiques cérébraux, *Rev. Neurol. (Paris)* **127**:241–251.

Dresse, A., and Niemegeers, C., 1961, La stimulation par l'apomorphine de certains centres nerveux: Est-elle sujette à tachyphylaxie? *Compt. Rend. Soc. Biol. (Paris)* **155**:1713–1715.

Düby, S. E., Cotzias, G. C., Papavasiliou, P. S., and Lawrence, W. H., 1972, Injected apomorphine and orally administered levodopa in Parkinsonism, *Arch. Neurol.* **27**:474–480.

Ernst, A. M., 1965, Relation between the action of dopamine and apomorphine and their *O*-methylated derivatives upon the CNS, *Psychopharmacologia (Berlin)* **7**:391–399.

Ernst, A. M., 1967, Mode of action of apomorphine and dexamphetamine on gnawing compulsion in rats, *Psychopharmacologia (Berlin)* **10**:316–323.

Ernst, A. M., 1972, Relationship of the central effect of dopamine on gnawing compulsion syndrome in rats and the release of serotonin, *Arch. Intern. Pharmacodyn.* **199**:219–225.

Ernst, A. M., and Smelik, P. G., 1966, Site of action of dopamine and apomorphine on compulsive gnawing behavior in rats, *Experientia* **22**:837.

Etevenon, P. R., Simon, P., Gabilly, E., and Boissier, J. R., 1970, Antagonism by apomorphine of the permanent catalepsy induced by bilateral diencephalic lesions in rats, *Res. Comm. Chem. Path. Pharmacol.* **1**:115–120.

Ettigi, P., Lal, S., Martin, J. B., and Friesen, H. G., 1974, Effect of sex, oral contraceptives, menstrual cycle and glucose loading on apomorphine-induced growth hormone secretion, *Proceedings of the Canadian Psychiatric Association*, 24th Meeting, Ottawa, October, 1974.

Everett, G. M., Morse, P., and Borcherding, J., 1971, Antagonism of oxotremorine symptoms by L-dopa and apomorphine, *Federation Proc.* **30**:677.

Farnebo, L. O., and Hamberger, B., 1971, Drug-induced changes in the release of ³H-monoamines from field-stimulated rat brain slices, *Acta Physiol. Scand. Suppl.* **371**:35–44.

Fekete, M., Kurti, A. M., and Pribusz, I., 1970, On the dopaminergic nature of the gnawing compulsion induced by apomorphine in mice, *J. Pharm. Pharmacol.* **22**:377–379.

Feldman, F., Susselman, S., and Barrera, S. E., 1945, A note on apomorphine as a sedative, *Amer. J. Psychiat.* **102**:403–405.

Fenger, H. J., Gudmand-Höyer, E., and Rasmussen, K., 1972, A modification of the apomorphine dumping test, *Scand. J. Gastroent.* **7**:743–746.

Ferrini, R., and Miragoli, G., 1972, Selective antagonism of dopamine by apomorphine, *Pharmacol. Res. Commun.* **4**:347–352.

Feser, A., 1873, Die in neuester Zeit in Anwendung gekommenen Arzneimittel, *Zschr. Prakt. Vet.-Wiss.* **1**:302–306.

Finch, L., and Haeusler, G., 1973, The cardiovascular effects of apomorphine in the anaesthetized rat, *Eur. J. Pharmacol.* **21**:264–270.

Frommel, E., 1965, The cholinergic mechanism of psychomotor agitation in apomorphine-injected mice, *Arch. Int. Pharmacodyn.* **154**:231–234.

Frommel, E., Ledebur, I. V., and Seydoux, J., 1965, Is apomorphine's vomiting action in man and dog equivalent to its chewing effect in guinea pig? *Arch. Int. Pharmacodyn.* **154**:227–230.

Fuxe, K., and Hökfelt, T., 1969, Catecholamines in the hypothalamus and the pituitary gland, *in Frontiers in Neuroendocrinology* (W. F. Ganong and L. Martini, eds.), p. 47, Oxford University Press, New York.

Fuxe, K., and Sjöqvist, F., 1972, Hypothermic effect of apomorphine in the mouse, *J. Pharm. Pharmacol.* **24**:702–705.

Garelis, E., and Neff, N. H., 1974, Cyclic adenosine monophosphate: Selective increase in caudate nucleus after administration of L-dopa, *Science* **183**:532–533.

Gessa, R., Tagliamonte, A., and Gessa, G. L., 1972, Blockade by apomorphine of haloperidol-induced dyskinesia in schizophrenic patients, *Lancet* **2**:981–982.

Ginos, J. Z., LoMonte, A., Wolf, S., Cotzias, G. C., 1972, Apomorphine: Its dopaminergic action and its spectrofluorimetric determination, *Federation Proc.* **31**:269.

Gold, R. M., and Proulx, D. M., 1972, Bait-shyness acquisition is impaired by VMH lesions that produce obesity, *J. Comp. Physiol. Psychol.* **79**:201–209.

Goldberg, L. I., 1972, Cardiovascular and renal actions of dopamine: Potential clinical applications, *Pharmacol. Rev.* **24**:1–29.

Goldberg, L. I., and Musgrave, G., 1971, Attenuation of dopamine-induced renal vasodilation by bulbocapnine and apomorphine, *Pharmacologist* **13**:227.

Goldberg, L. I., Sonneville, P. F., and McNay, J. L., 1968, An investigation of the structural requirements of dopamine-like renal vasodilatation: Phenylethylamines and apomorphine, *J. Pharmacol. Exptl. Ther.* **163**:188–197.

Goldstein, M., Freedman, L. S., and Backstrom, T., 1970, The inhibition of catecholamine biosynthesis by apomorphine, *J. Pharm. Pharmacol.* **22**:715–717.

Goldstein, M., Anagnoste, B., and Shirron, C., 1973, The effect of trivastal, haloperidol and dibutyryl cyclic AMP on [^{14}C] dopamine synthesis in rat striatum, *J. Pharm. Pharmacol.* **25**:348–351.

Goodwin, F. K., Dunner, D. L., and Gershon, E. S., 1971, Effect of L-dopa treatment on brain serotonin metabolism in depressed patients, *Life Sci.* **10**:751–759.

Gouret, C., 1973, L'épreuve des redressements à l'apomorphine chez la souris: son intérêt comme test de sélection des psychotropes, *J. Pharmacol. (Paris)* **4**:341–352.

Grabowska, M., Antkiewicz, L., Maj, J., and Michaluk, J., 1973a, Apomorphine and central serotonin neurons, *Polish J. Pharmacol. Pharm.* **25**:29–39.

Grabowska, M., Michaluk, J., and Antkiewicz, L., 1973b, Possible involvement of brain serotonin in apomorphine-induced hypothermia, *Eur. J. Pharmacol.* **23**:82–89.

Granchelli, F. E., Neumeyer, J. L., Fuxe, K., Ungerstedt, U., and Corrodi, H., 1971, Synthesis of hydroxyaporphines and a study of their possible dopamine receptor stimulating properties, *Pharmacologist* **13**:252.

Green, K. F., and Garcia, J., 1971, Recuperation from illness: Flavor enhancement for rats, *Science* **173**:749–751.

Gupta, G. P., and Dhawan, B. N., 1965, Blockade of apomorphine pecking with phenothiazines, *Psychopharmacologia (Berlin)* **8**:120–130.

Gupta, G. P., Saxena, R. C., Chandra, O., and Dhawan, K. N., 1969, Assessment of anti-reserpine and anti-apomorphine activities of some psychic energizers in pigeons, *Psychopharmacologia (Berlin)* **15**:255–259.

Harnack, E., 1874, Über die Wirkungen des Apomorphine am Säugethier und am Frosch, *Arch. Exptl. Path. Pharmakol.* **2**:254–306.

Hensiak, J. F., Cannon, J. G., and Burkman, A. M., 1965, N-Allylnorapomorphine, *J. Med. Chem.* **8**:557–558.

Hester, J. B., Rudzik, A. D., Keasling, H. H., and Veldkamp, W., 1970, 4'-Fluoro-4-(1,4,5,6-tetrahydroazepino(4,5-b)indol-3(2H)-yl)butyrophenones, *J. Med. Chem.* **13**:23–26.

Heykants, J. J. P., Lewi, P. J., and Janssen, P. A. J., 1970, On the distribution and metabolism of neuroleptic drugs. Part II. Pharmacokinetics of moperone, *Arzneim.-Forsch.* **20**:1238–1241.

Hill, H. F., and Horita, A., 1972, A pimozide-sensitive effect of apomorphine on body temperature of the rabbit, *J. Pharm. Pharmacol.* **24**:490–491.

Hökfelt, T., and Fuxe, K., 1972, Effects of prolactin and ergot alkaloids on the tuberoinfundibular dopamine (DA) neurons, *Neuroendocrinology* **9**:100–122.

Hökfelt, T., Fuxe, K., Johansson, O., and Ljungdahl, Å., 1974a, Pharmacohistochemical evidence of the existence of dopamine nerve terminals in the limbic cortex, *Eur. J. Pharmacol.* **25**:108–112.

Hökfelt, T., Ljungdahl, Å., Fuxe, K., Johansson, O., 1974b, Dopamine nerve terminals in the rat limbic cortex: Aspects of the dopamine hypothesis of schizophrenia, *Science* **184**:177–179.

Holtz, P., Stock, K., and Westerman, E., 1964, Pharmakologie des Tetrahydropapaverolins und seine Entstehung aus Dopamin, *Naunyn-Schmiedebergs Arch. Exptl. Pathol. Pharmakol.* **248**:387–405.

Horn, A. S., Cuello, A. C., and Miller, R. J., 1974, Dopamine in the mesolimbic system of the rat brain: Endogenous levels and the effects of drugs on the uptake mechanism and stimulation of adenylate cyclase activity, *J. Neurochem.* **22**:265–270.

Hornykiewicz, O., 1971, Pharmacology and pathophysiology of dopaminergic neurons, *Adv. Cytopharmacol.* **1**:369–377.

Janssen, P. A., Niemegeers, C. J. C., and Jageneau, A. H. M., 1960, Apomorphine-antagonism in rats, *Arzneimittel-Forsch.* **10**:1003–1005.

Janssen, P. A., Niemegeers, C. J. E., Schellekens, K. H. L., and Lenaerts, F. M., 1967, Is it possible to predict the clinical effects of neuroleptic drugs (major tranquillizers) from animal data? IV., *Arzneim.-Forsch.* **17**:841–854.

Kamberi, I. A., Mical, R. S., and Porter, J. C., 1971a, Effect of anterior pituitary perfusion and intraventricular injection of catecholamines on FSH release, *Endocrinology* **88**:1003–1011.

Kamberi, I. A., Mical, R. S., and Porter, J. C., 1971b, Effect of anterior pituitary perfusion and intraventricular injection of catecholamines on prolactin release, *Endocrinology* **88**:1012–1020.

Kaul, P. N., and Brochmann-Hanssen, E., 1961, Auto-oxidation of apomorphine, *J. Pharmac. Sci.* **50**:266–267.

Kaul, P. N., and Conway, M. W., 1971, Induction and inhibition of *in vivo* glucuronidation of apomorphine in mice, *J. Pharmac. Sci.* **60**:93–95.

Kaul, P. N., Brochmann-Hanssen, E., and Way, E. L., 1961a, Biological disposition of apomorphine. II. Urinary excretion and organ distribution of apomorphine, *J. Pharmac. Sci.* **50**:244–247.

Kaul, P. N., Brochmann-Hanssen, E., and Way, E. L., 1961b, Biological disposition of apomorphine. IV. Isolation and characterization of "bound" apomorphine, *J. Pharmac. Sci.* **50**:840–842.

Kazdova, E., Dlabać, A., Metysova, J., 1972, Methods for evaluation of long acting neuroleptic drugs in animals, *Activ. Nerv. Sup. (Prague)* **14**:126–127.

Kebabian, J. W., and Greengard, P., 1971, Dopamine-sensitive adenylcyclase: Possible role in synaptic transmission, *Science* **174**:1346–1349.

Kebabian, J. W., Petzold, G. L., and Greengard, P., 1972, Dopamine-sensitive adenylate cyclase in caudate nucleus of rat brain, and its similarity to the "dopamine receptor," *Proc. Nat. Acad. Sci. (U.S.A.)* **69**:2145–2149.

Kehr, W., Carlsson, A., Lindqvist, M., Magnusson, T., and Atack, C., 1972, Evidence for a receptor-mediated feedback control of striatal tyrosine hydroxylase activity, *J. Pharm. Pharmacol.* **24**:744–747.

Kellogg, C., and Lundborg, P., 1972, Ontogenic variations in responses to L-dopa and mono-amine receptor-stimulating agents, *Psychopharmacologia (Berlin)* **23**:187–200.

Kier, L. B., and Truitt, E. B., Jr., 1970, The preferred conformation of dopamine from molecular orbital theory, *J. Pharmacol. Exptl. Ther.* **174**:94–98.

Klawans, H. L., 1970, A pharmacologic analysis of Huntington's chorea, *Eur. J. Neurol.* **4**:148–163.

Klawans, H. L., Jr., and Rubovits, R., 1972, An experimental model of tardive dyskinesia, *J. Neural Transmission* **33**:235–246.

Klawans, H. L., Goetz, C., and Westheimer, M. A., 1972, Pathophysiology of schizophrenia and the striatum, *Dis. Nerv. Syst.* **33**:711–719.

Klawans, H. L., Goetz, C., and Weiner, W. J., 1973, Dopamine receptor site sensitivity in hyperthyroid guinea pigs: A possible model of hyperthyroid chorea, *J. Neural Transm.* **34**:187–193.

Kleinberg, D. L., Noel, G. L., and Frantz, A. G., 1971, Chlorpromazine stimulation and L-dopa suppression of plasma prolactin in man, *J. Clin. Endocrinol. Metab.* **33**:873–876.

Koch, M. V., Cannon, J. G., and Burkman, A. M., 1968, Centrally acting emetics. II. Norapo-morphine and derivatives, *J. Med. Chem.* **11**:977–981.

Koster, R., 1957, Comparative studies of emesis in pigeons and dogs, *J. Pharmacol. Exptl. Ther.* **119**:406–417.

Koster, R., 1964, Emetic and anti-emetic actions of glycine in dogs, *Arch. Int. Pharmacodyn.* **150**:384–400.

Kramer, S. G., 1971, Dopamine: A retinal neurotransmitter. I. Retinal uptake, storage and light-stimulated release of ^{3}H-dopamine *in vivo*, *Invest.Ophthalmol.* **10**:438–452.

Kramer, S. G., Potts, A. M., and Mangnall, Y., 1971, Dopamine: A retinal neurotransmitter. II. Autoradiographic localization of ^{3}H-dopamine in the retina, *Invest. Ophthalmol.* **10**:617–624.

Kunz, K., Benešová, and Tikal, K., 1971, Tryptophan–pyrrolase activity after chronic admin-istration of reserpine and apomorphine in rats, *Activ. Nerv. Sup. (Prague)* **13**:225–227.

Kuschinsky, K., and Hornykiewicz, O., 1972, Morphine catalepsy in the rat: Relation to striatal dopamine metabolism, *Eur. J. Pharmacol.* **19**:119–122.

Lahti, R. A., McAllister, B., and Wozniak, J., 1972, Apomorphine antagonism of the elevation of homovanillic acid induced by antipsychotic drugs, *Life Sci.* 11, Part 1:605–613.

Lal, S., 1974, Clinical orientations in the use of apomorphine and related compounds, *Proc. Am. Chem. Soc.*, 167th National Meeting, Los Angeles, California, April, 1974.

Lal, S., and Sourkes, T. L., 1972, Effect of various chlorpromazine metabolites on ampheta-mine-induced stereotyped behavior in the rat, *Eur. J. Pharmacol.* **17**:283–286.

Lal, S., and Sourkes, T. L., 1973. Ontogeny of stereotyped behavior induced by apomorphine and amphetamine in the rat, *Arch. Int. Pharmacodyn.* **202**:171–182.

Lal, S., Sourkes, T. L., Missala, K., and Belendiuk, G., 1972*a*, Effects of aporphine and emetine alkaloids on central dopaminergic mechanisms in rats, *Eur. J. Pharmacol.* **20**:71–79.

Lal, S., de la Vega, C. E., Sourkes, T. L., and Friesen, H. G., 1972b, Effect of apomorphine on human growth hormone secretion, *Lancet* **2**:661.

Lal, S., de la Vega, C. E., Sourkes, T. L., and Friesen, H. G., 1973a, Effect of apomorphine on growth hormone, prolactin, luteinizing hormone and follicle stimulating hormone levels in human serum, *J. Clin. Endocrinol. Metab.* **37**:719–724.

Lal, S., Martin, J. B., and Friesen, H. G., 1973b, Effect of apomorphine (Apo) and L-dopa on growth hormone (HGH) and prolactin (HPRL) secretion in man, *Clin. Res.* **21**:1025.

Lal, S., de la Vega, C. E., Garelis, E., and Sourkes, T. L., 1973c, Apomorphine, pimozide, L-dopa and the probenecid test in Huntington's chorea, *Psychiat. Neurol. Neurochir.* **76**:113–117.

Lal, S., Martin, J. B., de la Vega, C. E., and Friesen, H. G., 1975, Comparison of the effect of apomorphine and L-dopa on serum growth hormone levels in normal men, *Clinical Endocrinology* (in press).

Lamarre, Y., and Puil, E., 1974, Induction of rhythmic activity by harmaline, *Can. J. Physiol. Pharmacol.* **52**:905–908.

Larochelle, L., Bédard, P., Poirier, L. J., and Sourkes, T. L., 1971, Correlative neuroanatomical and neuropharmacological study of tremor and catatonia in the monkey, *Neuropharmacol.* **10**:273–288.

Laville, C., and Margarit, J., 1964, Métaclopramide et épreuve à l'apomorphine chez le rat, *Path. Biol.* **12**:726–727.

Lewi, P. J., Heykants, J. J. P., Allewijin, F. T. N., Dony, J. G. H., and Janssen, P. A. J., 1970, Distribution and metabolism of neuroleptic drugs. I. Pharmacokinetics of haloperidol, *Arzneim.-Forsch.* **20**:943–948.

Lieberman, A. N., Goodgold, A. L., and Goldstein, M., 1972, Treatment failures with levodopa in parkinsonism, *Neurology* **22**:1205–1210.

Liebman, J. M., and Butcher, L. L., 1973, Effects on self-stimulation behavior of drugs influencing dopaminergic neurotransmission mechanisms, *Naunyn-Schmiedebergs Arch. Pharmacol.* **277**:305–318.

Lorenzetti, O. J., and Sancilio, L. F., 1970, Morphine dependent rats as a model for evaluating potential addiction liability of analgesic compounds, *Arch. Int. Pharmacodyn.* **183**:391–402.

Lotti, V. J., 1971, Actions of various centrally acting agents in mice with unilateral caudate brain lesions, *Life Sci.* **10**, Part I:781–789.

Maj, J., Grabowska, M., and Gajda, L., 1972, Effect of apomorphine on motility in rats, *Eur. J. Pharmacol.* **17**:208–214.

Malmfors, T., and Thoenen, H. (eds.), *6-Hydroxydopamine and catecholamine neurons*, Elsevier, Amsterdam, 1971.

Manske, R. H. F., 1954, The aporphine alkaloids, *in The Alkaloids, Chemistry and Physiology* (R. H. F. Manske and H. L. Holmes, eds.), pp. 119–145, Academic Press, New York.

Martin, J. B., Lal, S., Tolis, G., and Friesen, H. G., 1974, Inhibition by apomorphine of prolactin secretion in patients with elevated serum prolactin, *J. Clin. Endocrinol. Metab.* **39**:180–182.

McConaghy, N., 1969, Subjective and penile plethysmograph responses following aversion–relief and apomorphine aversion therapy for homosexual impulses, *Brit. J. Psychiat.* **115**:723–730.

McConaghy, N., 1970, Subjective and penile plethysmograph responses to aversion therapy for homosexuality: A follow-up study, *Brit. J. Psychiat.* **117**:555–560.

McDowell, F. H., Markham, C. H., Lee, J. E., Treiiokas, L. J., and Ansel, R. D., 1971, The clinical use of levodopa in the treatment of Parkinson's disease, *in Recent Advances in Parkinson's Disease* (F. H. M. McDowell and C. H. Markham, eds.), pp. 175–201, Davis Company, Philadelphia, Pennsylvania.

McKenzie, G. M., 1971, Apomorphine-induced aggression in the rat, *Brain Res.* **34**:323–330.

McKenzie, G. M., 1972, Role of the tuberculum olfactorium in stereotyped behavior induced by apomorphine in the rat, *Psychopharmacologia (Berlin)* **23**:212–219.

McKenzie, G. M., and Boyer, C. E., 1974, Dissociation of the behavioral and biochemical changes currently attributed to postsynaptic dopaminergic receptor activation, *Proceedings of the Canadian Federation of Biological Sciences*, Hamilton, Ont.

McKenzie, G. M., and White, H. L., 1973, Evidence for the methylation of apomorphine by catechol-*O*-methytransferase *in vivo* and *in vitro*, *Biochem. Pharmacol.* **22**:2329–2336.

McKenzie, G. M., Viik, K., and Boyer, C. E., 1973, Selective blockade of apomorphine-induced aggression and gnawing following fenfluramine or raphe-lesions in the rat, *Federation Proc.* **32**:248.

Menon, M. K., Clark, W. G., and Aures, C., 1972, The central stimulant and potential anti-parkinsonism effects of 2(*p*-nitrobenzylthio)-imidazoline-(3H).HCl, *Eur. J. Pharmacol.* **19**:43–51.

Mims, R. B., Scott, C. L., Modebe, O. M., and Bethune, J. E., 1973, Prevention of L-dopa induced growth hormone stimulation by hyperglycemia, *J. Endocrinol. Metab.* **37**:660–663.

Missala, K., Lal, S., and Sourkes, T. L., 1973, *O*-Methylation of apomorphine and the metabolic prolongation of apomorphine-induced stereotyped behavior, *Eur. J. Pharmacol.* **22**:54–58.

Morita, S., 1915, Untersuchungen an grosshirnlosen Kaninchen. II. Die Wirkung verschiedener Krampfgifte, *Arch. Exp. Pathol. Pharmacol.* **78**:188–217.

Müller, E. E., Pecile, A., Felici, N., and Cocchi, D., 1970, Norepinephrine and dopamine injection into the lateral ventricle of the rat and growth hormone releasing activity in the hypothalamus and plasma, *Endocrinology* **86**:1376–1382.

Murphy, D., 1973, Mental effects of L-dopa, *Ann. Rev. Med.* **24**:209–216.

Nahorshki, S. R., Rogers, K. J., and Binns, J., 1973, Cerebral phosphodiesterase and the dopamine receptor, *J. Pharm. Pharmacol.* **25**:912–913.

Neumeyer, J. L., Neustadt, B. R., and Weinhardt, K. K., 1970, Aporphines V: Total synthesis of (±)-apomorphine, *J. Pharmac. Sci.* **59**:1850–1852.

Neumeyer, J. L., Neustadt, B. R., Oh, K. H., Weinhardt, K. K., Boyce, C. B., Rosenberg, F. J., and Teiger, D. G., 1973a, Aporphines. 8. Total synthesis and pharmacological evaluation of (±)-apomorphine, (±)-apocodeine, (±)-*N-n*-propylnorapomorphine, and (±)-*N-n*-propylnorapocodeine, *J. Med. Chem.* **16**:1223–1228.

Neumeyer, J. L., McCarthy, M., Battista, S. P., Rosenberg, F. J., Teiger, D. G., 1973b, Aporphines. 9. Synthesis and pharmacological evaluation of (±)-9, 10-dihydroxyaporphine [(±)-isoapomorphine], (+)-, (−)-, and (±)-1,2-dihydroxyaporphine, and (+)-1,2,9,10-tetrahydroxyaporphine, *J. Med. Chem.* **16**:1228–1233.

Nielsen, E. B., and Lyon, M., 1973, Drinking behavior and brain dopamine: Antagonistic effect of two neuroleptic drugs (pimozide and spiramide) upon amphetamine- or apomorphine-induced hypodipsia, *Psychopharmacologia (Berlin)* **33**:299–308.

Niemegeers, C. J. E., 1971, The apomorphine antagonism test in dogs, *Pharmacology* **6**:353–364.

Niemegeers, C. J. E., and Janssen, P. A. J., 1965, A comparative study of the inhibitory effects of haloperidol and trifluperidol on learned shock–avoidance behavioral habits and on apomorphine-induced emesis in mongrel dogs and in beagles, *Psychopharmacologia (Berlin)* **8**:263–270.

Nikki, P., 1969, Biogenic amines, cold-adaptation and halothane shivering in mice, *Ann. Med. Exptl. Fenn.* **47**:129–140.

Nybäck, H., Schubert, J., and Sedvall, G., 1970, Effect of apomorphine and pimozide on synthesis and turnover of labelled catecholamines in mouse brain, *J. Pharm. Pharmacol.* **22**:622–624.

Nymark, M., 1972, Apomorphine provoked stereotypy in the dog, *Psychopharmacologia (Berlin)* 26:361–368.

Pedersen, V., 1967, Potentiation of apomorphine effect (compulsive gnawing behavior) in mice, *Acta. Pharmacol. (Kbnh.)* 25:Suppl. 4, 63.

Peng, M. T., and Wang, S. C., 1962, Emetic responses of monkeys to apomorphine, hydergine, deslanoside and protoveratrine, *Proc. Soc. Exptl. Biol. Med.* 110:211–215.

Persson, T., and Waldeck, B., 1970, Is there an interaction between dopamine and noradrenaline containing neurons in the brain? *Acta Physiol. Scand.* 78:142–144.

Pi, W. P., and Peng, M. T., 1971, Functional development of the central emetic mechanism in the puppy dog, *Proc. Soc. Exptl. Biol. Med.* 136:802–804.

Pinder, R. M., Buxton, D. A., and Green, D. M., 1971, On the dopamine-like action of apomorphine, *J. Pharm. Pharmacol.* 23:995–996.

Pinder, R. M., Buxton, D. A., and Woodruff, G. N., 1972, On apomorphine and dopamine receptors, *J. Pharm. Pharmacol.* 24:903–904.

Poirier, L. J.. and Sourkes, T. L., 1972, Experimentally induced Parkinsonism, *in Neurotransmitters* (I. J. Kopin, ed.), Association for Research in Nervous and Mental Diseases, New York.

Puri, S. K., and Lal, H., 1973, Effect of dopaminergic stimulation or blockade on morphine-withdrawal aggression, *Psychopharmacologia (Berlin)* 32:113–120.

Quik, M., and Sourkes, T. L., 1974, Inhibition of adrenal tyrosine hydroxylase by apomorphine, *Pharmacologist* 16:213.

Quinn, J. T., and Kerr, W. S., 1963, The treatment of poor prognosis alcoholics by prolonged apomorphine aversion therapy, *J. Irish Med. Assoc.* 53:50–54.

Rajput, A. H., 1973, Levodopa in dystonia musculorum deformans, *Lancet* 1:432.

Randrup, A., and Munkvad, I., 1970, Biochemical, anatomical and psychological investigations of stereotyped behavior induced by amphetamines, *in International Symposium on Amphetamines and Related Compounds*, pp. 695-713, Raven Press, New York.

Rekker, R. F., Engel, D. J. C., and Nys, G. G., 1972, Apomorphine and its dopamine-like action, *J. Pharm. Pharmacol.* 24:589–591.

Richter, W., 1964, Estimation of vasodilator drug effects in mice by measurements of paw skin temperature, *Acta Pharmacol. (Kbnh.)* 21:91–104.

Roos, B. E., 1969, Decrease in homovanillic acid as evidence for dopamine receptor stimulation by apomorphine in the neostriatum of the rat, *J. Pharm. Pharmacol.* 21:263–264.

Rotrosen, J., Wallach, M. B., Angrist, B., and Gershon, S., 1972a, Antagonism of apomorphine-induced stereotypy and emesis in dogs by thioridazine, haloperidol and pimozide, *Psychopharmacologia (Berlin)* 26:185–194.

Rotrosen, J., Angrist, B. M., Wallach, M. B., and Gershon, S., 1972b, Absence of serotonergic influence on apomorphine-induced stereotypy, *Eur. J. Pharmacol.* 20:133–135.

Rozin, P., 1969, Central or peripheral mediation of learning with long CS-US intervals in the feeding system, *J. Comp. Physiol. Psychol.* 67:421–429.

Saari, W. S., King, S. W., and Lotti, V. J., 1973, Synthesis and biological activity of (6aS)-10,11-dihydroxyaporphine, the optical antipode of apomorphine, *J. Med. Chem.* 16:171–172.

Sandler, M., Carter, S. B., Hunter, K. R., and Stern, G. M., 1973, Tetrahydroisoquinoline alkaloids: *in vivo* metabolites of L-dopa in man, *Nature* 241:439–443.

Sasame, H. A., Perez-Cruet, J., DiChiara, G., Tagliamonte, A., Tagliamonte, P., and Gessa, G. L., 1972, Evidence that methadone blocks dopamine receptors in the rain, *J. Neurochem.* 19:1953–1957.

Sassin, J. F., Taub, S., and Weitzman, E. D., 1972, Hyperkinesia and changes in behavior produced in normal monkeys by L-dopa, *Neurology* 22:1123–1125.

Scheel-Krüger, J., 1970, Central effects of anticholinergic drugs measured by the apomorphine gnawing test in mice, *Acta Pharmacol. (Kbnh.)* **28**:1–16.

Schelkunov, E. L., and Stabrovskii, E. M., 1971, Relationship between depletion of norepinephrine in the brain and the hypothermic effect of apomorphine in mice, *Farmakol. Toksikol.* **34**:653–657.

Schlatter, E. K. E., and Lal, S., 1972, Treatment of alcoholism with Dent's oral apomorphine method, *Quart. J. Studies Alcohol.* **33**:430–436.

Schlosser, W., Horst, W. D., Spiegel, H. E., and Sigg, E. B., 1972, Apomorphine and its effects on the spinal cord, *Neuropharmacol.* **11**:417–426.

Schneider, H. P. G., and McCann, S. M., 1970, Release of LH-releasing factor (LRF) into the peripheral circulation of hypophysectomised rats by dopamine and its blockage by estradiol, *Endocrinology* **87**:249–253.

Schoenfeld, R., and Uretsky, N., 1972, Altered response to apomorphine in 6-hydroxydopamine-treated rats, *Eur. J. Pharmacol.* **19**:115–118.

Schwab, R. S., Amador, L. V., and Lettvin, J. Y., 1951, Apomorphine in Parkinson's disease, *Trans. Amer. Neurol. Assoc.* **76**:251–253.

Senault, B., 1968, Syndrome agressif induit par l'apomorphine chez le rat, *J. Physiol. (Paris)* **60**: Suppl. **2**:543–544.

Senault, B., 1970, Comportement d'agressivité intraspécifique induit par l'apomorphine chez le rat, *Psychopharmacologia (Berlin)* **18**:271–287.

Senault, B., 1971, Influence de l'isolement sur le comportement d'agressivité intraspécifique induit par l'apomorphine chez le rat, *Psychopharmacologia (Berlin)* **20**:389–394.

Senault, B., 1972, Influence de la surrénalectomie, de l'hypophysectomie, de la thyroidectomie, de la castration ainsi que de la testosterone sur le comportement d'agressivité intraspécifique induit par l'apomorphine chez le rat, *Psychopharmacologia (Berlin)* **24**:476–484.

Senault, B., 1973, Effets de lésions du septum, de l'amygdale, du striatum, de la substantia nigra et de l'ablation des bulbes olfactifs sur le comportement d'agressivité intraspécifique induit par l'apomorphine chez le rat, *Psychopharmacologia (Berlin)* **28**:13–25.

Senault, B., 1974, Amines cérébrales et comportement d'agressivité intraspécifique induit par l'apomorphine chez le rat, *Psychopharmacologia (Berlin)* **34**:143–154.

Sethy, V. H., and Van Woert, M. H., 1974, Modification of striatal acetylcholine concentration by dopamine receptor agonists and antagonists, *Res. Commun. Chem. Pathol. Pharmacol.* **8**:13–28.

Shaar, C. J., Smalsig, E. B., and Clemens, J. A., 1973, The effect of catecholamines, apomorphine and monoamine oxidase on rat pituitary prolactin release *in vitro*, *Pharmacologist* **15**:256.

Shamma, M., and Slusarchyk, W. A., 1964, The aporphine alkaloids, *Chem. Rev.* **64**:59–79.

Share, N. N., Chai, C. Y., and Wang, S. C., 1965, Emesis induced by intracerebroventricular injections of apomorphine and deslanoside in normal and chemoreceptive trigger zone ablated dogs, *J. Pharmacol. Exptl. Ther.* **147**:416–421.

Sheard, M. H., 1969, The effect of *p*-chlorophenylalanine on behavior in rats: Relation to brain serotonin and 5-hydroxyindoleacetic acid, *Brain Res.* **15**:524–528.

Shemano, I., and Wendel, H., 1964, A rapid screening test for potential addiction liability of new analgesic agents, *Toxicol. Appl. Pharmacol.* **6**:334–339.

Sheppard, H., and Burghardt, C. R., 1971, The effect of α, β, and dopamine receptor-blocking agents on the stimulation of rat erythrocyte adenyl cyclase by dihydroxyphenethylamines and their β-hydroxylated derivatives, *Mol. Pharmacol.* **7**:1–7.

Shields, K. G., Ballinger, C. M., and Hathaway, B. N., 1971, Antiemetic effectiveness of haloperidol in human volunteers challenged with apomorphine, *Anesth. Analg.* **50**:1017–1027.

Simon, A., and van Maanen, E. F., 1971, Apomorphine and phentolamine antagonism of dopamine and epinephrine, Federation Proc. 30:624.

Simon, P., Chermat, R., Fosset, M. Th., and Boissier, J. R., 1972, Inhibiteurs beta-adrénergiques et stéréotypies provoquées par l'amphétamine ou l'apomorphine chez le rat, Psychopharmacologia (Berlin) 23:357–364.

Smelik, P. G., and Ernst, A. M., 1966, Role of nigro-neostriatal dopaminergic fibers in compulsive gnawing behavior in rats, Life Sci. 5:1485–1488.

Smith, R. V., and Sood, S. P., 1971, In vitro metabolism of certain nornuciferine derivatives, J. Pharm. Sci. 60:1654–1658.

Smith, R. V., Cook, M. R., and Stocklinski, A. W., 1973, Analysis of apomorphine and norapomorphine in urine by thin-layer chromatographic fluorescence quenching, J. Chromatog. 87:294–297.

Sourkes, T. L., 1970, On the mode of action of L-dopa in Parkinson's disease, Biochem. Med. 3:321–325.

Sourkes, T. L., 1971, Possible new metabolites mediating actions of L-dopa, Nature (London) 229:413–414.

Sourkes, T. L., 1972a, Parkinson's disease and other disorders of the basal ganglia, in Basic Neurochemistry (W. Albers, G. J. Siegel, R. Katzman, and B. W. Agranoff, eds.), pp. 565–578, Little, Brown, Boston.

Sourkes, T. L., 1972b, Biochemical pharmacology, in Basic Neurochemistry (W. Albers, G. J. Siegel, R. Katzman, and B. W. Agranoff, eds.), pp. 581–606, Little, Brown, Boston.

Sourkes, T. L., 1972c, The early history of dihydroxyphenylalanine, in Dimensiones de la Psiquiatria Contemporanea (C. Pérez de Francisco, ed.), pp. 295–297, La Prensa Médica Mexicana, Mexico.

Sourkes, T. L., 1973, Enzymology and sites of action of monoamines in the central nervous system, Adv. Neurol. 2:13–36.

Sourkes, T. L., Poirier, L. J., and Lal, S., 1975, Diseases of the basal ganglia, in Molecular Pathology (S. B. Day and R. A. Good, eds.), C. C. Thomas, Springfield, Illinois, in press.

Späth, E., and Hromatka, O., 1929, Opiumalkaloids. X. Synthesis of dl-apomorphine dimethyl ether, Chem. Ber. 62B:325–332.

Sprince, H., Parker, C. M., Smith, G. C., and Gonzales, L. J., 1972, Alcoholism: Biochemical and nutritional aspects of brain amines, aldehydes, and amino acids, Nutrition Reports Internat. 5:185–200.

Srimal, R. C., and Dhawan, B. N., 1970, An analysis of methylphenidate induced gnawing in guinea pigs, Psychopharmacologia (Berlin) 18:99–107.

Stadler, H., Lloyd, K. G., Gadea-Ciria, M., and Bartholini, G., 1973, Enhanced striatal acetylcholine release by chlorpromazine and its reversal by apomorphine, Brain Res. 55:476–480.

St. Laurent, J., Leclerc, R. R., Mitchell, M. L., and Miliaressis, T. E., 1973, Effects of apomorphine on self-stimulation, Pharmacol. Biochem. Behav. 1:581–585.

Strian, F., Micheler, E., Benkert, O., 1972, Tremor inhibition in Parkinson syndrome after apomorphine administration under L-dopa and decarboxylase-inhibitor basic therapy, Pharmakopsychiatrie Neuro-Psychopharmakologie 5:198–205.

Struppler, A., and von Uexküll, Th., 1953, Untersuchungen über die Wirkungsweise des Apomorphin auf den Parkinsontremor, Zeitschr. klin. Med. 152:46–57.

Symchowicz, S., Korduba, C. A., and Veals, J., 1971, Inhibition of dopamine uptake into synaptosomes of rat corpus striatum by chlorpheniramine and its structural analogs, Life Sci. 10, Part I:35–42.

Tagliamonte, A., Tagliamonte, P., Perez-Cruet, J., Stern, S., and Gessa, G. L., 1971, Effect of psychotropic drugs on tryptophan concentration in the rat brain, J. Pharmacol. Exptl. Ther. 177:475–480.

Takaori, S., Nakai, Y., Matsuoka, I., Sasa, M., Fukuda, N., and Shimmamoto, K., 1968, The mechanism of antagonism between apomorphine and metoclopramide on unit discharges from nuclear structures in the brainstem of the cat, *Int. J. Neuropharmacol.* **7**:115–126.

Takaori, S., Fukuda, N., and Amano, Y., 1970, Mode of action of chlorpromazine on unit discharges from nuclear structures in the brainstem of cats, *Japan. J. Pharmacol.* **20**:424–431.

Tan, B. K., Leijnse-Ybema, H. J., and Brand, H. J. V. D., 1972, Levodopa in Huntington's chorea, *Lancet* **1**:903.

Tattersall, R. N., 1971, Emetics, *Practitioner* **206**:111–113.

Teitel, S., O'Brien, J., and Brossi, A., 1974, Aporphines and related tetracycles by enzymatic oxidative coupling, *Proceedings American Chemical Society*, 167th National Meeting, Los Angeles, California, April 1974.

Tesarova, O., 1968, Mechanism of thymoleptic drug action studied in the model of apomorphine depression, *Activ. Nerv. Sup. (Prague)* **10**:287–288.

Tesarova, O., 1972, Experimental depression caused by apomorphine and phenoharmane, *Pharmakopsychiatrie* **5**:13–19.

Tesarova, O., and Molcan, J., 1966, A contribution to the problem of experimental depression, *Activ. Nerv. Sup. (Prague)* **8**:551–552.

Ther, L., and Schramm, H., 1962, Apomorphin-Synergismus (Zwangsnagen bei Mäusen) als Test zur Differenzierung psychotroper Substanzen, *Arch. Int. Pharmacodyn.* **138**:302–310.

Thierry, A. M., Stinus, L., Blanc, G., and Glowinski, J., 1973*a*, Some evidence for the existence of dopaminergic neurons in the rat cortex, *Brain Res.* **50**:230–234.

Thierry, A. M., Blanc, G., Sobel, A., Stinus, L., and Glowinski, J., 1973*b*, Dopaminergic terminals in the rat cortex, *Science* **182**:499–501.

Thoa, N. B., Eichelman, B., and Ng, L. K. Y., 1972, Shock-induced aggression: effects of 6-hydroxydopamine and other pharmacological agents, *Brain Res.* **43**:467–475.

Tiffeneau, M., and Porcher, M., 1915, The apomorphine series, Diacetyl and triacetylmorphine, *Bull. Soc. Chim.* **17**:114–119.

Toldy, M., 1962, The effect of adrenergic agents on the excitability of the emetic center, *Activ. Nerv. Sup. (Prague)* **4**:402–404.

Tompkins, J. E., 1899, Apomorphine in acute alcoholic delirium, *Med. Rec.* **55**:56.

Tseng, L. F., and Walaszek, E. J., 1970*a*, Blockade of the dopamine depressor response by bulbocapnine, *Federation Proc.* **29**:741.

Tseng, L. F., and Walaszek, E. J., 1970*b*, Influence of alteration of catecholamine and serotonin levels on bulbocapnine-induced catatonia, *Pharmacologist* **12**:198.

Tseng, L. F., Wei, E., and Loh, H. H., 1973, Brain areas associated with bulbocapnine catalepsy, *Eur. J. Pharmacol.* **22**:363–366.

Turner, A. J., Baker, K. M., Algeri, S., Frigerio, A., and Garattini, S., 1974, Tetrahydropapaveroline: formation *in vivo* and *in vitro* in rat brain, *Life Sci.* **14**:2247–2257.

Ungerstedt, U., 1971*a*, Stereotoxic mapping of the monoamine pathways in the rat brain, *Acta Physiol. Scand.* Suppl. **367**:1–48.

Ungerstedt, U., 1971*b*, Striatal dopamine release after amphetamine or nerve degeneration revealed by rotational behavior, *Acta Physiol. Scand.* Suppl. **367**:50–67.

Ungerstedt, U., 1971*c*, Postsynaptic supersensitivity after 6-hydroxydopamine induced degeneration of the nigro-striatal dopamine system, *Acta Physiol. Scand.* Suppl. **367**:69–92.

Ungerstedt, U., 1971*d*, Adipsia and aphagia after 6-hydroxydopamine induced degeneration of the nigro-striatal dopamine system, *Acta Physiol. Scand.* Suppl. **367**:95–121.

Ungerstedt, U., 1973, Selective lesions of central catecholamine pathways: Application in functional studies, *in Neurosciences Research*, Vol. 5 (S. Ehrenpreis and I. J. Kopin, eds.), pp. 73–96, Academic Press, New York.

Ungerstedt, U., Butcher, L. L., Butcher, S. G., Andén, N. E., and Fuxe, K., 1969, Direct chemical stimulation of dopaminergic mechanisms in the neostriatum of the rat, *Brain Res.* 14:461–471.

VanderWende, C., and Spoerlein, M. T., 1973, Role of dopaminergic receptors in morphine analgesia and tolerance, *Res. Comm. Chem. Path. Pharmacol.* 5:35–43.

Van Heyningen, W. E., 1959, Tentative identification of the tetanus toxin receptor in nervous tissue, *J. Gen. Microbiol.* 20:310–320.

van Praag, H. M., and Korf, J., 1971, Retarded depressions and the dopamine metabolism, *Psychopharmacologia (Berlin)* 19:199–203.

van Rossum, 1966, The significance of dopamine-receptor blockade for the mechanism action of neuroleptic drugs, *Arch. Intern. Pharmacodyn.* 160:492–494.

Van Tyle, W. K., and Burkman, A. M., 1970, New method for assaying antiapomorphine activity in pigeons, *J. Pharm. Sci.* 59:1757–1759.

Van Tyle, W. K., and Burkman, A. M., 1971, Spectrofluorometric assay of apomorphine in brain tissue, *J. Pharm. Sci.* 60:1736–1738.

Vedernikov, Y. P., 1969, Interaction of amphetamine, apomorphine and disulfiram with morphine and the role played by catecholamines in morphine analgesic action, *Arch. Int. Pharmacodyn.* 182:59–64.

Vedernikov, Y. P., 1970, The influence of single and chronic morphine administration on some central effects of amphetamine and apomorphine, *Psychopharmacologia (Berlin)* 17:283–288.

Vogt, M., 1954, The concentration of sympathin in different parts of the central nervous system under normal conditions and after the administration of drugs, *J. Physiol.* 123:451–481.

von Uexküll, T., 1953, Ein Beitrag zur Pathologie und Klinik der Bereitstellungsregulationen, *Verhandl. Deutsch. Gesellsch. Inn. Med. Kong.* 59:104–107.

Von Voigtlander, P. F., and Moore, K. E., 1973, Turning behavior of mice with unilateral 6-hydroxydopamine lesions in the striatum: Effects of apomorphine, L-dopa, amantadine, amphetamine, and other psychomotor stimulants, *Neuropharmacology* 12:451–462.

Waldeck, B., 1971, Some effects of caffeine and aminophylline on the turnover of catecholamines in the brain, *J. Pharm. Pharmacol.* 23:824–830.

Weissman, A., 1966, Apomorphine elicitation of key pecking in a pigeon, *Arch. Int. Pharmacodyn.* 160:330–332.

Weissman, A., 1971, Cliff jumping in rats after intravenous treatment with apomorphine, *Psychopharmacologia (Berlin)* 21:60–65.

White, H. L., and McKenzie, G. M., Methylation of apomorphine by catechol-O-methyl transferase, *Pharmacologist* 13:313.

White, R. R., 1952, The use of apomorphine with scopolamine in labor, *Am. J. Obst. Gynec.* 64:91–100.

Wolfarth, S., Grabowska, M., Lacki, M., Dulska, E., and Antkiewicz, L., 1973, The action of apomorphine in rats with striatal lesions, *Activ. Nerv. Sup. (Prague)* 15:132–133.

Woodruff, G. N., 1971, Dopamine receptors: A review, *Comp. Gen. Pharmacol.* 2:439–455.

Woodruff, G. N., and Walker, R. J., 1969, The effect of dopamine and other compounds on the activity of neurones of *Helix aspersa*; structure–activity relationships, *Int. J. Neuropharmacol.* 8:279–289.

Yayura-Tobias, J. A., Diamond, B., and Merlis, S., 1970, The action of L-dopa on schizophrenic patients; a preliminary report, *Curr. Ther. Res.* 12:528–531.

York, D. H., 1972, Dopamine receptor blockade—a central action of chlorpromazine on striatal neurones, *Brain Res.* 37:91–99.

Zetler, G., and Thörner, R., 1973, Drug-induced catalepsy as influenced by psychostimulants, apomorphine, L-dopa and yohimbine, *Pharmacology (Basel)* 10:238–251.

INDEX

Hypothalamus
  and dopamine, 251
  and releasing factor, 254

Indomethacin
  inhibitory action of, 10, 14, 21, 32
Immunofluorescent technique, 215
Immunological procedures
  assay for olfactory marker proteins, 199,
    200-215
  assay for S-100 protein, 141-142
  identification of brain-specific markers,
    196

Jacobson's vomeronasal organ, 212, 214, 218

Kernicterus, 250
Krabbe's disease (GLD)
  clinical aspects of, 86-88
  fatty acid distribution in, 79
  and galactolipid hydrolase activity, 81-83
  and lactosidase, 80-81

Lactosidase
  and cerebrosidase, 80-81
  substrate for, 79
Linguomandibular reflex
  and apomorphine, 280
Lipogranulomatosis
  and ceramidase activity, 57-58
Luteinizing hormone (LH)
  and apomorphine, 284
  and PGE_2, 24

Magnesium
  stimulating ATPase activity, 157-187
Marker protein, olfactory, 193-238
  assay for, 199
  biosynthesis of, 212-213
  and carnosine, 235-237
  cellular localization of, 212-219
  characterization of, 219-224
  distribution of, 200-205

Marker proteins, olfactory *(cont'd)*
  effect of hormones on, 205-206
  function, approaches to, 224-226
  genetic influences, 205-206
  identification of, 198-199
  ontogeny, 206-207
  phylogenetic distribution of, 207-212
3-Methylhistidine
  and actin, 178, 179
N-ξ-Methyllysine
  and actin, 178, 179
α-Methyltyrosine
  and akinesia, 254
  and catalepsy, 254
  and experimental tremor, 255
  and learned behavior, 280
  and rotational behavior, 275-276
  and stereotyped behavior, 266, 268
Monoamine oxidase (MAO)
  and aggressive behavior, 275
  in dopaminergic transmission, 253, 268-
    269
Morphine
  in apomorphine synthesis, 256, 259
  and catalepsy induction, 269-270
  and cyclic AMP formation, 27
Multiple sclerosis
  and acid protease, 116
  and basic protein, 121
  and glial fibrillary protein, 152
  model of, 96
Myelin
  and basic protein, 95-126
  and cerebrosidase inhibitors, 85-86
  composition of, 99-101
  and encephalitogenic activity, 97
  enzymatic activities of, 100
  galactocerebrosidase activity in, 78, 82
  in GLD, 86
  proteins of, 100-101, 138
Myelin kinase
  and basic protein, 111
Myelin synthesis deficiency
  and galactocerebrosidase activity, 82
Myelinogenesis, 113-114
Myosin, brain (see stenin)
Myosin, muscle
  from actomyosin, 159-161, 168